A BASIS FOR THE THEORY OF MEDICINE

A BASIS FOR THE THEORY OF MEDICINE

By

A. D. SPERANSKY

Director of the Department of Patho-Physiology of the
All-Union Institute of Experimental Medicine

Translated and Edited by

C. P. DUTT, B.A. (Cantab.)

With the Collaboration of

A. A. SUBKOV

Senior Research Worker of the Timiryazev
Biological Institute

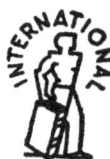

INTERNATIONAL PUBLISHERS

NEW YORK

CONTENTS

CONTENTS

LIST OF PLATES

PREFACE TO THE ENGLISH EDITION

DURING recent years it has often been remarked that the science of medicine is passing through a crisis. On a superficial view there would seem to be little basis for such a judgment. Each year sees the addition of tens of thousands of researches directly or indirectly affecting medicine; new methods of technique are continually arising, new fields of work are being opened up. In size of output and intensity of study there are few branches of science which can compare with medicine.

What is wrong then? An effort to answer this question leads inevitably to the conclusion that medicine has gradually and almost imperceptibly ceased to treat its subject matter in a synthetic form, substituting instead a comprehensive and often profound analysis of details. Specialisation, carried to an extreme degree, has almost become the hallmark of contemporary theoretical and practical medicine. As a result, medical science has been broken up into separate parts, both as regards subject matter and method.

Already, from time to time, many physicians have proclaimed the need for a return to a synthetic form of work. Such appeals, however, have not yielded any real results for they left undecided the question how exactly this was to be realised. A formal union of the isolated parts can be easily achieved by any method of work. But it has not led, and cannot lead, to the desired goal, and is even capable of introducing still more confusion into the subject by deliberately directing it along a wrong path.

Hence, the question remains one of the search for the essential principles for union. This demands a method capable of unifying not merely diverse but even contradictory phenomena. A consistent analysis must reveal the general laws underlying a mass of particular data. Then, at last, the investigator will be in possession of the "leading link," a grasp of which enables one, as Lenin remarked, to manipulate the whole chain.

For a number of years past, together with my collaborators, I have been engaged in research on the participation of the nervous system in the genesis of various pathological processes. The originally limited, special problem gradually assumed larger and larger dimensions, research widened out, embraced new fields and yielded new data of a varied nature. The appraisal of these data led so often to a conflict with many existing views that very soon we perceived the necessity of giving up the study of isolated questions. By the force of circumstances, we were compelled to pass to a revision of the conceptions of the basic processes of general physiology, from the point of view of the nervous component in their origin and history.

As a result, a system came into being capable not only of unifying around a common centre all the diverse data provided by pathology and the clinic, but also of advancing these branches of science along a characteristic and as yet almost untrodden path. The time has come when the matter can no longer be left in the exclusive possession of a limited circle of persons but imperatively demands the wide participation of scientific circles for testing what has been achieved, for judging the propositions that have been enunciated and, above all, for ensuring further progress. This has impelled me to embark on the publication of our views in the Soviet and foreign press.

I am very glad to welcome the appearance of an English translation of my book, since this will make it more widely accessible both to European and American readers.

A. D. SPERANSKY

Leningrad, July 14, 1935

PREFACE TO THE RUSSIAN EDITION

WHEN the material of a book is finally arranged and the book written, the order of exposition of the material appears to be the same as that of its collection. As a matter of fact, many years of work may elapse between two experiments which occupy adjacent places in the description, and between which there appears to be an uninterrupted internal connection. As the material accumulates, parts of it, arranged according to old systems, may be set out in a new order. In this process, the original starting point may lose its value and be done away with; the facts acquired earlier receive then a new significance and take up a new place in the logical order of the book.

The exposition of material obtained as the result of a long course of work *could turn out to come in advance of the cause which gave rise to the whole sequence.* Thus the historical order of succession in the production of the material does not coincide with the logical order of succession in the exposition of it. This holds good not only for biology but also for the so-called exact sciences. It is, of course, particularly evident in biology, which operates with highly complex processes.

Five years ago the author wrote a book entitled *The Nervous System in Pathology.* Very shortly afterwards it became clear that the book could not be republished in its previous form. The advance of research not only added something new to the data already available but necessitated a rearrangement of the entire material. In part, this occurred because particular questions were repeatedly made the subject of experiment and then set aside. Such processes as tetanus, rabies, epilepsy, tuberculosis and others, used by us as indicators in the study of various physiological mechanisms, were repeatedly made the subject of fresh experiments depending on the acquisition of new facts in other spheres. Since the basic idea of this work was to grasp the common elements in pathological processes that are externally dissimilar, each fact came under a cross-fire of criticism from other facts, frequently taken from very remote spheres. This made possible the noting of details that had previously escaped observation, but which now altered not only the general appearance of the phenomenon itself, but also its place in the series of other phenomena. In the above-mentioned book, it was still possible for me to set out the material in the order of the experiments; this has now become impracticable.

Beginnings and ends have so frequently changed places and have become so intricately entangled that a description of the material in historical sequence would make the line of thought appear disjointed, which in actual fact is not the case.

It was necessary either to renounce the possibility of seeing the material as a whole and to restrict oneself to the publication of separate facts or to pass to *a systematic exposition of the subject.*

The latter depends on two factors: on the quantity of new facts and on their co-ordination with already existing scientific systems.

For the solution of the first task, the volume of research was considerably increased and the work encroached upon all the basic departments of general pathology.

The second task proved to be much more difficult, and in certain respects simply impossible to fulfil since the new material could not be inserted in the framework of the old ideas. The original intention of giving merely a systematic exposition of the subject gave place to the necessity of *constructing a new system* and the question was shifted to the plane of methodological relations. Not only facts and general propositions had to be revalued, but also the methods and manner of the research itself. It can be understood that such a work could not be brought to a conclusion in a few years; nevertheless its fundamental features have been adequately defined.

It may be mentioned in passing that even now a number of difficulties in the way of systematic exposition still remain; the conclusions arrived at have proved to be so far from those generally accepted that to set out the subject directly, without any introduction depicting the work in its evolutionary course, would have involved the risk of being not understood or understood wrongly. Consequently it was necessary to keep to a mixed form: at the outset to demonstrate the course of the experiments, and only afterwards to pass to the systematic arrangement of the conceptions.

One of the defects of this form of exposition lies in a certain lack of correspondence in the treatment of the separate questions that are analysed in the beginning and at the end of the book, but this provides a striking example of the evolution of views in dependence on the evolution of the work.

As regards characterisation of the concrete forms and directions of experimental activity, it is necessary to say the following:

Although we carried out experiments with various chemical substances, toxins and viruses, we did not assume the special task of studying individually each process brought about by these agents. We merely had recourse to them at particular points in the course of research, as indicators for throwing light on those parts of the general question in which we were interested.

Hence, in this book also, which represents a summary of our work, I do not unite together the separate observations made at various times and with various purposes. In the reactions evoked by various agents we frequently saw so much similarity that it was impossible to distinguish them, and we turned our attention to the study of the mechanisms lying at the basis of this unity.

The usual form of work both in the laboratory and in the clinic does not ensure an exhaustive treatment of the subject. The clinic, by the nature of its position, is deprived of the right of extensive, and particularly of unhampered, experiment, while the laboratory investigates each pathological process separately as a special and independent entity.

This, of course, is also necessary and has its advantages. But in that case, everything taking place in the organism has to be looked at from the very beginning and is inevitably connected with the properties of the "causal agent." In actual fact, however, it may happen that a certain phenomenon in rabies can be more easily understood by the study of epilepsy, and in scarlatina by observation of tetanus. If each pathological process in each appropriate case is approached as an indicator of a definite physiological process and is included in the arsenal of other methodological means which contemporary science has at its disposal, then it will be seen that the virus of rabies can play the same role in the solution of one particular problem as the string galvanometer in the solution of another.

In spite of the fact that the questions touched upon in this book have already a history of many years behind them, it must be admitted that at the present time they are still in their infancy. Only too frequently it is still necessary to be content here with compiling a series of indirect data, seeking out unexpected occasions for experiment and conducting the research itself in circumstances as complicated as the solution of an equation with a number of unknown quantities. It will be evident from the materials presented that only simultaneous work on a number of associated questions, often very dissimilar in externals, has enabled us to discover the requisite conditions and, at least in part, to advance the subject over the dead point.

This work has been carried out during ten years in the laboratories and clinics under my guidance in the Institute of Experimental Medicine and the Institute of Surgical Neuro-Pathology in Leningrad, with the participation of a large number of specialists in different subjects who have collaborated with me in the provision of the necessary material. Each of them, besides giving his labour, has also introduced much that is individual, thereby making possible the gradual extension of the limits of the research.

In the shaping of this book, much assistance has been given me by my collaborators Dr. I. A. Pigalev, and Dr. C. I. Lebedinskaya, and also by Dr. N. E. Lebedev and my wife. I take this opportunity of acknowledging my deeply felt thanks.

A. D. SPERANSKY

Leningrad, September 1934

THE NERVOUS MECHANISM OF COMPLEX
CONVULSIVE STATES

CHAPTER I

CONSEQUENCES OF FREEZING PORTIONS OF THE CEREBRAL CORTEX IN DOGS

THE origin of these researches was as follows. In 1923-24, while working in the physiological laboratory of I. P. Pavlov at the Institute of Experimental Medicine, I participated, among other things, in the surgical activities of the laboratory, preparing animals for future special investigations. Naturally, like others, I encountered the unpleasant fact that many of the animals (dogs), after removal of different portions of the cerebral cortex, not infrequently died from epilepsy. It is true that one can counteract this phenomenon, but by no means in all cases. In addition, a new trepanning, with excision of the cicatrice, gives what is physiologically a new dog that cannot serve for the continuation of old experiments begun on it. Hence I set myself the task of working out a method of disconnecting limited portions of the cortex in such a way as to leave intact both the dura mater and the soft membranes.

I took as my starting point the instability of nerve tissue in the face of sharp changes of temperature. Experimental work in this direction had already been carried out in the period of physiology when the theory of the localisation of functions in the cerebral cortex was still new and alluring. Thus, in 1883, in Goltz's laboratory, Openchowski carried out research on the local effect of cold applied to the cerebral cortex. The results of this work were published by him in a short communication printed in *Cpt. rend. Soc. Biol.*, Vol. 2. To obtain a restricted or extensive effect of cold he applied to the cortex a glass apparatus cooled by means of ether vapour. The work was carried out on rabbits and dogs. In the latter, the development of convulsive attacks was observed in two cases. In rabbits, symptoms of anaesthesia were observed, and certain pathological forms of movement on the opposite side of the body. Openchowski also obtained convulsive phenomena by the cooling and partial freezing not only of the motor, but also of the occipital areas of the cortex. Hence, he came to the conclusion that there are no special epileptogenous zones or centres in the cortex of the hemispheres. As regards the solution of the basic task of his investigation—the application of cold for the purpose of studying the localisation of cortical processes—he remained dissatisfied, since he considered the effect of cold to be superficial. Later, other investigators also studied the influence of cold on nerve elements. Thus, Trendelen-burg established a number of data providing evidence that even simple cooling of the cortex results in prolonged disorganisation of its functions.

It was established that sufficiently intense freezing of a portion of the cortex kills the nerve elements in it. At the same time, other more stable structures can withstand such destruction of their normal state. We must expect that if freezing of the cortex is carried out through the dura mater without damaging the latter but only exposing it over a limited area, then both the dura mater and the soft membranes will suffer less than the cortex.

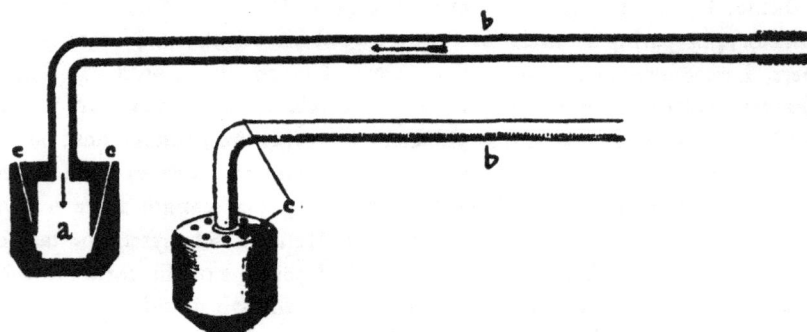

Fig. 1. Apparatus for Freezing the Cerebral Cortex
a) Thick-walled metal chamber. b) Tube for incoming vapour. c) Openings
for exit of vapour from the chamber

It was not difficult to realise this in practice. The cerebral cortex of the dog has a relatively elementary character. The sulci and convolutions throughout almost their whole extent have the form of arcs, beginning at the frontal pole and ending at the temporal. The variations are also simple. This renders possible sufficiently accurate reference of definite parts of the cortex to corresponding places of the skull of the dog. It is convenient to protect adjacent parts of the brain by trepanning over a restricted area, strictly within the limits of that area of the cortex which it is proposed to exclude.

Having constructed some pieces of apparatus based on the principle of the freezing microtome, of various sizes and forms, and having provided them with openings for the exit of carbon dioxide in such a way that neighbouring parts (muscles, skin) would not suffer, I proceeded to carry out the experiments.[1]

The first dog which was subjected to the operation of freezing a small portion of the cortex in the visual zone died in the course of 24 hours, with

[1] A. D. Speransky. *Zhurn. Exp. Biol. i Med.*, No. 7, 1926; *Ann. de l'Inst. Pasteur*, Vol. 40, 1926.

the exhibition of severe epileptic convulsions during more than 12 hours. Repetition of this experiment in a second, third and fourth case had the same results.

In all cases the general character of the illness developed not immediately but after a definite interval of time—from one to five hours. The dog emerges from narcosis without any special phenomena as regards the nervous system. Very soon, tonic spasms develop in various groups of muscles, after which comes clonic twitching, also in various groups of muscles and separate muscles. Following on this, or simultaneously, rhythmic convulsions and other complex movements take place and, finally, a typical epileptic seizure in its classical form sets in. These attacks are repeated at various, often remarkably accurate, intervals of time; they become more and more frequent and lead to a condition which can be defined as *status epilepticus*. Then coma supervenes. In this state the animals die, some 12-50 hours after the operation.

The post-mortem examination reveals that the external part of the dura mater is hæmorrhagic, but entire and firm; its internal surface is smooth and shining. There is no growth of connective tissue either on it or between it and the surface of the brain. The pia mater is permeated with blood throughout the whole extent of the hemisphere. At the point where freezing has taken place, the substance of the brain is visibly changed, appearing as a sharply demarcated patch of a dark cherry colour. The vessels in this portion undergo thrombosis. The size and shape of the dark portion corresponds almost exactly to the size and shape of the apparatus. In cross-section it is found that the alteration of the brain substance extends to a depth of 2-4 mm. In this region, the cortex is converted into a pulpy mass of a cherry colour which can be abraded from the surface of the section like the pulp of the spleen in cases of acute swelling. (Plate 1.)

Subsequently, a number of such experiments were performed, and it was possible to establish the following results:

1. The location of the portion of cortex subjected to freezing does not play any essential role in the development of the resulting picture of the illness. Freezing different points of the cortex (excluding motor points) in the accessible parts of the occipital and temporal areas yields approximately the same picture.

2. If freezing is carried out on any portion of the cortex of the dog, and this portion is afterwards removed, then no convulsive or other phenomena of motor agitation develop afterwards. The animal quickly recovers without complications.

3. On the other hand, if one waits for the appearance of pronounced symptoms after freezing (such as usually occur after some hours) and then

the corresponding portion of the cortex is removed, this does not save the animal from the further development of the illness, although the latter changes its course and general character.

4. Freezing a portion of the cortex in a dog which had been subjected a month previously to the operation of section of the *corpus callosum* causes the development of epileptic seizures and other convulsive phenomena on both sides of the body simultaneously and equally.

5. More detailed observation has demonstrated that the first symptoms to appear after freezing, and the last to vanish, in the general picture of the illness are not cortical but subcortical.

For purposes of illustration I will give an extract from the records.

RECORD No. 5

Dog. Male. Weight 18 kg.

On August 12, 1925, trepanning was carried out, and also freezing of a portion of the cortex through the undamaged dura mater by the application to the latter of the freezing apparatus, cooled to a very low temperature.

The operation was concluded (and the wound sewn up) at 11.05 a.m.

12.15 p.m. Tonic spasm of the extensors of the fore extremities. Twitching of muscles of the face and tongue.

12.35 p.m. Movement of all the extremities as in running; the dog lies on its side with head and body resting on the ground and in this position "runs," coordinating the movements of its extremities absolutely correctly and consistently—right foreleg and left hind leg, then left foreleg and right hind leg. These movements are carried out uninterruptedly, increasing in speed or slowing down.

1.10 p.m. The first epileptic attack. Tonic-clonic convulsions affecting the whole musculature of the body, head and extremities. Heavy attack. Foam at the mouth. Defecation and urination. Duration of the attack—1½ minutes. Immediately after the conclusion of the attack, "stationary running" is resumed.

1.20 p.m. The attacks are renewed after 3-5 minutes. "Running" during the intervals. Between the attacks (and of course during them) there is no reaction to external (even painful) stimuli. At times, tonic spasm of the flexors of the hind extremities occurs. At such times the movement of "running" is carried out only by the fore extremities, the hind ones are pressed to the body and in this position twitch awkwardly.

1.30 p.m. *Status idem.*

2.15 p.m. The beginning of an attack either with tonic spasm of the hind extremities or with tonic spasm of the lower jaw (with forced opening of the mouth). This is followed by rapid masticatory movements and further by general tonic-clonic convulsions. Much frothy mucus.

3.30 p.m. Intervals of 5-6 minutes between the attacks. The mucoid froth is secreted in such quantity that the whole floor of the chamber is covered by it. During the intervals, the dog lies immovable. "Stationary running" has ceased.

4.30 p.m. The intervals between the attacks become longer, the attacks themselves shorter and less pronounced.

7.15 p.m. Since 4.48 p.m. there was only one convulsive attack. Coma. In the beginning—laboured breathing of the expiratory type, afterwards the breathing is regular and deep, but slow.

7.28 p.m. Heavy attack of epileptic convulsions lasting 2¹/₂ minutes. Convulsive panting at the outset.

7.35 p.m. A new attack lasting 2 minutes.

8.05 p.m. Epileptic seizure, followed by a second after a short interval of time (3 minutes) then a third and so on.

8.55 p.m. *Status epilepticus.*

10.40 p.m. *Status epilepticus.* The convulsions affect all muscular groups but are more feebly expressed.

11.15 p.m. Coma. Breathing very slow, regular and deep.

August 13, 1.35 a.m. Death. Breathing gradually becomes slower but remains regular and deep to the end. The dog lived 14 hours 30 minutes after the operation. Weight at death 15.7 kg.

In order to complete the picture I shall give some notes from other records and summaries compiled in regard to various symptoms.

1. Practically all the records report considerable flow of saliva. Sometimes it assumes enormous proportions (forming pools on the floor around the muzzle of the dog; at times the whole floor is covered by frothy mucus). In some cases the saliva is liquid like water, in other cases it is thick and mucilaginous. On turning our attention to this phenomenon, we found that the mucilaginous mass was secreted from the oral cavity while the watery liquid, devoid of mucus, came from the nostrils. In some cases this flow was very abundant.

Further investigation showed that we have here an admixture of cerebrospinal fluid, which during the seizures flows abundantly into the lymphatic system of the nasal cavity and is excreted through the stomata onto the surface of the mucous membrane. Further details of this phenomenon will be given below.

2. In the intervals between the separate attacks no comatose condition was observed but "stationary running" or very strong motor agitation usually occurred. During the latter the dogs incessantly run about the room, stumbling against objects, not reacting to pain or to the impossibility of overcoming the obstacles encountered. During this time they frequently exhibit "proud appearance," with widely distended eyes, head held very erect, the ears laid back and a dancing gait ("Spanish trot"). As a rule, in all serious cases the comatose state is observed between groups of epileptic seizures. Usually 2-3 such groups occur during the course of the illness. The longer the epileptic state, the more protracted is the comatose period. Coma invariably supervenes before death, sometimes for a short period, sometimes for several hours (5-6). Breathing until the end is regular and deep, gradually slowing down. In some cases Cheyne-Stokes breathing was observed.

3. In regard to the order of development of the symptoms, the first to appear is usually tonic spasm of the flexors of the hind extremities. It is interest-

ing to note that this symptom is the most constant, and persists, with interruptions, throughout the course of the illness; and in cases which terminate in recovery of health, it is the last to disappear (it may be retained more than two weeks). Sometimes the first symptom of the illness is a clonic convulsion of one particular muscle or group of muscles, rhythmic convulsions (nictation, nystagmus, twitching of the tongue, ear and one or all of the toes of the fore or hind paws). Following on this, irregular tonic and clonic convulsions develop in various groups of muscles; at the same time the rhythmic convulsions are continued and even intensified. Subsequently, either the above-described strong motor agitation or "stationary running" takes place. Finally, the epileptic seizure begins. Sometimes one or two such seizures occur at the beginning of the illness, after which there is a pause of 2-3 hours during which there are no seizures but other convulsive phenomena develop and intensify. Then the epileptic period is resumed.

4. The latent period, before the appearance of the first symptoms of the illness, varies. It depends in part on the size of the portion frozen and on the duration of action of the cold, and in part, apparently, on the individual properties of the animal. The period before the first symptoms appear varies from 30 minutes to 5 hours, and before epilepsy—2-13 hours.

5. "Stationary running," described above, is usually observed shortly before the beginning of the epileptic state and in the intervals between attacks. It may also be the chief symptom in cases where epileptic attacks do not develop. Thus, dog No. 11 "ran" for 14 hours without interruption, with faster or slower tempo of movement but without any essential alteration, right up to the time of death.

6. Reaction to external stimuli depends on the phase of the illness. During the period when only irregular tonic or local clonic contractions are to be observed, reaction to stimuli is usually retarded but correct. At the outset there is reaction to contact, change of position, etc., afterwards to noise and calls. Frequently a considerable time (several seconds) elapses between the stimulus and the response to it. Sometimes the stimulus has to be repeated several times for the reaction to be obtained, but the latter remains correct, *i.e.*, it corresponds to the character and strength of the stimulus. Later on, it can become not only lively but also excessive. During the periods of epileptic seizures, "stationary running" and coma, there is no reaction to any kind of stimulus, even destructive ones.

7. In cases which last for a long time and end in death or recovery, disorganisation of mastication and swallowing, and of the functions of the tongue, was observed. The external manifestation of this is that the act of eating is disorganised in such animals. Sometimes the dog required 12 minutes to lap

up 150 c.c. of milk, without stopping once during the whole time. Attention was attracted to the awkward movements of the tongue and jaws and the "loud" swallowing.

8. During the illness, the animal often takes up awkward postures in the form of a cross, spiral or circle, etc.; these postures are retained by the animals for a considerable period.

9. We repeatedly observed also that the illness exhibited a form absolutely typical of Jackson's or Kozhevnikov's local epilepsy. Sometimes the whole illness proceeded in this fashion and ended in recovery. More frequently, however, the forms of local epilepsy characterised only a certain period of the illness, and were followed by general epilepsy and the death of the animal.

10. The weight of the animals rapidly decreased. Thus, dog No. 5 lost 2.3 kg. in 14 hours, dog No. 9 lost 2 kg. after 13 hours, and dog No. 10 lost 2.75 kg. after 50 hours, and so on. This is explained by the large loss of saliva, and partly of urine and exhaled water vapour.

11. In a number of cases the stomach of the dog was found after death to contain a considerable quantity of turbid fluid, of acid reaction, almost devoid of mucus. During the comatose period intensified peristalsis was frequently observed.

12. Sometimes peculiar forms of illness were met with, such as those described by my collaborator Dr. L. N. Fedorov.[1] We diagnosed this case as laryngo-epilepsia. The following is the history of the illness in this dog.

Dog No. 21. Male, rufous. Weight 10 kg.

September 11, 1926. Operation of freezing performed in visual zone of the left hemisphere. Area of freezing *ca.* 2¹/₂ sq. cm. Duration of freezing 100 seconds.
9.40 a.m. Operation concluded.
12.00 noon. First epileptic seizure. Previous to it the phenomena of general motor agitation and tonic convulsions in various parts of the body were observed.
September 12, 9.20 a.m. During the past 24 hours there were several groups of epileptic attacks, dying down during the night and occurring only rarely towards morning (after 1-2 hours). Feeble tonic-clonic convulsions in various groups of muscles proceed without interruption. The usual motor agitation is absent.
11.30 a.m. A convulsive attack of a type not previously observed began to develop. This starts suddenly in the form of a short yelp. The whole body is held tensely rigid. Loud, short yelps follow one another. Then the general tonus weakens and at the same time the short barking comes to an end, but the marked difficulty in breathing persists for about 1-2 minutes longer. Inspiration is prolonged, noisy, with whining as in croup. Expiration is much less laboured and therefore quicker, but also noisy. The difficulty of breathing gradually grows less. After some time (5-10 minutes) the dog breathes normally. Following this there is another sudden development of tonic convulsions of the whole body, short barking in the form of yelps, and on its cessation difficulty in breathing in the form described above. This

[1] L. N. Fedorov. *Zeitschr. f. d. ges. exp. Med.,* Vol. 72, No. 1-2, 1930.

state persisted for about 3 hours, after which there were no attacks of epileptic convulsions in any form.

September 13. During the whole day only tonic convulsions of separate muscular groups and general weakness was observed.

The dog reacts feebly and slowly, but correctly, to external stimuli. It attempts to drink milk, performing awkward movements with the tongue and jaws. The act of swallowing is very difficult. Swallowing is noisy and the greater part of the milk runs back into the bowl.

During the following days the phenomena of general weakness are intensified.

The dog is artificially fed. On September 18, a paralytic condition of the muscles of the neck was observed; when placed on its feet the dog could stand for some time, but the neck hung down feebly and the head retained whatever position happened to be adopted on placing the dog on its feet.

The dog died on September 19.

CHAPTER II

SUBCORTICAL PHENOMENA IN THE CONSTITUTION OF THE EPILEPTIC ATTACK

In weighing up the data regarding the external symptoms of disease in our dogs, the following characterisation has to be given: freezing separate portions of the cerebral cortex gives rise to a definite sequence of phenomena proceeding in the manner of a progressively developing illness. The latter expresses itself in a gradually increasing excitation of the nervous system both in the motor and in the secretary and receptor spheres. The most pronounced changes are observed in the motor sphere. These changes are manifold and clearly marked. They include all forms of hyperkinetic disturbances met with in the clinic.

Even the most superficial examination shows that we are confronted here with something more than phenomena which could be ascribed to isolated damage to the cortex. The general tonus, constituting the fundamental background of the disease, "frantic running," "Spanish trot," "stationary running," disorganisation of swallowing and other bulbar phenomena, forced attitudes, special forms of convulsions as described above, such as laryngo-epilepsia—*all this clearly indicates that cerebral regions lying below the cortex have been drawn into the process.*

The frozen portion itself, or its immediate periphery, is the source from which the process arises. This cannot be doubted, because its extirpation before the manifestation of the illness prevents the appearance of the latter. However, although it has its origin here, the process quickly passes beyond the limits of the cortex. Motor disturbances, the origin of which is connected with various nerve structures, arise at the same time, becoming superposed on one another and passing into that highest form of motor excitation which is termed an epileptic seizure. From this moment it is difficult to observe any plan or order in the motor syndrome.

Careful observation, however, has shown us that in the majority of cases the epileptic state is preceded by *a preparatory period which develops in a regular fashion.* This aroused the desire to analyse the whole picture of the epileptic attack into its constituent elements. Attempts of this nature were also made previously; but so far clarity on this question has not been reached.

The method employed by us has the following specific features. 1. The illness does not develop immediately. Various parts of the brain are included gradually, making it possible to observe the development of separate symptoms which in the clinic may exist independently. 2. Owing to this, the whole process follows the type of a progressive illness, concentrating into hours what the clinic observes during months and years.

In addition, the freezing method makes it possible to alter the relations between the cortex and the underlying regions of the brain by the use of various means.

The matter can be summarised as follows. The starting point from which the whole process develops is the cortex in the immediate neighbourhood of the frozen portion. It is natural to suppose that the greatest effect is exercised on the parts of the brain immediately connected with the cortex of the particular hemisphere selected for freezing. By combining the extirpation of various areas with altering the position of the frozen portion of the cortex of both hemispheres, we secure that the freezing exercises the desired degree of influence on the underlying regions. One may expect that by this means the order of superposition of the various nerve actions on one another can be altered and thus their separate elements made more accessible to observation.

As pointed out above, the most pronounced changes take place in the motor sphere. The connection of the cortex with the motor area of the underlying regions is, of course, very complex, but it is most clearly expressed in the zone of the motor cortical analyser, i.e., in the zone of motor functions. Consequently the separation of the cortex from the motor areas of other regions of the brain is best of all carried out by means of extirpation of the motor cortex. However, other regions of the cerebral hemispheres also have some particular relation to the motor areas of the underlying parts. Hence the removal of the entire hemisphere on one side already constitutes the next succeeding degree of alteration of the relations in which we are interested. In exactly the same way it can be presumed that freezing a point of the cortex of a hemisphere after preliminary removal of the motor cortex in the same hemisphere will not give the same results as freezing carried out in the region of the opposite intact hemisphere, etc.

In proceeding to the actual fulfilment of this plan, it is possible to draw up four forms of experiment.

First form. Extirpation of the motor cortex of one hemisphere and freezing a portion of the cortex of the other.

Second form. Extirpation of the entire cerebral hemisphere on one side and freezing a portion of the cortex of the other hemisphere.

Third form. Extirpation of the motor cortex of one hemisphere and freezing a portion of the cortex of the same hemisphere.

Fourth form. Extirpation of the motor cortex of both hemispheres and freezing a portion of the cortex of one of them.

These experiments were performed by my collaborator Dr. L. N. Fedorov.[1]

In all cases freezing was performed on the more easily accessible visual cortex of the hemispheres.

The results of our observations were formulated as follows:

First Form of Experiment

Trepanning was carried out in the motor area on one side, this area of the cortex was removed, the flow of blood was staunched and the wound sewn up. After 1-2 months, when the dog had completely recovered and the effects of destruction in the motor area had passed away, trepanning was performed *in the visual zone of the healthy hemisphere* and a portion of the cortex was frozen in the usual way.

Observation showed that the development and course of illness in these dogs differ very little from the ordinary. The only difference is that the tonic spasms begin earlier and are more sharply exhibited on the side opposite to that of the removal of the motor cortex. In this case also, strong motor agitation is observable up to the moment of appearance of the epileptic attacks, with sharply increased reflex excitability towards all stimuli at the outset, while later on all response to stimuli disappears. This period coincides with the development of the condition termed by us "frantic running" and "Spanish trot." This condition is interrupted by the epileptic attacks but is immediately resumed on the cessation of the attacks. The epileptic attacks themselves are also almost indistinguishable from the usual, but the tonic convulsions are more strongly marked on the side opposite to that of the removal of the motor cortex. Clonic contractions, however, occur on both sides, only to a different extent. A constant symptom, also, is the pronounced "visual aura," manifested in the motor action of "attention," such as pricking up the ears, etc. Not all these dogs die.

Second Form of Experiment

Here the preliminary operation consisted of complete removal of one hemisphere. About six months to a year afterwards, the operation of freezing was carried out on a small portion of the visual cortex of the healthy hemi-

[1] L. N. Fedorov. *Zeitschr. f. d. ges. exp. Med.*, Vol. 72, Nos. 1, 2, 1930.

sphere. Here also the syndrome proved to be closely similar to that just described, except that, during the whole illness, especially at the beginning and
end, tonic convulsions on the side opposite to that of the extirpated hemisphere, were more pronounced. During the first epileptic seizure, the extremities on this side remain stretched out like sticks and only twitch strongly.
At the same time, clonic spasms occur on the other side of the body. As a result
of the difference of the motor state of the two halves of the body, the animal
turns over several times during the attack, and on its termination remains
fixed for some time in the "ring posture."

As the attacks become more frequent, the general motor agitation during
the intervals grows stronger. The dog "runs" lying on its side, but the constant tonus of one-half of the body disturbs the co-ordination of the movements and "running" is performed only by the extremities of the healthy side.
As a result the dog performs circus movements, lying on one side and pivoting
around itself.

With the development of the epileptic state, the general motor agitation also
increases and finally reaches the form of "frantic running." Then for some
time an interesting phenomenon is observable. *The movements become temporarily unfettered.* The animal suddenly acquires the capacity to co-ordinate
them and marches forward with a dancing step on the tips of its toes, blunder-
ing against objects and not reacting to any stimuli. Suddenly this state is interrupted by tonic convulsions. The dog falls down, and almost immediately
an epileptic attack starts.

This can be explained in the following way. With the strengthening of
the excitation of the subcortical apparatus of the brain, the subcortical mechanisms of complex motor actions are released and the automatic character of
these motor actions is liberated. In these dogs, the visual or auditory aura
(expressed in the motor manifestations of the phenomenon of "watchfulness") is always clearly marked.

Third Form of Experiment

The preliminary operation was the removal of the motor area of the
cortex in one hemisphere. After 2-3 months, the usual operation of freezing
a portion of the cortex was performed *in the visual zone of the same hemisphere.*

Soon after the termination of narcosis, a pronounced increase of reflex
excitability to all stimuli was observed. The reflex reaction was incorrect and
excessive. Any kind of stimulation evoked an attack of tonic convulsions,
expressed more strongly on the side opposite to that where the motor cortex
had been removed. Very soon, irregular clonic twitching of various groups

of muscles develops, followed by periods of agitation. The dog leaps and runs forward, or more frequently in a circle. During these periods, it is practically *impossible to note any difference between the right and left halves of the body and extremities—they act alike.* During the same period, frequent attempts to defecate are sometimes observable. Two or three times the dog actually defecates, but thereafter merely performs repeatedly the external movements of the act.

Later, a number of special phenomena make their appearance. Fits of general motor agitation, in the form of frantic running in a circle, begin with pronounced and prolonged aura. The dog jumps about with its ears pricked up, it gazes fearfully and fixedly at something behind it, it whines and leaps as if attempting to escape from danger. Rapid "running" in a circle begins, accompanied all the time by champing movements of the jaws, which gradually increase in frequency, causing the teeth to chatter as in shivering. Frothy mucus accumulates around the muzzle. After making some circles round the room the dog falls down and the fit of agitation temporarily ceases.

The subsequent attacks are clearly epileptic and proceed in a very characteristic way. In our previous experiments we were accustomed to observe that in those cases when the dog was standing on its feet at the moment of the onset of the epileptic attack, it immediately fell down; while in those cases when it was lying on the ground, the convulsive attack only altered the posture. Here we observe exactly the opposite. If the dog is lying on the ground in some accidental posture, it jumps to its feet, and the above-described "aura" appears, after which the animal suddenly starts to spin round frenziedly. The whole body is rigid and trembles, the head is thrown back, the jaws champ, there is froth around the muzzle. The movement is performed in such a small circle that the hind quarters remain in one place and the whole body revolves round them. The fore extremities are thrown upwards and while still in the air succeed in making some small movements. As a result of throwing up both the fore extremities at once, the dog sometimes falls down, but it immediately gets up and the attack continues in the same form. On the conclusion of the attack, laboured panting (up to 200 breaths per minute) persists for a long time. During the attack there is no reaction to any kind of stimulus. After the attack, the reaction is incorrect and excessive. Such a state sometimes lasts for hours. The epileptic attacks gradually become more frequent, but the convulsive phenomena become more and more feeble. The dog now remains prostrate all the time. Then comes a short period of coma and death. The dogs invariably die.

Fourth Form of Experiment

The motor area of the cortex of one hemisphere is removed 5-6 months before the experiment, followed by removal of the same area of the other hemisphere 1-2 months before freezing.

After freezing the cortex in such dogs the illness develops slowly. A considerable period elapses before the first symptoms, *i.e.*, tonic convulsions, make their appearance. Shortly afterwards a period of generally heightened excitability ensues, with the complicated form of movement which was defined above as aura. Later, convulsive attacks begin. These must necessarily be regarded as epileptic. At the outset they are comparatively feeble and consist in sudden increase of tension in all the muscles of the body and extremities, sometimes with suspension of breathing. During the first attacks, one observes only isolated "champing" movements of the jaws. The intervals between the attacks last one hour, or even two hours. Subsequently the attacks become somewhat more frequent, and in the intervals the dog, as it were, acquires freedom of movement. It frequently shudders convulsively, scratches itself, and sometimes carries out movements as in defecation, gradually passing into a state of general motor agitation. It "runs" without taking account of obstacles, stumbling against persons and objects and not reacting to pain. This state is interrupted during the epileptic seizures, but these consist only in a sudden development of general tonus. At this period the tonus is very strong, the whole body held with maximum muscular tension, the head thrown back and the extremities stretched out like sticks. The only clonic form of convulsive movements in this case is the champing movement of the jaws (mastication). The number of such attacks quickly diminishes and they disappear, and afterwards the motor agitation also passes off. Phenomena such as could be brought under the conception of *status epilepticus* do not develop. The general tonic tension is retained for a fairly long time. Not all the dogs die.

Further observations (experiments of my collaborator V. S. Galkin[1]) have shown that the same phenomena can also be produced by freezing the cortex of normal dogs. By careful analysis it becomes clear that the convulsive character is only externally irregular. It consists almost wholly of separate compound motor actions, each of which is most precise and even harmonious. In many cases among normal dogs also it is easy to observe at the beginning of the illness the periodical appearance of 1) short champing (mastication), 2) sudden frantic running, 3) the external features of the act of defecation, repeated many times, 4) periodical and stereotyped licking of the sexual organs or the

[1] V. S. Galkin. *Arkh. Biol. Nauk*, Vol. 31, No. 6, 1931; *Zeitschr. f. d. ges. exp. Med.*, Vol. 77, Nos. 3, 4, 1931.

purely external action of searching for insects, without the dog even touching its skin, 5) rhythmic scratching, etc. The picture includes motor actions, expressing some particular emotion, *e.g.*, fear, attention, watchfulness. In all these cases, the attacks retain the form of fits, *i.e.*, they begin suddenly, proceed with a very definite rhythm and equally suddenly come to an end. Not infrequently the rhythm of these reactions is so constant that one can schedule them in advance, convincing oneself, watch in hand, of the accuracy of the prediction. Previously also, this had been repeatedly noticed by us (experiments of my collaborator K. A. Efimov). As an example I shall quote one of these observations made by Dr. V. S. Galkin.

Dog No. 583. Male, black. Weight 8 kg.

June 2, 1930. Freezing in the usual place, 2 minutes. Operation concluded 12.05 p.m.

From 1.05 p.m. to 3.35 p.m., *i.e.*, 2^1/$_2$ hours, 45 attacks lasting 1-2 minutes each with short interruptions, *i.e.*, genuine epileptic state.

4.05 p.m. Attacks cease. The animal lies on its side or on its back, with its paws in the air. It reacts incorrectly. Now and again it jumps up and carries out circus movements on the operated side.

4.30 p.m. At a whistle or shout, the whole body twitches violently. The dog lies on its back with legs bent at all joints and spastically pressed to the body.

5.45 p.m. An attack which can be characterised as *"petit mal"*; stupor for several seconds, slight twitching of the facial muscles, nystagmus in the widely distended eyes, twitching of the hind extremities. Saliva in a thin thread.

5.55 p.m. Another attack lasting several seconds, with champing movements of the jaws; immediately after the attack the dog runs about, stumbling against objects.

Subsequently, during 5 hours (until 10.55 p.m.) the attacks occur in absolutely regular rhythm. The attacks are repeated at intervals of 10 minutes (so accurately that they can be verified by a watch), each lasting for some seconds, at 8.05, 8.15, 8.25, 8.35, 8.45, 8.55, 9.05, 9.15, 9.25 p.m., etc.

After that the rhythm is slightly lost: 10.55, 11.06, 11.19, 11.33, 11.45, 11.59 p.m. and 0.13 a.m.

Besides their accurate rhythm, the attacks are remarkable on account of their stereotyped character—each one exactly like the last. The dog lies down on its right side. The fore extremities are tonically extended, the eyes wide open, the eyeballs motionless. Judging by the general appearance of the animal, one would say it is on guard. The head, held tonically rigid, stretches upwards. Small movements of the jaws, distinct champing, a slight thread of saliva at a corner of the mouth, twitching of the ears and nose. The attack lasts some seconds and during it the animal winks exactly 3 times; then it winks a fourth time and immediately after that the attack comes to an end: the head droops, the animal jumps up, shudders and begins to run rapidly in a circle. The whole attack lasts some seconds. In the intervals the dog is restless.

We have in our possession also a series of other observations, similar to those described. In some cases the accurate rhythm referred to the genuine epileptic attacks, in others—to the *phenomena of scratching, the motor action of defecation or chorea-like convulsions.*

Experiments of interest in this connection were carried out by my collaborators, N. A. Astapov, A. A. Vishhnevsky and M. S. Skoblo, on cats under light ether narcosis. The animals received subarachnoidally (by suboccipital injection) a 25 per cent solution of alcohol in acetone. The quantity of the solution was 0.1 c.c.

After 2-3 minutes, narcosis passes off. Shortly afterwards the animal begins to scratch its ear, usually with the hind paw. Sometimes the first symptom is "washing." Gradually, both forms of complex motor movement become intensified to such an extent as to become compulsory. This is especially evident in cases where the movement is not accompanied by any real effect, *i.e.*, when it is carried out in the air without contact with the skin. On the other hand, there are cases when the scratching and washing reaches a level amounting to self-mutilation. The movements are then performed so energetically that hair is torn from the ears and face, and the skin is covered with blood. During the interval, the phenomenon can easily be provoked by any stimulus—nocuous, auditory, or tactile. The whole ends in a general attack of tonic-clonic convulsions, *i.e.*, an epileptic attack. Here also, in the general picture of the attack, we frequently meet with simultaneous exhibition of a whole series of compound automatic movements.

As has been pointed out, the irregular picture of the general convulsions can be analysed into its constituent elements by artificial means. Then the clear-cut forms of separate motor actions are revealed. Here also we include aura, at least its motor part, since in dogs we are, naturally, unable to judge of the sensory aura, hallucinations and similar phenomena. However, it is quite possible that the process of excitation includes also the sensory part of the subcortical cerebral areas. Not being corrected by normal relations with the cortex, they lose their physiological significance and manifest themselves in the form of pure emotions in the same way as the motor actions under the same conditions, losing their importance and becoming purposeless and automatic.

Finally, in some cases we encounter merely fragments of these acts. Here some particular part of a complex movement is repeated in a stereotyped form. If it is carried out in a definite rhythm, then we are confronted by a chorea-like disease.

The opinion that epilepsy is a disease of subcortical origin (especially as regards some forms of it and individual special cases) has been expressed on many occasions. Khorosko explains in this way cases of Kozhevnikov's epilepsy, on the basis of clinical data and pathological analysis. The same treatment of epileptic attacks is given by Spiller, Wimmer, Knapp and Starling. Hartenberg, who systematically develops this view, regards the convulsive process as a manifestation of the cessation of cortical inhibition of the lower cerebral regions. The same view is adhered to by Dandy, although he points out that after the removal of the cortex in dogs he could artificially produce only tonic convulsions.

I think tha· this depended on the time which elapsed in his experiments between the removal of the cortex and the basic experiment. I myself have often carried out on dogs the operation of removing the hemispheres on both sides. In all cases where this was done in one operation, the animals died within a short period. Some of them remained in a state of complete prostration and heavy shock, passing imperceptibly into death. Others, on the other hand, experienced a state of violent motor agitation, barking persistently and without interruption, baring their teeth and carrying out a number of other awkward but expressive movements. Laboured breathing was always observed in these animals. This state lasts for a comparatively short time and also terminates in shock and death. Consequently, with such dogs it is only possible to perform acute experiments, which, of course, do not enable any decisive conclusions to be drawn.

Academician I. P. Pavlov has noted that if the removal of the cortex of the hemispheres in dogs is carried out by portions and on several occasions, then the animals stand the operation much better and, with suitable care, live for a long time. In one such case I observed heavy tonic-clonic convulsions in the form of attacks following rapidly on one another and completely typical of epileptic attacks. In this case the whole of the left hemisphere and five-sixths of the right had been removed. There remained only a small portion of the latter, belonging to the region of the skin analyser. The whole motor area of this hemisphere, the parietal, occipital and temporal parts, had already been removed some months before. The remaining fragment of the cortex did not exceed four square cm. in area and was strongly altered as the result of the several preceding extirpations of the surrounding parts. It could, of course, be the starting point of stimulation, but there is no reason to suppose that it was responsible for all the phenomena of the complex motor picture which we observed. The latter developed in other parts of the brain.

Recently I observed a similar case a second time, in a still more pronounced form.

Both hemispheres were removed entirely from one of the dogs in the course of several operations. The animal was in good condition and for many months had been serving as an object of experiments in I. P. Pavlov's labo-

ratory by the method of conditioned reflexes. Suddenly one evening the dog
exhibited motor agitation which quickly passed into a convulsive state. The
character of the convulsions was entirely typical of epilepsy: general tonus
followed by uninterrupted clonic twitching of the muscles, powerful and
extensive "stationary running" movements, constant champing, a large
amount of mucoid froth, repeated defecation. The whole terminated in
status epilepticus, coma and death within 12 hours.

In regard to this dog it was not only impossible to speak of the presence
of any cortical regions, whether as a whole or in part, but it was even doubtful
whether there had been any separate cellular elements of the cortex capable
of functioning. This, however, did not prevent the development of a typical,
"classical," epileptic state. I venture to think that the case mentioned decides
the question categorically and does not allow of any other interpretation.

From the experiments described at the beginning of this chapter it is
evident that the manifestation of the symptoms in the form of fits is typical
not only in cases of the so-called "classical" epileptic seizures. Many of the
other reactions described above also come in fits; this testifies merely to that
internal rhythm which is characteristic in general for the activity of the nervous system.

We conclude that all those individual elements that can be separated by
analysing the motor processes constituting an epileptic attack, are compound
automatic movements. These actions, or (to use Pavlov's terminology)
higher un-conditioned reflexes, have been definitely referred by the well-
known experiments of Sherrington to the subcortical cerebral regions. Situated here in the form of potential compound processes, they develop in the
normal animal under the influence of impulses which proceed from the appropriate receptor organs and are corrected by the cortex. In these conditions
they correspond according to time and intensity with the stimulus received
from outside. In the conditions of our experiments, not being upheld by normal relations with their receptor organs and the cortex, they make their
appearance in the form of purely motor actions and are now only subject to the laws of rhythmic activity of the nervous system. It is on this account
that the rhythm is so exact.

But it is due to the same reason that irregularity arises. Separate, harmonious motor actions are superposed on one another, interfere with each
other and finally attain that degree of intensity which we note as a general
convulsive attack, as an epileptic attack. In some cases, when the prodromal
period is very short, the illness begins directly with epileptic seizures. Here the
indispensable degree of excitation of the regions concerned is reached, not
gradually, but all at once.

CHAPTER III

THE CORTEX

THE analysis of the material put forward justifies us in regarding so-called subcortical phenomena as fundamental in the constitution of epileptic attacks.[1] Practically the whole external picture of the process can be summed up by this description.

What is the role played by the cortex?

Both clinicians and experimenters consider that its participation in the origin of epileptic attacks is indubitable. This is testified to by cases of traumatic or scar epilepsy (e.g., by Foerster's clinical observations on the influence of the localisation of cortical change› upon the epileptic manifestations), by experiments on stimulation of the cortex by electric currents, and by absinthe epilepsy which can be produced by the application of this substance to the exposed motor areas of the cortex (L. A. Orbeli and D. S. Fursikov). Finally, our experiments with freezing bear witness to the same thing. Consequently, the question is not whether the cortex participates, but of the form of this participation.

First of all, are we confronted here with excitation of the cortex or, on the contrary, with its inhibition? In the first case it must be admitted that the excitation at definite points of the cortex reaches an intensity at which the underlying cerebral regions pass out of its control and lose their normal connection with it. In the second case, the process must be likened to the experiments of removal of the hemispheres with consequent cessation of the permanent inhibitory activity of the cortex (I. M. Sechenov).

Both views have their adherents, but both rest on indirect data. Thus the question has remained unsettled.

We have now at our disposal some new material for arriving at a judgment in the matter.

In the course of other investigations we have frequently undertaken the extraction of the cerebro-spinal fluid in dogs. This operation is carried out under narcosis by means of suboccipital puncture. In the majority of cases

---

[1] In using the expression "subcortical phenomena" or "subcortical areas," I do not have in mind any exactly defined morphological structure. Where this is the case, the reservation is made in the text. Here by the word "subcortex" is to be understood regions of the brain lying below the cortex.

the maximum quantity of fluid is withdrawn (6.0-12.0 c.c.). At the beginning, when such extraction was not accompanied by operations on other parts
of the body, we did not get any bad effects. We even obtained an impression
of its complete harmlessness. Subsequently this view had to be given up.

On one occasion, immediately after withdrawal of the maximum quantity
of fluid, we rapidly introduced into the substance of the flexors of the knee
about 8.0 c.c. of tetanus toxin, and this resulted in the development,
while the dog was still on the operating table and while *still under narcosis*,
of a powerful attack of epileptic convulsions. After some minutes the attack
was renewed, *status epilepticus* quickly developed, followed by the death of
the animal. Analogous cases began to recur under the same conditions. Later
on, when we proceeded to inject various substances immediately into the
centripetal end of the severed nerve trunk, such cases became a common
occurrence in the experience of the laboratory. They always appeared under
the same conditions, but not in all experiments, only in a certain percentage of
them. The external description and primary analysis of these phenomena
were given at the time in an article by my collaborators I. A. Pigalev and
L. N. Fedorov.[1] At the beginning, all the workers in my laboratory who
made use of the above-mentioned method lost in this way a certain percentage
of animals, which impelled us to attempt to penetrate more deeply into the
nature of this process. We succeeded by degrees in establishing some of the
conditions determining it.

A large number of experiments with chemical trauma of nerve trunks
showed us that this operation is not accompanied by the development of a
convulsive state in dogs, provided that there has been no preliminary extraction of a maximum volume of cerebro-spinal fluid.

It also became clear that the qualitative nature of the substance introduced
into the nerve (toxins, croton oil, phenol, formalin, acids, bile) plays practically no role in this process. Cases of fatal epilepsy were observed after the
injection into the nerve, not only of strongly, but also of weakly stimulating
substances, such as an emulsion of fresh nerve tissue from the same animal.
Another reason making it impossible to speak of the action of the substance
itself was that the convulsive attacks frequently began immediately after the
injection. Moreover it was shown that, other conditions remaining the same,
the introduction of many of these substances into the blood was not accompanied by the development of the above-mentioned state. Thus the effect had
to be ascribed to the reflex mechanism.

The choice of nerve does not have any essential importance in obtaining

[1] I. A. Pigalev and L. N. Fedorov. *Zeitschr. f. d. ges. exp. Med.*, Vol. 70, Nos. 3, 4, 1930.

this reflex. We observed the development of convulsive phenomena in experiments with the sciatic, vagus, trigeminus and other nerves.

The convulsions, once begun, frequently persist with short pauses until the animal's death, which ensues after several hours. These convulsions are absolutely typical of so-called "classical" epileptic seizures. A certain proportion of the animals, after undergoing a number of attacks, completely recover later.

It is impossible to calculate exactly the percentage of cases in which the above-described means will bring about the development of the epileptic state. Sometimes we observed it twice, or even three times, in the course of a single day, but after that a week elapsed in which all similar experiments ended satisfactorily. Thus, one further condition was noticed. It became obvious that withdrawal of the cerebro-spinal fluid and subsequent stimulation of the nerve was not sufficient for the reflex development of the epileptic state in dogs. The presence of some kind of general background is also necessary here, without which the reflex is extinguished.

Later we began to observe the same process under somewhat other conditions. While undergoing investigation of the consequences of transection and chemical trauma of nerves, many dogs in our laboratory lived for a long while. In the injured place a neuroma develops, i.e., a point of permanent irritation of the nervous system is created. If the cerebro-spinal fluid is extracted from these dogs under narcosis without a second trauma of a nerve, then the epileptic state frequently develops in the form such as has been described. It begins while they are still under narcosis and in the majority of cases lasts until death.

My collaborator N. F. Bokhon observed the same process, without causing neuromata of the centripetal end of a severed nerve. The basic aim of his experiment was to study the forms of development of neuro-dystrophic processes in cases where the primary irritation is applied to one of the auxiliary nasal cavities. He began his observations with the frontal sinus, which was irritated by the injection into it of 2-3 drops of croton oil. The operation was conducted under conditions ensuring against the irritant coming into contact with any of the covering tissues (skin, muscle). In these dogs inflammation of the frontal sinus quickly developed as well as other phenomena which only gradually disappeared. In some cases, the extraction of the cerebro-spinal fluid from such animals, under narcosis, 2 to 10 days after the first operation, also caused development of the epileptic state.

To sum up, we obtained the following results: extraction by itself of the cerebro-spinal fluid from a normal dog does not cause the development of the epileptic state. Damage by itself to the nerve also does not bring about such consequences. *The epileptic effect is the result of the combination of both operations and, moreover, in the presence of complex narcosis.*

What are the mutual relations of all these components?

For the solution of this problem, we took the following two considerations as our starting point.

The first is based on the data obtained by analysis of the external manifestations of the epileptic seizure. As has been pointed out, the whole picture of it is covered by the conception of the excitation of cerebral regions lying below the cortex.

The second and more important consideration is that, under the conditions mentioned, we repeatedly observed in dogs the development of epileptic convulsions while still on the operating table, before the sewing up of the wounds had been completed, *i.e.,* while in a state of narcosis (morphine-ether-chloroform). If the convulsions appeared later, they nevertheless followed within a short interval of time (5-20 minutes after the operation). In this period, the effect of our complex narcosis had by no means come to an end.

Both features provide reason for thinking that the development of the process interesting us is preceded by functional dissociation of the cortex from the underlying parts. In this case, the excitation evoked by the nerve trauma, on reaching the subcortical parts, not only does not die out but acquires the character of a protracted process, which continues rhythmically until complete exhaustion, *i.e.,* until the death of the animal.

In the experiments described, the role of narcosis emerged so clearly that it involuntarily caused attention to be concentrated on it. We saw that the general character of the illness after freezing the cortex is in all respects similar to the picture of our reflex epilepsy. The consequences of both forms are almost the same, with the difference that after freezing, the illness begins later, passes through definite stages, gradually increases and lasts longer, whereas in the reflex form described, the illness begins immediately with epileptic seizures; but once the seizures have begun, the processes are indistinguishable until the death of the animal. In both cases the convulsions bear the stamp of classical epilepsy, appear periodically in the form of seizures, and in the intervals between them it is possible to observe the motor agitation, complex automatic movements, "aura" phenomena, etc., which we already know. Finally, reflex epilepsy also frequently brings the dog into a comatose condition passing into death.

Since narcosis thus plays an essential role in the mechanism of reflex epilepsy, we thought it necessary also to find out its significance in the process developing after freezing the cortex.

Until recently, all our experiments on freezing the cerebral cortex in dogs (as in general all other operations on them) were carried out under complex narcosis, beginning with subcutaneous injection of morphine (2 per cent solution, 1.0 c.c. for each 4 kg. of weight of the animal). After some minutes, vomiting and defecation take place, the dog becomes limp, and in this condition is brought onto the operating table where narcosis is continued by a mixture of ether and chloroform. Between the injection of morphine and the inhalational narcosis, 15-30 minutes usually elapsed. This form of narcosis in dogs is very convenient in many respects and quite harmless. It has been used for decades in I. P. Pavlov's laboratory, whence I adopted it.

The effect of this narcosis, gradually becoming weaker, continues for some hours after the operation, while the effects of inhalational narcosis alone, with ether, chloroform or a mixture of both, but without morphine, already passes off after ¼-1 hour. After this period the dogs react quite normally, walk correctly and even eat. Bearing in mind that after freezing a portion of the cortex the illness does not begin at once but in the course of the 2 or 3 hours immediately following, it follows that it takes place against a background of the still-continuing effect of the morphine.

What role does the morphine play in the development of this process? What change is produced in the development of the general picture of the illness if this condition is excluded and the operation of freezing is carried out under inhalational narcosis alone (chloroform-ether)?

To answer these questions, experiments were performed by my collaborator V. S. Galkin.[1]

As a result it was found that freezing the cortex almost lost its property of evoking the illness, to the careful observation of which so much labour had been devoted and the description of which had required so many pages.

All the 10 dogs that were first taken for this experiment remained alive. In 7 of them, from the beginning to the end of the observations, lasting continuously for several days, there were no symptoms of illness at all. They did not differ from normal dogs which had been subjected to no more than a short period of inhalational narcosis. Some of them already took food within one hour after the operation, all of them walked excellently and reacted absolutely correctly. Neither at the beginning nor later on were any signs of motor agitation observed in them. In one of the 10 dogs, there was a short period of twitching of the facial muscles on the side opposite to the one operated on. Convulsions in the form of epileptic seizures developed in 2 dogs, and in one of them there were only two such attacks. The other dog underwent several

[1] V. S. Galkin. *Arkh. Biol. Nauk*, Vol. 31, No. 6, 1931; *Zeitschr. f. d. ges. exp. Med.*, Vol. 78, Nos. 3, 4, 1931.

attacks at long intervals, but by the evening it had already completely recovered and afterwards remained healthy. In this dog, phenomena of motor agitation in the intervals between the attacks were also absent.

Under the previous conditions of the experiment, *i.e.*, with the employment of morphine, all 10 dogs would have developed the above-described typical disease with insignificant and unessential departures from the general standard. Out of this number, at least five or six would have died, and possibly all ten of them. It must be added also that this group happened to contain some dogs of hunting stock, which, according to our previous observations, always experience the effects of cerebral freezing particularly acutely.

The number of these experiments was later considerably increased. The results were the same. Almost all the dogs remained alive (in our material, more than 80 per cent). In 60-70 per cent of these animals, no pathological phenomena at all developed. The epileptic form of convulsions was observed very rarely, usually at the very beginning of the experiment, shortly after freezing, when the symptoms of inhalational narcosis had not yet passed off. The attacks were usually few in number, only 2-5, and afterwards they ceased.

In order to obtain convincing proof of the correctness of the observations made, the following experiment was performed. Under the old experimental conditions (with the employment of morphine) epileptic attacks among normal dogs made their appearance during the first 2-5 hours. The very latest time noted by us after several years of work was 14 hours. Now we decided to employ morphine not previously but subsequently. Some experiments were made with freezing under inhalational narcosis alone, without morphine. When it had become sufficiently evident that this experiment had not produced the development of the pathological process interesting us, *i.e.*, after the lapse of 10-48 hours, we gave the dog a subcutaneous injection of morphine in the usual dose. As a result we obtained a series of cases of typical development of the illness, ending with the epileptic state, coma and the death of the animal. The whole illness proceeded as if freezing had been carried out, not previous to, but coincidently with the injection of morphine. It was discovered also that the earlier the morphine was introduced, the more accurately the result was obtained. However, there were cases of fatal epilepsy, on injection of morphine 24 hours after freezing, in dogs which before this showed absolutely no signs of illness. In exactly the same way it was easily possible to obtain a renewal of convulsive phenomena and epileptic attacks in those animals which, having passed through a short period of illness, had emerged from this state. It was sufficient to make an injection of morphine to re-establish the whole picture but now in a considerably more serious form, continuing until the death of the animal.

It is interesting to note that a dog, which had previously appeared normal in the strictest sense of the word, sometimes had a serious epileptic seizure within the fourth or fifth minute after the morphine injection. If this experiment were to be shown to an outside observer, without communicating the preliminary conditions to him, he would be compelled to ascribe to the morphine properties analogous to absinthe or other such so-called convulsive poisons, which in actual fact would be incorrect.

In what exactly the mechanism of the effect of morphine on the central nervous system consists is not known. The usual effect of morphine in the case of the dog is depression, the depth of which is in proportion to the dose; but it has been shown that morphine can produce excitation and convulsions in the dog when introduced directly into the brain (Smirnov) or subarachnoidally (MacGuigan and E. Ross).

Is it morphine, or the manner of its introduction, which produces this effect?

We carried out a large number of experiments by injecting bile into the cerebral cortex of dogs (experiments of my collaborator V. S. Galkin). It is sufficient to introduce one drop of this substance for convulsions to make their appearance within a few minutes. Afterwards they persist without interruption for many hours and not only do not grow weaker but become progressively more intense. It is well known that all substances introduced into the brain immediately begin to be secreted from there into the circulatory and lymphatic system. Thus the quantity of bile in the brain decreases but the effect of its action continuously increases until the time when coma and death supervene (all the dogs die).

It is clear that we are faced here, not with an irritating agent, but with a process of irritation. The process proceeds in a manner entirely analogous to that observed on freezing the cerebral cortex. In the latter case, in order to prevent subsequent development of the disease, it was found necessary to extirpate the frozen portion before the moment of development of pathological symptoms. If the disease had once developed, removal of the point of primary irritation did not arrest the process.

Later on, we experimented with other substances besides bile. Some of them produced the same consequences. In these experiments we encountered the following series of phenomena, enabling us to proceed to a consideration of the general question of the mechanism of action of so-called convulsive poisons.

Withdrawal of cerebro-spinal fluid, especially in large quantities, is one of the means of increasing the permeability of the brain vessels. It is natural to suppose that under such circumstances "nerve poisons" introduced into the blood would have a markedly increased effect. It was found that the question is by no means so simple. Under externally identical experimental conditions, dissimilar effects were obtained. With some substances there was an increased effect, with others the effect diminished. The same thing applies also to the animals experimented on. The same experiment carried out on the dog and on the cat, or on the cat and the rabbit, ended quite differently in each case.

Our first observations of this kind were made with absinthe. We used a preparation (*essence d'absinthe cultivée*) received from Professor V. P. Ossipov, thoroughly investigated by him and accurately dosed.

The method used was as follows (the experiments were carried out by my collaborator A. S. Vishnevsky [1]). Dogs were selected in pairs according to weight and growth. From one of them, under light inhalational narcosis (chloroform-ether), the maximum amount of cerebro-spinal fluid was extracted. The other dog, in order to equalise the conditions of the experiment only underwent narcosis. Within 25-30 minutes both dogs had completely recovered, and then in both of them an exactly similar dose of the above-mentioned preparation of absinthe was introduced into the blood. Convulsions immediately developed in both animals, but their character was different in each case. While the control dog experienced a series of typical epileptic attacks with violent tonic-clonic convulsions, in the experimental dog the convulsions bore the character of strychnine cramps. Clonic phenomena were either absent or unclearly expressed. The picture consisted of general tetanus of the muscles of the body, head and extremities. The result was entirely similar to that obtained by L. A. Orbeli and D. S. Fursikov with dogs in which, after removal of the cortex of the big hemispheres, the same preparation of absinthe had been introduced into the blood.

These two authors are inclined to ascribe this effect to the absence of the cortex as the organ in which a definite part of the reaction proceeds, namely, its clonic phase. *In point of fact, however, one must take into account here the fact of the operation itself, the irritation arising from the region of the cicatrice, etc. This alters the reacting object. The forms of response to various kinds of irritation will now not be the same as previously.*

A second difference between the results in the control and the experimental dog was that a certainly fatal dose of our preparation (0.13 c.c. per kg. of weight) in the majority of cases proved not fatal for the latter animal.

The effect obtained is comprehensible only if it is assumed that in the

---

[1] A. S. Vishnevsky. *Arkh. Biol. Nauk*, Vol. 26, No. 4-5, 1926.

experimental dog the absinthe encounters a nervous system differing from the normal. As a result of interference, the mutual relations of the separate nervous parts have altered and the mechanism of the convulsive process has correspondingly changed.

From this it inevitably follows that the convulsive effect in itself does not depend only on the immediate action of absinthe on the appropriate nerve areas. To this must be added a number of essential combinations within the nerve network, the creation of definite relations between the parts of the latter.

In individual cases the effect of the action of a particular substance can even not be exhibited at all, as is shown by the following experiments (experiments of my collaborators N. A. Astapov and I. P. Bobkov). The animals experimented on were cats and dogs, the substance used was alcohol. The method used was the same as in the experiments with absinthe. The cats and dogs were selected in pairs. In one animal of each pair, the cerebro-spinal fluid was extracted; other conditions for the control and experimental animal were carefully equalised. Some 25-30 minutes after the withdrawal of the fluid (in the control animal the same period after light narcosis) a 25 per cent solution of alcohol was introduced into the stomach by means of a tube (for cats, on the basis of 6.0 gm. of pure alcohol per kg. of weight, for dogs slightly different proportions).

The experiment had the following results. The control, normal cat within a few minutes began to stagger about on its feet, fell on its side and could not get up again, even on painful stimulation. Immediately afterwards complete narcosis took place. The experimental cat during all this time still walked about quite freely, only slightly tottering on its legs. The narcotic state in its case either did not take place at all or was delayed for several hours in comparison with the control. There were cases where the animals went through the whole experiment on their feet and up to the end reacted to stimuli although not quite correctly.

In the case of dogs, the matter was different. Here it was the experimental animal that suffered first: narcosis began earlier and sometimes lasted for many hours longer. Some of these dogs died in the course of the days following the experiment.

It is interesting to note that in all the experiments the most pronounced result was obtained when a certain period (25-60 minutes) elapsed between the extraction of the cerebro-spinal fluid and the introduction of the particular substance used in the experiment. If the preparation was introduced immediately after the extraction, then there was no clear difference between the experimental and control animal. Consequently, the process which gradually develops in the nervous system after the withdrawal of the fluid plays a part here.

There is absolutely no doubt that under these conditions the alcohol penetrates into the brain region in greater quantity than normally, as a result of which the effect on dogs of the same dose of alcohol is intensified. In the cat this not only does not accelerate the onset of narcosis but clearly retards it. In exactly the same way, morphine, introduced into the blood of the dog, produces narcosis which undoubtedly arises as a consequence of morphine penetrating into the brain. If, however, it is injected directly into the brain, we get, instead of narcosis, heavy and prolonged convulsions.

In view of all these facts, is it possible to regard narcosis as a simple lowering of the functions of the nervous system? Is it not a process arising as a result of the creation of a special combination, and perhaps even of active relations, between various parts of the nervous system?

Besides this, all the material put forward, bears witness to the fact that *so-called nerve poisons have not any constant and independent properties.* Their action is determined by a number of conditions, for the basic factor here is the state of the irritated object itself—those incessantly changing mutual relations of its separate parts.

I shall permit myself to give one more example, providing an especially clear illustration of this thesis.

Absinthe is the classical means for obtaining epileptic convulsions. I think it can hardly be doubted that it is precisely the central nervous system that participates in this process. When our preparation of absinthe was introduced into the blood of a cat, to the amount of 0.2 c.c., it immediately, even after a few seconds, evoked epileptic attacks. These attacks frequently culminated in death in the course of the following 10-30 minutes. Since only a comparatively small part of the amount of absinthe taken finds its way into the brain, it would be natural to suppose that the injection of a full dose of absinthe (0.2 c.c.) directly into the subarachnoid spaces of a cat would produce death even during the first epileptic seizure. In actual fact nothing of the sort occurs (experiments of my collaborator K. P. Golysheva[1]). *The cats in this case not only did not die but did not even develop convulsions.* In some instances, after a considerable interval of time, 10-20 minutes, there could be observed tonic phenomena, some forms of compound automatic motor actions and only rarely genuine clonic spasms. But it remained unclear here whether we were confronted with the result of the action of the absinthe which had been introduced into the brain region, or whether our absinthe had been secreted into

[1] K. P. Golysheva. *Arkh. Biol. Nauk*, Vol. 32, No. 4, 1932.

the circulatory and lymphatic system and only penetrated into the brain together with the blood.

Later some experiments were carried out on cats and dogs by introducing absinthe directly into the substance of the cerebral hemispheres. The effect of this method was hardly different from the effect of subarachnoid injections. Convulsions either did not develop, or were retarded by 10 or more minutes in comparison with the control. Only injection of absinthe into the motor cortex or its immediate neighbourhood brings about the appearance of some convulsive actions, but they are feeble and not comparable with the usual picture of absinthe epilepsy.

There is one further curious detail. The application of a small piece of cotton-wool soaked in absinthe to the motor cortex in the dog produces a more pronounced convulsive effect than the injection of absinthe into the same region. *But in both cases the effect is immeasurably lower than that obtained on injection of absinthe into the blood, although the relative quantity of the acting substance is here, of course, considerably greater.* It was found also that with this method of using absinthe the latent period of irritation is considerably longer than in cases where absinthe is injected into the blood. Consequently, here also it is again unclear by what means precisely the convulsive effect is obtained.

It is one thing when the substance is conveyed into the cell through the blood, and another thing when the cell is irritated directly by the same substance. In the latter case also the form of reaction should be different, because through the blood the substance simultaneously draws various elements into the process. *Each of the parts suffering can begin its own process* and already serves as a physiological stimulus for processes in a number of new regions. All this gives reason for doubting that nerve structures participating in the creation of the general picture of the epileptic attack are brought into an active state merely by the poisonous substance itself.

Now, what determines the final effect? Is it a property of morphine, or the manner of its introduction, or the state of the organism itself at the moment of acting on it?

It is clear that all three factors are of significance simultaneously. Since the last two are not constant, it is comprehensible that experiments externally identical may end differently. In our experiments with freezing the cortex in dogs the fundamental role of morphine is not that of evoking convulsions. *Morphine does not possess this property, and in general does not possess any properties independent of all the other conditions.* The convulsive effect of morphine here is bound up with the fact that, after a portion of the cortex has been frozen, *the dog has already become a different animal.* In this new combination, only the morphine has remained unchanged. After this, what grounds are there for ascribing to it definite and constant properties?

In a normal dog, morphine produces depression of the higher regions of the central nervous system which, in its turn, to a certain extent liberates the underlying parts of the brain from inhibitory influences. However, for obtaining a convulsive effect this alone is insufficient. When the freezing of a portion of the cortex is added, then we have a cortex with lowered functions, upon which the freezing has produced a point of irritation which represents an additional stimulus for the excitation of the subcortical areas. *The same irritation, arising from the same cortical zone, will not result in convulsive effects, if the inhibitory influences of the remaining cortical parts are not removed.*

Consequently, in the mechanism of the development of the epileptic attack, it is possible to note the presence of a minimum of two factors, coinciding in time: *the irritation of nerve areas connected with the formation of complex motor actions and some degree of lowering of the cortical activity.*

The source of irritation in these cases is by no means the cortex alone. The examples of reflex epilepsy given above demonstrate that the requisite irritation can arise in many other places. Then, during the whole period of the attack, from start to finish, the participation of the cortex will be passive, which, however, does not bring about any change in the external picture. This is evidence, once again, that the elements *entering into the composition* of the epileptic seizure are not derived from the cortex.

Freezing a limited portion of the cortex damages to some extent the state of its other regions. Hence, as we have seen, in a certain percentage of cases, freezing alone can result in the development of convulsive phenomena, but in the majority of cases it is not sufficient, and then morphine comes to the assistance, depriving the subcortical cerebral regions of the remaining means for their natural defence.

Foerster studied in man symptoms of the first phases of epileptic seizures, the starting point of which was some alteration in the cortex of the big hemispheres. He noticed that with a given localisation of the disease, the initial symptoms were very constant. But the focus from which the irritation spreads exerts its influence on the general picture of the convulsions only at the beginning, during the period when the process proceeds within definite morphological and functional limits. As the irritation increases, or, what is the same thing, as the general excitability is heightened, the local convulsions pass into general convulsions. Generalising, one may say that the process draws in a large number of other automatic mechanisms. The specific picture characteristic of the first brief stage is now lost and the seizure *passes into the standard form.*

If irritation remains localised, then the process is limited to local convulsive action in the form of nictation, twitching of the ears, tongue, toes, etc. In such cases we have the manifold symptoms of local epilepsy. Under appropriate conditions they can pass into an epileptic attack. The clinic is well acquainted with phenomena of this nature. Recently my collaborator S. I. Lebedinsky succeeded in reproducing them experimentally.

The experiment was made as follows. Under light ether narcosis, an injection of 2 mg. of atropine in a 1 per cent solution was made in a rabbit by means of a suboccipital puncture. Shortly afterwards it was possible to observe a specific convulsive symptom in the form of periodical shaking of the ears and head. The movement is very easily provoked by touching the ear. If the tactile stimulation is repeated several times with short pauses of less than a second, it ceases to evoke the above-mentioned motor effect. But the process is only inhibited, for on waiting for a few seconds and then again touching the ear of the rabbit, one obtains the phenomenon of induction, *i.e.,* not a local convulsive effect but a genuine, even if comparatively short-lived, epileptic seizure. This phenomenon can be repeated several times in the course of the following 30-60 minutes.

Interesting data can be obtained by comparing the general picture of complex convulsive states with the general picture of rabies at various stages of both these processes.[1]

Rabies, produced by fixed virus, usually begins with phenomena due to disorganisation of co-ordination. The gait is altered, becoming staggering, drunken. During the whole initial period of the illness, however, the behaviour of the animals, at least in dogs, remains practically normal. They respond to calling, approach tottering on their legs, wag their tails, caress, and distinguish between attractive food (sausage) and unattractive food (black bread), etc.

Later the illness passes into the stage of spastic paralysis, and frequently even during the first 8-12 hours we find the dog in a characteristic attitude on its side, with extremities stretched out like sticks, the head thrown back and rigid extension of the spinal column (opisthotonus). These phenomena are intensified reflexly on any external stimulation—sharp sounds, touching or sudden illumination. Simultaneously there is nearly always considerable flow of saliva, sometimes squinting, and in rabbits, grinding of the teeth (convulsions of the jaw muscles). The stage of spastic phenomena is followed by

[1] A. D. Speransky. *Ann. de l'Inst. Pasteur,* Vol. 41, 1927.

feeble paralysis and then the animal dies. All these symptoms do not present anything characteristic or specific and can be observed in varying degrees in many diseases of the nervous system: in tetanus, in strychnine and other poisoning, and at particular moments of that characteristic process which we observe in dogs on partial freezing of the cortex.

At the beginning of our work on the infection of dogs by *"virus fixe"* we regarded the stereotyped character of all the phenomena as a specific syndrome of rabies. Later, we had to change this view. It was found that *the stereotyped character of the picture was connected with the mode of infection*, or more correctly with the place at which the process began. The usual method is to introduce the virus directly in the cerebral region of dogs; introduction of the virus [1] into the blood and other tissues, even into nerve trunks, only rarely results in illness. At the present time, however, we have been able to obtain a constant means of infecting dogs by Leningrad and other stocks of *virus fixe* through nerve trunks. The number of dogs developing rabies when infected in this way is about the same as when they are infected through the brain (the appropriate method is described in another chapter).

On observing such dogs, it was found that the initial symptoms of the disease vary, depending on the place where the virus penetrated from the periphery (*n. vagus, n. hypoglossus, n. ischiadicus,* etc.). Thus the order of inclusion of separate nerve parts into the process is reflected also in the external features of the disease. But this holds good *only for its first stages*. Very quickly the above-mentioned difference is wiped out and "fixed" rabies develops in its standard form.

The external manifestations of disease in "street" rabies are considerably more complicated and manifold; on the other hand the impairment of the cerebral regions lying below the cortex is here still more pronounced. The distinguishing feature of the external picture of "street" rabies consists in the exhibition of an additional period which is entirely, or almost entirely, absent in "laboratory" rabies. It is characterised by *excitation of the nerve apparatuses of compound automatic movements,* such as mastication, swallowing, locomotor actions (which sometimes compel the dog to run considerable distances), aggressive reactions, etc. The disturbance of co-ordination begins much later, and from this time the picture of the disease in street rabies is in no way different from that of rabies produced by infection with *virus fixe.*

In our experiments, we were also able to observe directly the correspondence in the external picture of street and laboratory rabies. This was in the case of dogs in which, 18 hours after subdural inoculation with *virus fixe,* there was further introduced also subdurally, a small quantity (about 3.0

[1] Leningrad stock of *"virus fixe."*

c.c.) of antirabic serum. The same dose of serum was repeated after two days. On the sixth day (the normal incubational period for dogs) the animal had not become ill, nor on the seventh or following days. It became ill on the twelfth day after inoculation, *i.e.*, after an incubational period twice the normal.The disease began with general agitation. At the slightest noise (knocking, opening the door, entering the room) the dog jumped up, glanced around and attempted to run away. In doing so, the animal fell down, as a result of incipient disorganisation of co-ordination, but after falling continued to run while lying on its side. Very quickly, this is supplemented by clonic convulsions, abundant salivation and, finally, *an uninterrupted convulsive state, reminiscent of* status epilepticus, *broken sometimes by the above-described "stationary running."* This state lasted 12 hours and only then passed into a picture of spastic and afterwards feeble paralysis, such as is characteristic of the laboratory form of rabies (*virus fixe*). Following this the animal died.

What happened here? After the measures taken, there was a prolongation of the incubational period. It approached that which is usual for street rabies on direct infection through the brain. As a result, the process assumed the character of an intermediate disease, uniting together features characteristic of both forms of rabies.

If we compare these data with those obtained from the analysis of the constituent parts of the epileptic attack, it is not difficult to note the great resemblance. Observations throughout many years have shown that it is sometimes very difficult to distinguish them from one another. This appears especially clearly at particular moments of observation. One involuntarily comes to the conclusion that the nervous mechanism of both processes is identical, that *rabies is an epileptic seizure extended in time.*

In spite of the fact that analysis of the processes entering into the picture of the epileptic seizure itself, and also of its preliminary and subsequent stages, inevitably leads us to actions of complex automatic movements—the view of the leading role of the cortex in the origin of clonic convulsions is still maintained very stubbornly (Gordon Holmes, D. Collier). Recently, N. I. Propper carried out a series of experiments on dogs in order to prove the same thesis. The author produced the convulsive process by applying the electric current of the lighting supply to the head of the animal for several seconds (one electrode being on the lower jaw, the other on the *protuberantia occipitalis*). Having established the usual picture of the convulsive attack brought about by this means, the author proceeded to an additional extirpation of various parts of the nervous system with the object of observing the changes which would thereby be produced in the complex convulsive syndrome. As a result, it was found that the picture of the epileptic attack can be destroyed by very *diverse means*. The greatest effect in altering the clonic phase of the attack is obtained in the period immediately following extirpation of the motor cortex. After that the difference gradually disappears. Injury to the cerebellum and excision of parts of the peripheral trunk acted in almost the same way. However, the author draws the conclusion from this of the "predominant role of the cortex in the construction of the clonic phase of the epileptic attack." He reduces the role c the subcortex to the construction of the tonic phase.

The experiments of N. I. Propper are undoubtedly interesting, but they prove only one thing: *if a local injury is inflicted on the nervous system at any point of it, this is reflected in some degree also on its other parts.* If the author had taken as an indicator, not the symptoms of the convulsive picture, but, for example, the qualitative and quantitative features of the secretion of gastric juice, the effect would have been approximately the same. In this case also, he would have obtained a change to one side or the other, with the same tendency to gradual equalisation. There is no doubt that different parts of the nervous system are not equivalent, and that an injury inflicted at one spot will have more pronounced consequences for one particular group of reactions and less pronounced ones for another. But this takes place not only as a result of direct exclusion of parts entering into the mechanism of the given reaction, but also because the injury alters the reacting capacity of the entire object as a whole. The proofs of this statement have already been given above. The material in the following chapter is intended especially to throw light on this question.

CHAPTER IV

THE THRESHOLD OF EXCITABILITY IN CONVULSIVE PROCESSES

In order to understand the working of a particular nerve mechanism, it is not sufficient to know its constituent parts and the order of their inclusion in the process. A stimulus arising at one point of the nervous system passes through a series of stages in the centripetal and centrifugal directions. The final results depends, not only on each of the links taken separately, but also on the state of the whole chain. It is what is called tonus, *i.e.*, the degree of working readiness, and is measured by the threshold of stimulation.

The tonus of the nervous system is determined by two basic factors. One is the chemical background against which the process takes place. The other is connected with the functional state of the nerve structures taking part in the reaction. This factor *embraces not only the totality of the producing or active elements themselves, but also the maintenance by these elements of normal connections with others that have no immediate relation to the process concerned.*

Any nerve cell, wherever it may be situated, is a receptor apparatus for any other nerve cell if it can be connected with the latter directly or indirectly by the transferred stimulus. The general sum total of such unconsidered influences is reflected in the state of excitability of the working parts. In order that the subcortical cerebral regions, which express high degrees of this excitation through epileptic attacks, should be in a state of the requisite tonus, it is necessary that their connections with other nerve regions should not have been destroyed.

At definite moments of activity a cortical cell is as much a receptor apparatus for the cells of the subcortical parts as an olfactory or auditory receptor. In this sense the ablation of the motor cortex can only be compared with the injury of a receptor apparatus, olfactory, auditory or visual. As a result of the operation, some parts of the subcortical regions are deprived of constant, normal stimulation and their tonus, with which the threshold of stimulation is connected, is bound to be lowered. They have become different cells and previous stimulating agents will not have the former power over them.

Put in this form, the question is easily susceptible of experimental test, and this was carried out by us in the following way (experiments of my collaborator V. S. Galkin [1]).

Under narcosis we laid bare the frontal sinuses in a dog, and their inner osseous lamina was cautiously trepanned above the upper extremity of the *bulbus olfactorius*, damaging the dura mater as little as possible. The latter was removed by means of a narrow sharp lancet throughout the whole extent of the *lamina cribrosa*, which in the dog is somewhat bent and stands almost vertically to the base of the skull. At the same time the olfactory nerves were severed outside the membranes of the brain, and in this way there was almost no flow of blood within the cranial cavity. Trauma of the frontal lobes was also avoided, since it is known that such trauma may lead in the dog to the development of the epileptic state. In the post-operational period, subcutaneal emphyseuma of the head is sometimes noticed, but this usually passes off fairly quickly.

Simple observation of such animals often reveals the difference between their behaviour before and after the operation. Some of them are dull, many of them sleep. In contact with new surroundings they do not display the usual lively orientational reactions. Sometimes the dogs become noticeably thinner and may even die in a state of exhaustion. The majority, however, recover from the consequences of the operation fairly easily.

After various periods, from some days up to 2-3 months, the experiment of freezing a portion of the cortex was carried out in the usual way, under general narcosis with invariable preliminary introduction of our usual dose of morphine. Observation showed that convulsive phenomena, which, under usual conditions, are the most prominent feature of the illness, in this new form of experiment are much less pronounced. The process developed more slowly and rarely attained a higher degree of the convulsive state.

It has already been mentioned that the epileptic attacks in normal dogs usually begin 1-2-5 hours after freezing. Only on one occasion, among many dozens of observations, did the first epileptic attack take place after 14 hours. Normal dogs are frequently already dead at the end of 15-20 hours after the operation. In the present case, however, we observed a late development of epilepsy. Sometimes the retardation was considerable. Thus, we observed the first epileptic attack in our dogs after 20, and even after 40, hours from the time of freezing.

In the intervals between the attacks, external manifestations of disease were scanty. The period of motor agitation, which previously was the exclusive source of varied material for observation, was almost absent here. At the beginning tonic convulsions were noticed in various groups of muscles but

[1] V. S. Galkin. *Arkh. Biol. Nauk*, Vol. 32, No. 2, 1932; *Zeitschr. f. d. ges. exp. Med.*, Vol. 81, No. 3-4, 1932.

they were feeble and inconstant. Nor does death by any means take place in all cases. In this respect our experimental material can be divided into two groups.

The first group includes animals where either a short period of 1-2 days, or, on the contrary, a very long period, 4-5 months, elapsed between the operations of severing the olfactory paths and of freezing the cortex. About 50 per cent of the dogs in this group die after the freezing of the cortex.

The second group comprises animals in which the interval between the two operations amounts to 2-5 weeks. These dogs, as a rule, remain alive after freezing the cortex. Moreover, convulsive phenomena, particularly in the form of epileptic attacks, hardly occur among them at all. Cases were observed fairly often when these animals exhibited no pathological phenomena of any kind.

Such cases also occur among the animals of the first group, but much more rarely. We can look for an explanation of this difference in the fact that, with a short interval between the two operations, the deprivation of normal excitation through the olfactory organs is replaced by irritation from the region of the fresh operational trauma. When, however, the interval is prolonged, then either scars develop in the frontal regions of the brain or the animals compensate for the missing olfactory receptor by using the auditory, visual, tactile and other receptors to a greater extent than normally.

Such were the general data of our observations.

In addition, during the period of the experiment genuine peculiarities were noticed belonging only to this particular form of experiment. In a number of dogs it was found that after freezing the cortex there developed, *not a convulsive state, but sleep*, deep sleep lasting one, two or even three days. Such consequences of an operation had never been met with before during several year's work.

That it was actually sleep, and not coma or a similar condition, is clear from the fact that the animal could be awakened. It is true that this requires considerable exertion. The dog must be shaken and put on its feet several times, before it finally takes several steps. On such occasions, it looks for a more secluded spot and creeps under the table, stool or the steam radiator. Thus, its behaviour cannot be considered automatic. Left in peace it immediately falls asleep again, but gets up for defecation, drinking and ultimately for eating. In general, it produces the impression of a dog deprived of its hemispheres, in which case also sleep is often the usual condition during the first weeks, interrupted for short periods by somatic reflexes.

Among some of the animals, epileptic attacks develop during sleep and without any preliminary preparation, and are immediately followed again by sleep. More than once, we found that epileptic attacks made their appearance during sleep under the influence of external stimuli. Thus, on one occasion, in transferring a dog from one building to another, it was accidentally dropped. Immediately a typical epileptic seizure developed. Soon after this, another seizure was evoked in this dog, also by external stimulation. These attacks formed the only convulsive part of the syndrome of the illness; all the rest of the time the only symptom was sleep. Subsequently we made several more such observations.

After various periods, the dogs' somnolent state gradually diminishes and disappears; they recover and afterwards can be considered healthy. Sometimes, however, the sleep passes imperceptibly into coma followed by death.

In the next experiment, we passed from the olfactory to the auditory and visual receptors. The exclusion of the auditory receptor was carried out by means of bilateral destruction of the cochlea and of the visual receptor by severing the visual nerves.

The cessation of visual stimuli has almost no influence on the development of pathological phenomena after freezing the cortex. In any case it is difficult to make a proper estimate of it. The consequences, however, of the loss of the two cochleæ are in part similar to those observed after the destruction of the olfactory receptor but are much less pronounced. Convulsions and other phenomena of motor excitation are frequently met with in this case. In one instance, however, instead of the convulsive state, we had here also the development of prolonged and deep sleep.

It is interesting to note that all our dogs in which the cochleæ were destroyed died within a certain period after the operation of freezing the cortex. Thus it was found that the nerve trauma brought about by the destruction of the cochlea is more important for the vital processes than the trauma due to section of the olfactory nerves, although in the first case the brain is in no way subjected to trauma. The whole operation is carried out from the tympanic cavity through the *foramen rotundum*, takes very little time (not more than 15 minutes) and does not require the use of a chisel. In the course of the following days, the dogs recover and, apart from deafness, differ in no way from normal. However in these cases, a second nerve trauma in the form of freezing a portion of the cortex proved fatal. What apparently plays a role here is that the primary damage directly affects the *medulla oblongata*.

The data obtained raised the question as to what would be the consequence of excluding all at once a whole group of fundamental receptors—olfactory, visual and auditory (experiments of V. S. Galkin[1]). It was found

[1] V. S. Galkin. *Arkh. Biol. Nauk*, Vol. 33, No. 1-2, 1933; *Zeitschr. f. d. ges. exp. Med.*, Vol. 88, Nos. 3, 4, 1933.

that in this case there were no signs of excitation in the post-operational period, but the dogs simply did not wake up after narcosis: it was impossible to observe in them the transition from narcosis to sleep. During the first days, only violent stimulation could arouse the animals for some minutes from their state of immobility. In that case, a short but powerful excitation was exhibited, in the form of an irregular motor reaction similar to the reaction of children when awakened from deep sleep. After that the dogs fell asleep again. Observations carried out without interruption for days and nights together showed that the animals could remain in one posture for 15-20 hours or even longer.

For a long while the animals have to be fed artificially, since they do not take food, and if food is put into their mouths they at once reject it. During all this time, everything proceds satisfactorily in the region of the operation wounds, which heal rapidly by first intention. Artificial feeding has to be continued more than a month. We carried it out once a day and always at exactly the same hour. Gradually, a time reflex is established in the dogs and they begin to take food, feebly and awkwardly, but independently. At the same hour they defecate and urinate, *excreting at one time the whole 24 hours' quantity of urine*. During the first two weeks, if the dog is not forcibly put on its feet, it defecates lying down. In spite of the fact that the animal finally begins to take food independently, all the rest of its behavior remains unchanged. As before, after eating and defecation the dogs immediately go to sleep again and do not change their attitude for many hours. Sleep continues for almost whole days and nights at a time.

Some of these dogs lived more than a year after the operation, and during the whole time the basic form of their "behaviour" was sleep. Only gradually is some simple life routine established, taking from sleep a very small amount of time (eating, licking themselves, stretching themselves). Thus, the loss of extero-ceptive stimuli gradually passed into an almost unchanging state of inhibition. This state depended in fact on the general lowering of tonus and not on any other causes produced by the operation. This is confirmed by the following characteristic case.

On one occasion, the operation of excluding smell, sight and hearing was performed on a young, very lively and active dog which was suffering from a skin disease with very strong itching (*acarus folliculorum*). The animal incessantly scratched itself not only in the waking condition but also during sleep. When the above-mentioned receptors were cut out one after another, its behaviour did not change. The animal remained active, played and quarrelled with its neighbours, took food independently and occupied the normal amount of time in sleep.

But as soon as the skin disease began to heal and the itch disappeared, the dog at once lost all its liveliness and began to pass whole days in sleep. The other vital manifestations changed correspondingly—the taking of food, time of defecation, etc. As soon as the healing was interrupted and the disease reappeared, the animal once again became lively and sociable. Thus the missing stimuli were made up for here by the heightened functioning of the skin receptor. As long as this was the case, the general tonus was also maintained at the necessary level and the behaviour of the animal remained normal.

I described above the reasons why we regard the nervous mechanism of epileptic attacks as closely allied to the nervous mechanism of rabies. Here was an occasion for verifying this by a new form of experiment (experiments carried out by my collaborators V. S. Galkin and A. M. Cheshkov.[1]).

On several dogs an operation was performed consisting of separation of the dura mater from the *lamina cribrosa*, thereby tearing all the olfactory nerves passing through the *lamina*. Some time after the dogs had recovered, we inoculated them subdurally with "street" virus of rabies. Within 2-3 weeks, all the animals fell ill, but the disease took a course as if they had been inoculated, not with street virus, but with *virus fixe*. In addition, while in the case of fixed rabies it is possible to notice a few active pathological symptoms, especially during the initial period, here, from the very beginning of the illness, *the dogs remained lying down, immobile, and died while in this state of somnolence*. At the same time also, the period of the illness was shortened. Street rabies in dogs usually lasts 3-4 days, sometimes even considerably longer. In these cases, however, the disease ended in death in the course of 20-30 hours. In only one dog did we observe a very short period of agitation, but it was a unique case in which several months had elapsed between the operation of disconnecting the olfactory receptor and infection. As has been pointed out, we found the same thing in experiments with epilepsy. Thus, all the phenomena observed in our experiments with epilepsy were repeated here even to minute details.

I have already mentioned above that, during the first weeks after removal of the cortex of both hemispheres, dogs usually pass the greater part of their time in sleep. Subsequently this gradually passes off. The observations carried out in the laboratory of I. P. Pavlov (S. I. Lebedinsky and I. S. Rosenthal) have shown that after a certain period the number of hours of the waking state and of sleep approximate to the normal. Here, also, a primitive life routine is finally established.

All this does not imply that we see a full analogy between the conse-

[1] V. S. Galkin and A. M. Cheshkov. *Arkh. Biol Nauk*, Vol. 32, No. 3, 1932; *Zeitschr. f. d. ges. exp. Med.*, Vol. 82, Nos. 3, 4, 1932.

quences of the operation of removing the motor cortex and of excluding smell or hearing. The phenomena developing in the latter case are undoubtedly different. *But their reflection on another process taken by us as an indicator proved to be the same.* Consequently, if after the removal of any particular nerve region, we find that a number of symptoms are omitted from the conplex picture, this does not signify at all that the given symptoms constitute a direct and immediate function of the elements removed. It is necessary here to take account of the fact that the remaining parts become altered and this alteration is the stronger, the more intimate their connection with the region which has suffered. Moreover, from the example of the experiments of L. N. Fedorov [1] described above, we saw that in dogs subjected to freezing after extirpation of the motor cortex on one side, the difference in the motor state of the two halves of the body was noticeable only in the first period of the illness. As the convulsive phenomena increase, this difference decreases, and finally the moment comes when the motor effects on the right and left sides of the body become equal. How could this happen if, by extirpating the cortex, we actually abolished the producing elements?

Finally, let us recall that even removal of both hemispheres does not save the dog from the possibility of the subsequent development of a complex convulsive picture, absolutely typical of the epileptic state. In the final resort, it is this, and not the temporary change in the picture of the process after partial extirpations, that decides the matter.

The nervous system is an organ which cannot be altered locally. Local interference affects the whole nervous network; these changes pass away gradually and not completely, and give rise to a number of adaptations to the new artificial norm. The nervous system is a new object after the local lesion, and it reacts to stimuli in a new fashion. For the question raised here, the important point is that the object preserves its capacity for developing the complex convulsive syndrome in all its details, in spite of the absence of the corresponding cortical regions.

Of the particular features observed, one which presents interest is that of sleep, which we obtained instead of the convulsive state in a number of instances. Whatever may be said about the pathological nature of this phenomenon, it must be regarded as genuine sleep, since external influences interrupted it and then the behaviour of the dog approximated to the normal. In human pathology, a complex of symptoms is known, bearing the name narcolepsy, which very many consider closely related to epilepsy (Westphal, Fischer, Collier). Others maintain its independent character (Aby). Collier points to the fact that, in the course of the illness, attacks of narcolepsy are

[1] L. N. Fedorov. *Zeitschr. f. d. ges. exp. Med.,* Vol. 72, No. 1-2, 1930.

equivalent to genuine epileptic seizures and can alternate with them, as a basic reason for uniting these processes. In the material described by us, one may find a confirmation of this view. There is every reason to believe that either of these reactions can appear, depending on the state of excitability of the various parts of the nervous system of the given animal.

The last point deserving of separate consideration concerns the conditions for the development of *status epilepticus*. Not everything is clear as to the origin of this form. The view is generally current that the process mentioned is the result of toxœmia. The chief grounds for arriving at this conclusion are furnished by observations on eclampsia, which is always accompanied by considerable chemical changes in the blood and tissues and produces morphological changes in the organs similar to those in the case of poisoning. The data obtained here are applied also to all other forms of *status epilepticus*.

Collier draws attention to the fact that in all cases of *status epilepticus* observed by him (they all ended in death), fatty degeneration of the heart was found on autopsy. He considers that this can only be the result of acute toxœmia.

There is no doubt that in epileptic attacks the changes are not only related to the functioning of the motor areas of the nervous system. The changes here are much more extensive; they embrace many regions of the nervous system, including the so-called vegetative or autonomic centres. Thus, Cushing observed the development of epileptic attacks in dogs after removal of the pituitary gland. In so doing there is always trauma or irritation of the region of the *tuber cinereum* and *infundibulum*, *i.e.*, parts of the nervous system connected in the closest fashion with metabolic processes. We also obtained this effect in dogs by irritation of the posterior part of the *tuber cinereum* by means of a small glass sphere placed in the region of the *sella turcica*. If, instead of the glass sphere, we place in this region a pea which has been soaked in alcohol, *i.e.*, if in addition to the mechanical irritant we add a chemical one, then an epileptic state develops in the majority of the dogs. Subsequently, they exhibit various pathological changes of a dystrophic character, in almost all tissues and organs, which is evidence of the serious and deeply penetrating destruction of physico-chemical equilibrium in the organism. *These changes gradually progress, but without convulsive phenomena being renewed.*

One and the same irritation is capable of evoking simultaneously an active condition in various parts of the nervous system. These processes can mutually support one another, as is partially borne out, for example, in the phenomena of eclampsia. Nevertheless, it must be admitted that *status epilepticus* can exist also independently; otherwise, the cases described above of fatal epilepsy after extraction of the cerebro-spinal fluid with subsequent nerve trauma would remain completely inexplicable. Here, it is precisely *status epilepticus* that develops, usually suddenly, in an animal which half an hour before was absolutely healthy.

The conclusion that must be drawn is that *status epilepticus*, as a separate variety of the convulsive state, is not caused by toxœmia alone. The origin of this form is bound up with the basic property of the nervous system, namely the rhythmical character of its functioning. *If the strength of the irritation attains a certain degree, then the process evoked by it occurs of itself.*

This does not mean that the chemical background plays no role whatever in the development of *status epilepticus*. But each individual attack is also connected with this background. In many cases, the significance of toxœmia, as the fundamental factor in the origin of *status epilepticus*, can perhaps be substantiated. But there exist also forms where it is impossible to admit the existence of any preliminary toxic process. The chemistry of the blood is not the only factor responsible for the renewal of convulsive attacks, once these attacks have already begun.

Collier's reference to fatty degeneration of the heart as a clear sign of toxœmia cannot have any decisive significance. A direct causal connection between the two has not been proved. The study of the role of the nervous system in various pathological processes furnishes us daily with proofs that, in the development of many forms of degenerative phenomena at the periphery, the basic factor is the initial disease of the nervous system.

It remains to add a few words to conclude the question of the role of the cortex and subcortex in the origin of complex convulsive states, and in particular of epileptic attacks. The mutual relations here will be clear if we form an accurate conception of what we are dealing with at each given moment. It is necessary to separate the conception of the *composition* of the epileptic attack from the conception of its *genesis*. In the first case, we are satisfied with conceptions of localisation, *i.e.*, of a certain independence and definiteness of the functions of separate morphological groups, and we permit ourselves to say that the composition of the epileptic attack is a function of the subcortical cerebral regions.

For the solution of the question of genesis, these conceptions prove useless. For now we are no longer concerned with cortex, subcortex and other conventional subdivisions of the nervous system, since all parts of the latter can be brought into an active condition by irritation arising at any nerve point.

THE ROLE OF THE CEREBRO-SPINAL FLUID IN THE GENESIS OF SOME FORMS OF ENCEPHALITIS

CHAPTER V

ENCEPHALITIS AS ONE OF THE CONSEQUENCES OF FREEZING A PORTION OF THE CEREBRAL CORTEX IN DOGS

PROLONGED observation of the process developing in dogs as a result of freezing a portion of the cortex has demonstrated that the matter is by no means always restricted to the phenomena immediately following the experiment. The investigation of the remote results, however, is rendered difficult owing to the animal's death, which, in the majority of cases, forms the culmination of the experiment. The dogs usually die quite soon, and then the observations remain perforce within the limits of acute experiment. However, even from the very beginning of our work, we also had animals which recovered after they had passed through a certain proportion of the acute symptoms of the disease. Later on, as has been pointed out, the special means adopted by us frequently arrested, altered or even prevented the illness. Gradually we accumulated a considerable number of such animals. Their fate then became the subject of special observation.

It was found that their fate was not uniform. Taking all the animals together, we can divide them into 4 groups as regards the consequences of the experiments.

The first and largest group consists of dogs which die immediately after the experiment or, more correctly, during the experiment itself.

The second group comprises those animals which recover rapidly and afterwards remain healthy for such long periods that we can consider them to have definitely recovered.

The third group is made up of dogs which, after a certain period of apparent health, lasting from 1-3 weeks up to several months, suddenly fall ill, with a relapse of the convulsive state, in the course of which they usually die.

Finally, there is a fourth group of animals which pass out of the convulsive period into a new form of illness. It is this numerically small group which is now the subject of our special consideration.

The transition takes place imperceptibly. At the beginning, the epileptic attacks in the dog grow weaker and subsequently they disappear. Tonic cramps persist for some time and now stand out even more markedly since they are not obscured by other phenomena in the complex convulsive picture. Gradually, the general tonus also decreases and is expressed, for the most part, in spastic gait. This last may be retained for a long time, one or two weeks or even more. The animal grows noticeably thinner, becomes listless, spends much time lying down, refuses to take food, so that sometimes artificial feeding is necessary to maintain its life. Very soon paresis sets in, generally in the muscles of the hind extremities. In some cases, paralysis also overtakes the processes of chewing and swallowing. Flow of saliva is usually observed throughout the course of the illness. Sometimes a general picture arises similar to that of bulbar paralysis (in part this has already been mentioned above). If the illness is protracted, then very soon it is possible to observe also the development of dystrophic phenomena, expressed in local or general loss of hair, dryness of the integuments, eczema, sores and other non-healing, ulcerous skin diseases. The process terminates in the death of the animal.

Microscopical examination of the central nervous system in such dogs, carried out by my collaborator Dr. S. I. Lebedinsky, showed that alterations are to be found in many regions. It is possible to observe also parenchymatous changes, sometimes even destruction of nerve cells; the chief changes, however, are interstitial, in the form of round-celled infiltrates into the brain substance, with the formation of "cuffs" around the blood vessels. In protracted cases, the round-celled infiltration is noticed also under the ependyma of the ventricles. Sometimes one finds multiplication of the cells of the ependyma itself, disposed in several layers and forming outgrowths in the direction of the ventricles of the brain.

Some 10-15 days after the operation, the portion of the cortex which has been immediately subject to freezing forms a hollow on the surface of the brain. It is rough and, as it were, eaten out. Later, at this place a flat, closed cavity, or cyst, containing a small quantity of transparent fluid, is sometimes formed between the membranes.

Already from this short description it is clear that the general picture of the pathologo-anatomical changes in the brain of a dog, which has died at the end of a considerable period after the operation of partially freezing the cortex, does not present any specific peculiarities. It is the general picture of encephalitis. It can be observed in pathological processes of the most varied origin. In the first place, rabies must be included here, the external manifestations of which have much in common with the clinical picture just described. These anatomical changes, not merely in character, but partly also in situation, are reminiscent of epidemic encephalitis, progressive paralysis and some other processes in man. Long ago, I. P. Pavlov described an interesting form of disease occurring in dogs, in which the duodenum was withdrawn and fixed under the skin of the stomach through a wound in the abdominal wall. After some time, these animals developed a number of symptoms analogous to those observed in our dogs in which a portion of the cortex has been frozen; *viz.*, the formation of ulcerations, emaciation, other forms of dystrophic phenomena, spastic gait, paralysis and death. Pathologo-anatomical examination of the brain substance of these dogs revealed changes analogous to those just described.

Thus we see that all these processes of a very varied nature possess something in common. There is no doubt that in the final analysis *we are dealing here with encephalitis, the course of which depends, not so much on the irritation which has evoked it, as on the properties of the diseased substratum.*

In attempting to make a realistic estimate of these properties, it is necessary, in the first place, to consider the question of the circulation, which suggests itself both on account of the character of the morphological alterations enumerated and their situation in close proximity to the blood vessels and medullary cavities containing cerebro-spinal fluid.

If the round-celled infiltrate is regarded as one of the forms of the organism's reaction to damage, then it must be recognised that in the given case the elements of the central nervous system were threatened with damage from the direction of the blood vessels and cavities.

Inflammatory reaction in tissues is by no means only produced and maintained by microbes or foreign chemical irritants. The tissues and fluids of the organism, with a change in their biological properties, may themselves become irritating agents for other elements and produce in them inflammatory forms of local reactions.

In observing the local phenomena of inflammation, we naturally begin to look for their cause somewhere in the vicinity. Consequently, the first question which has to be raised is whether in the present case the blood may not be the source of irritation.

This must be answered in the negative. In all the instances described above, where the action gives rise to the general picture of encephalitis, the infiltration of the brain substance is by no means exhibited around all the blood vessels. Far from this being the case, in some processes, such as epidemic encephalitis, these changes have a specific localisation. It is absolutely impossible to assume that the injurious agent should by accident always penetrate through the same particular branches of the blood vessels.

It remains to look for another cause. There is no doubt that this cause must be in close proximity to the wall of the blood vessel. The sole suitable structures are the adventitious spaces and interstices surrounding the blood vessels of the brain. These spaces are accessible to the cerebro-spinal fluid. In spite of certain objections, it is apparently necessary to regard them also as normal channels of its circulation.

Among the indirect proofs that the adventitious spaces of the medullary vessels can be the source of local irritation of nerve tissue must be included the fact of round-celled infiltration of parts of the brain adjacent to the ventricles. But the ventricles do not contain anything beyond cerebro-spinal fluid and, consequently, it is precisely in the latter that the source of irritation must be looked for. The round-celled infiltrate, in the form of "cuffs" along the course of certain blood vessels of the brain, does not essentially differ in any way from the reactive changes under the ependyma of the ventricles. The content of the adventitious spaces also can only be cerebro-spinal fluid. Thus the analogy in the origin of various sources of inflammation in encephalitis suggests itself automatically. The cerebro-spinal fluid undoubtedly plays a part here.

Being the liquid medium of the brain, the sole form of its lymph known to us, it flows into general collectors from various sources. Even in the normal organism, the composition of the cerebro-spinal fluid cannot be identical in all the pathways of its circulation. This has already been established in regard to its big collectors, the ventricles and the subarachnoid spaces. Diverse pathological processes very often bring about a change in the composition of the cerebro-spinal fluid, as was known even to early investigators (Wiedal, Sicard and Lesné). By now an enormous literature devoted to this question has already accumulated.

It must be recognised that, together with local pathological changes of the medullary substance, a local change in the composition of the cerebro-spinal fluid also takes place. It follows from this that cerebro-spinal fluid in various adventitious spaces of one and the same central nervous system may possess the properties of an irritating agent in a varying degree.

We are therefore justified in comparing the changes of the medullary substance around the vessels in encephalitis with the phenomena of lymphangoitis developing at the periphery, for instance in inflammatory processes of the foot or hand.

As early as 1925, these considerations impelled me to begin a series of experimental investigations on the role of cerebro-spinal fluid in the origin of toxic and infectious encephalitis.

CHAPTER VI

THE ROLE OF CEREBRO-SPINAL FLUID IN THE PROCESS OF DISINTEGRATION OF BRAIN SUBSTANCE

On one occasion, in the very first period of our work, the following experiment was performed. When the whole picture of the illness after the operation of freezing had developed in one of the dogs and the animal was on the point of death, the diseased portion of the brain (a piece of $1\frac{1}{2}$-2 cm. in diameter and 3-4 mm. in thickness) was extirpated and placed under the dura mater of another, healthy dog.

Some time later (3-4 months) this animal was killed. On dissection it was found that the fragment had disappeared without leaving any traces, either on the surface of the cerebrum or on the dura mater. The experiment was repeated with approximately the same result. On dissection, we either found no traces of tissue reaction or they were very weak.

It was possible that the cerebro-spinal fluid was in some way concerned in this phenomenon. This impelled me to try and find out whether this fluid exercises any influence on the destruction of brain substance *in vitro*. The experiments were carried out as follows.[1]

The cerebro-spinal fluid of a dog was extracted under sterile conditions and placed in a test-tube. To the fluid was then added a small piece of brain cut out of the cerebral cortex of a dog (or mouse). As a control, another test tube with the same brain substance was filled with physiological salt solution. Both tubes were placed in a thermostat at 40°C. and shaken fairly frequently and vigorously.

Even after a few hours it was possible to note a difference. The piece of brain in the test tube with cerebro-spinal fluid had enlarged in size and its uncovered surface membrane had ceased to be smooth. On shaking, small particles were detached from it and the liquid became turbid. In the test-tube with physiological salt solution, the brain fragment during the same period did not change in size or only to a very insignificant extent. The liquid remained transparent. On shaking, hardly any particles became detached, or if they did, this operation required great labour.

---

[1] A. D. Speransky. *Zhurn. Exper. Biol. i Med.*, No. 7, 1926; *Ann. de l'Inst. Pasteur*, Vol. 40, 1926.

The above-described phenomena can also be observed if a small piece of the spinal cord of a rabbit is taken instead of the brain fragment. After opening the spinal column, two pieces of equal size are cut from the spinal cord together with the dura mater. One is placed in cerebro-spinal fluid, the other in physiological salt solution. Within some hours, the medullary substance in the vessel with cerebro-spinal fluid has swollen and protrudes on each side of the covering of the dura mater like a fringe. Thus the whole piece takes on the form of an hour-glass.

We concluded from these facts *that the disintegration of brain substance takes place more rapidly in cerebro-spinal fluid than in physiological salt solution*. A definite selective process was also established by these experiments. It is only the brain tissue that swells up and disintegrates. The medullary membranes and blood vessels do not change.

These observations were published by me in 1926. Since then they have been the subject of experimental work on several occasions.

Thus, in 1929 and 1930, C. Rizzo and Mario Gozzano published the results of their observations on this question. Starting out from the method described by me, they made a large number of experiments both in the form employed by me and in other variations. For some experiments they took fresh brain tissue, for others, pieces of fresh brain, which had been cut out and subjected to preliminary freezing, or, on the other hand, boiled in water. As control fluids, they used physiological salt solution and blood serum. It was found that in all cases where it was possible to observe disintegration of the piece of brain substance in cerebro-spinal fluid, micro-organisms were always present in large quantity. The addition of antiseptic substances to the cerebro-spinal fluid prevented the multiplication of germs in it, but at the same time put a stop also to the process of disintegration of the brain substance.

The authors ascribe the changes in the brain fragment to the activity of micro-organisms and not to the process of autolysis in the proper meaning of the word. They deny that the cerebro-spinal fluid has any special properties in this process and put it on the same level as all the other fluids used by them as controls.

At the time, in describing the results of my observations, I pointed out that we were still unclear whether the cerebro-spinal fluid plays an independent role here or whether it only forms the medium in which processes of disintegration of nerve substance can proceed in an optimal fashion. What we noted at that time was the fact that the disintegration of brain substance in this medium took place better than under other, more artificial, conditions. We still adhere to this view.

In 1931, Dr. Aldo Rivela Greco, of the Nerve Clinic in the University of Genoa, published the first part of his researches on the same subject. The author begins by confirming our observations regarding the rapid disintegration of particles of brain substance placed in the cerebral submembranous spaces of a living animal.

Later, he decided to repeat our experiments *in vitro* and also to perform new ones. As controls, he used not only physiological salt solution or Ringer's solution but also artificial cerebro-spinal fluid and blood serum from man or from dogs. The author summarises the results of his observations in the following form.

1. In the tests with cerebro-spinal fluid and nerve tissue, it was possible even after a short time to observe opalescence and afterwards turbidity. This process proceeds more rapidly with a piece of spinal cord than with cerebral cortex. Preliminary freezing of the piece taken also accelerates this disintegration.

2. In the control tests, with physiological solution, Ringer's solution, artificial cerebro-spinal fluid and blood serum, there was no speedy exhibition of opalescence and subsequent regular turbidity. A weak degree of opalescence in these liquids could be seen only after several days from the beginning of the experiment. The same was the case in regard to the fragment of nerve tissue. In the control tubes it retained its shape unchanged for a long time, merely slightly swelling on some occasions.

3. Being interested in the conditions hindering the appearance of the above phenomena, the author found that this could be achieved by heating the cerebro-spinal fluid to 70°C. for half an hour, by putting it in a water-bath at boiling temperature for 10 minutes, by freezing, and also by filtration through collodion. As a final result, he considers that the "difference in the tests with cerebro-spinal fluid and those with control fluids is obvious."

4. In all the tests—both those with cerebro-spinal fluid and the control— the author always found a large quantity of micro-organisms. He does not determine the degree of their influence on the autolysis of nerve tissue. While regarding their participation in this process as indubitable, he, nevertheless, does not regard this as the cause of the phenomenon.

It seems to me that in weighing up the data brought forward, the fact of the presence of micro-organisms both in the tests with cerebro-spinal fluid and in the controls is worthy of attention. Among the controls were liquids containing proteins and carbohydrates. These liquids, consequently, also formed nutritive media for micro-organisms not inferior to cerebrospinal fluid. Nevertheless, the disintegration of nerve tissue in them occurred much more slowly than in the latter.

Special relations undoubtedly exist between medullary substance and cerebro-spinal fluid. This is testified to by various facts. Thus the brain, even shortly after death, begins to alter in weight, becoming heavier. At the same time the cerebro-spinal fluid gradually disappears from the submembranous spaces and reservoirs.

In 1924, H. Böning confirmed the fact of the posthumous disappearance of cerebro-spinal fluid from the submembranous spaces owing to the saturation of the brain substance by it.

All anatomists are familiar, also, with the fact that preservation of the human brain demands rapid fixing, especially in summer, otherwise it rapidly softens, the disintegrative process beginning not with the external parts, but from within, in those portions which are most closely contiguous to the cerebral ventricles filled with cerebro-spinal fluid.

During the course of our work we verified our observations once more under somewhat different conditions.

The experiments were made by my collaborator V. S. Galkin.[1] Physiological salt solution and Ringer's solution were used as controls. At the beginning, the usual operation of freezing was carried out. After some hours (1-3) the portion subjected to freezing was cut out under narcosis, and in the form of similar small pieces, about 1 c.c. in volume, put in test-tubes with the above-mentioned liquids. The same thing was done in control experiments with pieces of normal brain. Under these new conditions, the experiment proceeds in an absolutely clear-cut way, *leaving no doubt that the autolysis of nerve tissue takes place much more rapidly and completely in cerebro-spinal fluid than in an artificial medium.* The following point was also demonstrated: if two small pieces are taken—one from a normal portion of brain, and the other from a frozen portion of the same brain, the autolysis of which has already commenced within the living organism—and both these pieces are placed in test-tubes with cerebro-spinal fluid, then the disintegration of the frozen portion proceeds much more rapidly.

Recently, A. Rivela Greco and his collaborators have carried out a number of supplementary researches on the same question. Some new details were established in the course of them. Thus, it was found that the neurolytic process proceeds much more feebly if cerebro-spinal fluid is added to the test-tube in greater quantity than usual. The author regards this as in correspondence with what generally holds good in the chemistry of enzymes. The energy of their action is directly connected with the quantity of substrate and not with the quantity of ferment (Rondoli). Dr. Lazzeri has carried out research with the object of establishing the time necessary after withdrawal for the

[1] V. S. Galkin. *Zeitschr. f. d. ges. exp. Med.*, Vol. 84, No. 3-4, 1932; *Arkh. Biol. Nauk*, Vol. 34, No. 5-6, 1933.

cerebro-spinal fluid to lose its neurolytic capacity. Dr. P. Meco communicated to the Congress of Neuro-Pathologists at Modena his observations on the neurolytic activity of cerebro-spinal fluid taken from 240 patients suffering from various diseases (quoted from A. Rivela Greco).

One of my collaborators, A. E. Zakharova,[1] has been occupied with the determination of the neurolytic properties of the *humor aquea* of the eye, the composition of which closely resembles that of the cerebro-spinal fluid. The comparison was made both with artificial media and with cerebro-spinal fluid from the same animal. The conclusions at which she arrived can be formulated thus: 1) a freshly-cut piece of brain is disintegrated in the fluid of the anterior chamber of the eye of dogs and cats in absolutely the same way and in approximately the same period as in cerebro-spinal fluid; 2) the *corpus vitreum* acts in the same way as the fluid of the anterior chamber but the process here proceeds more slowly.

Of a series of other observations of ours, resembling those described, I will permit myself to bring forward the following.

It was shown by Wassermann and Takaki that tetanus toxin, when mixed with triturated fresh brain substance, loses its toxic properties. If it is true that primarily the protein substances of the brain are disintegrated in cerebrospinal fluid, then it must follow that if a mixture of brain and toxin is put in this liquid, the brain should be destroyed and the toxin set free.

The possibility of separating toxins from substances connected with them has already been proved, both in regard to tetanus toxin (Marie and Morax, 1902, and Marie and Tiffenau, 1908) and in regard to cobra poison (Calmette). The cobra poison was separated from anti-toxin serum. The effect was obtained by the employment of various physico-chemical agents which did not destroy the toxin (drying, maceration, heating, papaine).

Our experiments were carried out with pigs and rabbits (experiments of A. V. Ponomarev[2]). A portion of the mixture of brain substance and tetanus toxin was divided into two equal parts. To one part was added cerebro-spinal fluid from a dog, bull or man, to the other physiological salt solution, and both mixtures were placed in a thermostat for several hours at a temperature of 38°C., after which they were introduced under the skin of two animals of the same weight. The period in the thermostat must not be prolonged, since this produces separation of the toxin even without cerebro-spinal fluid. In general it is best to keep both mixtures in the thermostat for 4-6 hours. Animals injected with the mixture without cerebro-spinal fluid reacted only

[1] A. E. Zakharova. *Arkh. Biol. Nauk*, Vol. 34, No. 5-6, 1933; *Zeitschr. f. d. ges. exp. Med.*, Vol. 93, Nos. 1, 2, 1934.

[2] A. V. Ponomarev. *Arkh. Biol. Nauk*, Vol. 26, No. 4-5, 1926.

by phenomena of local swelling (at the place of injection). The animals which received the mixture treated with cerebro-spinal fluid developed local tetanus, or even died, exhibiting the complete and typical syndrome of tetanus. Another form of the experiment consisted in introducing into the subarachnoid space of a dog a mixture of brain with a large quantity of toxin, but inactive when injected subcutaneously. This also brought about the separation of the toxin with all the resulting consequences.

CHAPTER VII

THE TOXICITY OF CEREBRO-SPINAL FLUID

WHATEVER view be taken of the part played by cerebro-spinal fluid in the disintegration of brain substance, there is no doubt that the fluid changes its composition during the process, and as a result can become toxic. Its toxicity, however, cannot be looked upon as absolute. The important point is not only the presence of unusual constituents in the cerebro-spinal fluid, but also the existence of a number of other factors which influence the reaction of these unusual constituents with the living nerve elements.

The experience of a large number of investigators has established that when animals are inoculated with cerebro-spinal fluid from healthy persons, or persons suffering from various nervous diseases, the fluid exhibits a varying degree of toxicity. The fluid taken from sick persons is more toxic (Wiedal, Sicard and Lesné, and subsequently others as well). Up to the present time, it has remained unclear what exactly gives the cerebro-spinal fluid its toxicity, whether the starting point itself which has produced the disease, or whether also products of disintegration and pathological metabolism. To decide the question, an experiment is necessary in which this aspect of the matter would be free from doubt. Hence the determination of the toxicity of the cerebro-spinal fluid taken from our dogs was of definite interest. For the purpose of elucidating this question, the following series of experiments were carried out (experiments of my collaborator I. S. Rosenthal).

The operation of freezing was performed in a dog on a portion of the cerebral cortex large enough to bring about death. Shortly after the dog died, or shortly before its death, we extracted several grams of cerebro-spinal fluid. Simultaneously, in another (normal) dog, extraction of the same fluid was carried out under light inhalational narcosis (ether and chloroform, without morphine), and the fluid from the first dog was then injected into the normal dog subarachnoidally.

In the vast majority of cases, this leads to definite disturbances. Nervous phenomena of medium severity usually develop, in the form of tonic, and sometimes also local clonic, convulsions, spastic gait, general motor agitation and subsequent depression.

Two cases deserve special description. On one occasion, a large healthy dog was inoculated subarachnoidally with the cerebro-spinal fluid from two smaller dogs. Both these latter dogs had been given a "lethal dose" of freezing the day before. At the beginning of the experiment one of them had just died, the other was on the point of death. From the normal dog, 7.0 c.c. of cerebro-spinal fluid was withdrawn and 9.0 c.c. of the fluid from the sick dogs was introduced. The general picture of the resulting illness proved to be fairly severe. The symptoms were the same as those described above, i.e., tonic and local clonic convulsions, flow of saliva, agitation and subsequent depression. The difference was that in the former case the pathological symptoms very soon completely disappeared, while in this case the pathological phenomena persisted for several weeks and ended with the death of the animal. Spastic phenomena right until the end were so sharply marked that the walking of the animal was sometimes interrupted by its falling down as a consequence of awkward jumping movements, for the most part of the hind extremities. The initial period in each new movement was difficult, chewing and swallowing were disturbed, the animal was in a state of depression.

The second case was the following. All the experiments just described were carried out with adult animals. But on one occasion we introduced subarachnoidally into two puppies cerebro-spinal fluid from a dog that had died after "freezing." In the period immediately following, no symptoms of disease were observed, other than slight depression. Subsequently also, nothing abnormal was observed in the behaviour of these puppies except that one of them began to lose weight. Five weeks later, this one becomes ill. At the beginning, it is listless and will not eat. Gradually the general picture of motor agitation develops. The dog is in constant movement, it sometimes literally rushes about the room, running against objects. The gait is sharply spastic, the extremities making awkward jumping movements. At the same time "hallucinations" develop: the animal in running about suddenly comes to a stop, it gazes fixedly at one spot, its hair bristles up, it leaps to one side with a yelp and hides itself in a dark corner. Shortly afterwards, the dog quietens down and again begins to wander about the room. Then the whole picture described above is repeated. Very soon, circus movements make their appearance. The phenomena of agitation, in the form of the above-described "hallucinations," persist for rather more than a day, but the spastic phenomena intensify every day. The dog ceases to react correctly, even from the second day of the illness, so that it has to be fed by pouring water and milk into its mouth. Then the motor agitation begins gradually to diminish and the behaviour of the dog becomes almost normal. The dog remains lying down, curling itself up, and adopting a comfortable position; it chooses the warmest corner of the room and, later, when another dog is placed with it in the same cell it snuggles itself against it. At this period, slight but almost uninterrupted trembling occurs, emaciation progresses, and on the seventh day from the beginning of the illness the dog dies. During the whole course of the illness there was flow of saliva, which began to diminish only during the last two days. Inoculation of a rabbit with the brain did not produce rabies.

Microscopic examination revealed infiltration of the walls of the blood vessels of the brain and medullary substance in the neighbourhood of the vessels, the absence of Negri bodies in the *cornu Ammonis*, infiltration of the superficial parts in the region of the cerebral ventricles and a slight growth of ependyma.

Recently, another of my collaborators, V. S. Galkin, observed something almost analogous. We had already concluded that the case was a "street" form of rabies, *but it ended with recovery of health.* Twice we have observed the same form of disease in adult dogs also. At the beginning, the dogs grew thinner. Later, after a fairly long period, there were symptoms of motor agitation, flow of saliva, disturbance of chewing and swallowing, paralysis and death. The whole illness lasted in one case about ten days, in the other more than two weeks. The period of agitation was considerably shorter than the period of depression and lasted one day. There is no doubt that the disease would have ended in death much earlier if we had not had recourse to appropriate measures (warming, artificial feeding, cardiacs).

Looking at the general picture of the disease in these, and also in other, animals, especially at certain moments of it, it would be easy to take it, now for the consequences of freezing the brain, now for street rabies, now for rabies from *virus fixe*, now for tetanus and now again for poisoning by various alkaloids. And although the very protraction of the disease as well as its variable character pronounced against rabies, all the same we carried out an investigation of the brain for virus, but naturally with negative results.

In these experiments we succeeded also in making a further observation which proved useful in later investigations. We usually extracted the cerebro-spinal fluid from a healthy dog before injection and introduced in its place the fluid of a dog that had died from "freezing." On one occasion we succeeded in withdrawing from the healthy dog only 2.0 c.c. of fluid in all. In this case, after inoculation with "toxic" fluid, hardly any disturbances were observed.

We made this the subject of special observation. It was found that if only a small quantity of cerebro-spinal fluid is extracted as a preliminary from the normal dog, then, after injecting "toxic" fluid into it, no pathological phenomena develop. If, as a preliminary, as much cerebro-spinal fluid is withdrawn as can be extracted, then after the introduction of "toxic" cerebro-spinal fluid the phenomena described above almost invariably develop.

We carried out a large number of such experiments, injecting into the subarachnoid space of dogs and rabbits the products of incomplete disintegration of brain substance after the extraction of cerebro-spinal fluid. We obtained these products by placing an emulsion of brain tissue in cerebrospinal fluid in a thermostat for various periods and subsequently sterilising it by fractional pasteurisation. In these experiments, the above-described fact stood out very clearly. *If we introduced the emulsion into healthy dogs without preliminary evacuation of the membranous sac, we hardly ever obtained any pathological symptoms. If, however, the same quantity of substance was introduced into the emptied membranous sac, then the symptoms described above developed.* This is especially observable in rabbits.

It must be mentioned that on the injection of brain emulsion, or the products of its disintegration, into the subarachnoid space of dogs, the development of convulsive phenomena is always much more weakly expressed than in cases of direct freezing. Consequently the presence in the brain itself of a portion which has been altered by freezing has incomparably greater consequences. This is comprehensible, for we have here, in addition to the products of disintegration of the portion destroyed by freezing, a focus of irritation in the immediate vicinity of this portion; this focus is responsible for the excitation of other parts of the nervous system.

All the facts here brought forward establish that, after freezing a portion of the cerebral cortex in a dog, the cerebro-spinal fluid acquires toxic properties and is capable of producing a number of pathological symptoms in healthy dogs. The general picture of the disease is by no means uniform. We have seen many cases where, under externally similar conditions of experiment, one dog succumbed while others exhibited only insignificant and transient symptoms. Consequently, the poisonous substances formed by this means in the brain cannot be compared to other poisons, *e.g.*, toxins. *Their toxicity is relative* and wavers markedly, depending on many causes. This is the reason why, not only the immediate, but also the remote consequences of our experiments varied in different animals. The products of the disintegration of nerve tissue, such as we are dealing with here, can, of course, also be termed "neuro-toxins," but there is no particular need to do so. Numerous reservations would be indispensable here, since it is impossible to attach specific properties to them. *They can be replaced by various other substances,* producing the same immediate and remote effects, and doing so with considerably greater constancy than "neuro-toxins."

As we have seen, the action of the latter is to a certain extent connected with the conditions of circulation in the region of the central nervous system.

But it is not only substances arising in the brain that find their way into the cerebro-spinal fluid. Many other irritating agents can penetrate into it from outside by various paths. In their distribution, the role of the circulation must also be taken into account. It was natural to test this question on such processes as tetanus and rabies.

Tetanus toxin is a specific nerve poison. It is considered that both in cases of spontaneous illness and on artificial introduction into the tissues, it reaches the central nervous system by travelling along the nerve trunk.

The question whether the cerebro-spinal fluid takes any part in distributing the toxin has been tested repeatedly, but without any uniform decision being arrived at. Some authors (Moschowitz) succeeded in determining its presence in the fluid, others did not (Sicard).

In our experiments (carried out by my collaborator A. V. Ponomarev[1]) we did not make it our aim merely to determine the presence or absence of the toxin in the cerebro-spinal fluid. Our aim was also to see how the course of the disease is influenced by the presence or absence of the toxin in the subarachnoid space of the diseased animals.

The experiments were made as follows. In two dogs of like weight and growth, we introduced simultaneously similar quantities of tetanus toxin under the skin of the leg (in other cases into the muscles), so that the phenomena of "local tetanus" should develop within 40-50 hours. *Shortly before the appearance of the "local" symptoms*, we extracted from one of these dogs by suboccipital puncture the maximum amount of cerebro-spinal fluid that it was possible to withdraw (7.0-12.0 c.c.). Following this, the extraction was repeated twice daily, in the morning and in the evening. Thus the membranous sac of the dog was maintained in an "empty" condition. No extraction of fluid from the control dog was carried out, but since the first dog was given narcosis for the operation of making the puncture and extracting the fluid, the control dog also received narcosis at the same times. It was found that the phenomena of "local" tetanus developed approximately equally in both the experimental and the control animal. But the subsequent picture of the disease was sharply different in the two cases. In the control dog the local phenomena were followed by "general" phenomena in the usual order. In the dog in which, from the moment of the appearance of local symptoms, daily emptying of the membranous sac had been carried out, the development of general tetanus was delayed by 24-48 hours or more. In connection with this also, the life of the experimental dogs was prolonged by 2-5 days (in one case even by 10 days), beyond that of the controls.

Of course, repeated extraction of the cerebro-spinal fluid, even if carried

[1] A. V. Ponomarev. *Arkh. Biol. Nauk*, Vol. 26, No. 4-5, 1926.

out twice a day, does not guarantee that the membranous sac of the brain is actually maintained in an empty condition. It frequently happens that after each 12 hours it is possible to obtain almost the same quantity of fluid as on the first extraction. There is no doubt, however, that the conditions of its circulation, and, depending on this, the conditions of the functioning of the nervous system also, are altered. As a result, the course of the process taken by us as an indicator is also altered.

The development and course of rabies justifies us in seeking here the same peculiarities that we observed in the processes analysed above.

On dissecting animals killed by tetanus, the virus can be discovered in various parts of the nervous system. The latter, as we say, "invades" it. The mechanism of this invasion remains unclear. The facts adduced above allow us to presume that the circulation of the cerebro-spinal fluid can bring about the distribution of the virus in the central nervous system. Hence we decided to perform some experiments with rabies on the same plan as those with tetanus toxin (experiments of my collaborator A. M. Cheshkov[1]).

At the beginning, the animals used for the experiments were rabbits in which extraction of the cerebro-spinal fluid was carried out previous to inoculation. It is easily possible to extract 0.6-1.5 c.c. from a rabbit weighing 1.5-2.5 kg. Immediately after this, trepanning was carried out and the virus introduced under the dura mater in the protuberant part of the cerebral hemisphere (by the usual Pasteur-Roux method). The control animals received the same dose of virus at the same time, only without preliminary withdrawal of fluid. The inoculation was carried out with Leningrad stock *of virus fixe* in the form of a 1 per cent emulsion.

Looking through the records of the inoculation department of the Institute of Experimental Medicine for the preceding years, we reached the conclusion that, in work with this virus, rabbits as a rule become ill at the end of the fourth day. As the result of our experiments it was found that almost all the rabbits, in which the cerebro-spinal fluid had been extracted previous to inoculation, became ill somewhat later than the controls. The delay varied from 5-12 hours, in rare cases it was even more.

In consequence of the shortness of the latent period of the disease in rabbits, we transferred our observations to dogs. A test showed that, on subdural inoculation with our virus, the latent period of the disease in dogs is almost constant and lasts for about six complete days. In these experiments, after extraction of the cerebro-spinal fluid, we performed trepanning in the parietal region and introduced there under the dura mater a 1 per cent emulsion of virus in a volume of 0.3-0.4 c.c. Here also, in all cases without exception a

[1] A. M. Cheshkov. *Arkh. Biol. Nauk*, Vol. 27, No. 4-5, 1927.

retardation of the initial symptoms was obtained. Moreover this retardation was longer than in the rabbits: the experimental animals became ill 15-24 hours later than the controls.

An essential condition for this prolongation of the incubational period is a definite volume of the virus and also inoculation under the dura mater in the region of the protuberant surface of the cerebral hemisphere. The volume of liquid in which the virus is introduced must not be more than 0.5 c.c. (less is better). The actual content of virus in this volume does not play any essential part. The emulsion can be 1, 2 or 3 per cent. It is important that the quantity of liquid should not be more than can be retained by surface tension in the narrow, crevice-like space between the dura mater and the surface of the hemisphere. If the same quantity of virus is introduced suboccipitally and, moreover, in a greater volume of liquid (3.0-4.0 c.c.) then no prolongation of the incubational period takes place. On the contrary, some diminution of it is even observed. Here we have a repetition of the phenomenon noted above in the experiments on subarachnoid introduction of products of the disintegration of brain substance after extraction of a large quantity of cerebro-spinal fluid: the effect produced is both accelerated and intensified.

It was discovered also that extraction of the fluid must precede inoculation. All subsequent extractions do not play any essential role. In all cases, single or repeated extraction of cerebro-spinal fluid begun later than 12-14 hours after infection exerts no influence on the length of the incubational period.

The cerebro-spinal fluid, while being the liquid medium of the brain, at the same time serves also as the pathway along which the distribution of the virus takes place. Contact alone between the virus and the undamaged surface of the brain is not sufficient for infection. Virus introduced in a small quantity (3-5 drops) in the space between the membranes, after emptying this space of fluid, does not get into the brain but remains on the spot for some time. The gradual accumulation of fluid moves it, and it becomes possible for the virus to spread, at first in the submembranous space and later also in the central nervous system.

The accumulation of cerebro-spinal fluid takes place slowly. Moreover, the rate of accumulation of fluid varies from one individual to another within fairly wide limits; hence the retardation observed by us was also not uniform. In some animals it exceeded a complete day and night, in others it was limited to some hours. There is no doubt that predisposition to the infection itself plays no part here, since animals infected through the brain in the usual way develop the disease with striking exactness.

To decide definitely the question of the participation of cerebro-spinal fluid in the distribution of rabies virus through the brain, yet another series of experiments was undertaken as follows (experiments of my collaborator A. M. Cheshkov). We made it our aim to separate part of the subdural space and to carry out infection in the chamber thus isolated. For this purpose we made use of an observation that had been previously made by me on dogs with electrodes *à demeure* in various regions of the cerebral cortex. It was noticed that an electrode, insulated by celluloid, whch passes between the dura mater and the surface of the brain, often becomes very quickly fixed by connective tissue, the growth of which is usually restricted to the region of the electrode and does not go beyond its limits.

A ring was prepared of fine silver wire and covered with celluloid. The operation was carried out as follows.

We laid bare the lateral surface of the cranium under narcosis and incised some of the covering bones in the region of the *fossa temporalis*. The ring was introduced through a cut in the dura mater in its interior portion, and was moved along the surface of the hemisphere backwards to the postero-

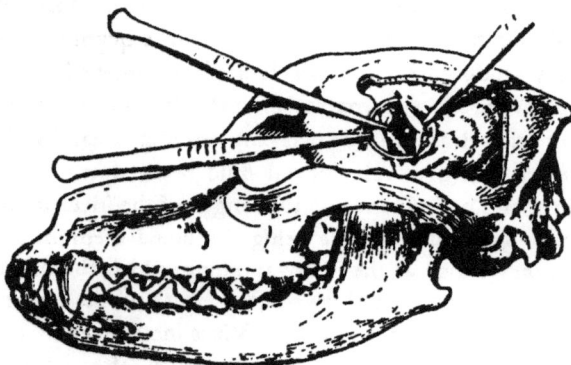

Fig. 2. Introduction of a Ring through a Cut in the Anterior Part
of the Dura Mater

superior corner of the opening in the bone, where it remained free. We disposed the ring in such a way that part of its circumference was exactly level with the postero-superior corner of the bony edge. This is of assistance subsequently, when the dura mater has become much calloused, in accurately determining the position of the ring on the surface of the brain. The cut in the dura mater is sewn up with two or three stitches. Afterwards, the *m. platysma* and skin are sewn up.

By means of this method we several times actually obtained a peripherally compressed crevice-like cavity forming a compartment with walls composed of the dura mater on one side and the *arachnoidea* on the other. Later, however, we gave up the use of silver rings, since they easily sink into the brain substance, producing sores. We substituted for the wire a cotton or silk thread soaked in celluloid. This also greatly facilitated a second important factor—the introduction of the ring under the dura mater which must be carried out without any trauma of the surrounding parts.

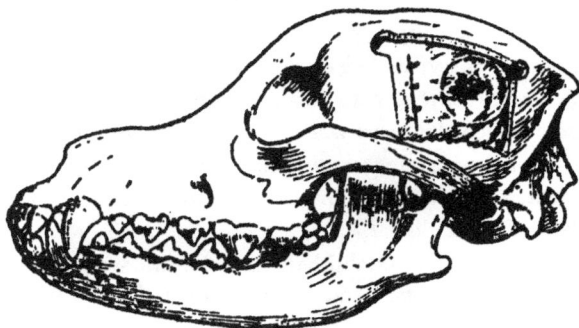

Fig. 3. Position of the Ring after Suture of the Dura Mater

Within 15-20 days, the ring has already become sufficiently firmly fixed. After the period mentioned, we made a cut in the soft tissues as far as the dura mater which by this time has considerably grown in thickness. The latter circumstance enables us to push the injection needle, bent at an angle, through the dura mater in a lateral direction. Thanks to this, the substance introduced into the compartment after the removal of the needle cannot flow back again. The passage of the needle through the substance of the dura mater must be carried out as cautiously as possible, since the slightest damage to the *arachnoidea* is sufficient to enable the virus to penetrate directly into the brain. It is best to make use of the ring 15-20 days after the first operation. Before this time, the union is not sufficiently strong. It is also not good if the inoculation is carried out 1½-2 months after the formation of the isolated compartment. In this case, secondary communications have almost always been formed, in the form of sinuous canals between the cavity of the compartment and the remaining part of the subdural space. After the introduction of the virus [1] the needle is withdrawn and the skin wound sewn up.

As a result it was found that the incubational period was prolonged in many cases. Even if the ring is not sufficiently fixed, *the incubational* period may be lengthened by 1-5 days.

In one case the incubational period reached 90 days. It is interesting to

[1] A 1, 2, or 5 per cent emulsion of *virus fixe* is introduced in an amount of 0.2 c.c. In preparing the emulsion it is essential to remove all the larger particles.

note that some of the biological properties of the virus were altered by its remaining in the isolated compartment for such a long period. Thus, an emulsion of the brain of this dog, immediately after its death, was injected into the brain of a rabbit. This rabbit became ill after 18 days. The brain of this rabbit, inoculated into another one, produced the disease after an incubation of five complete days. And it was only a third inoculation which produced an incubation of not quite four days, such as is normal in the rabbit for Leningrad virus. As a result of the virus (*virus fixe*) remaining isolated so long, its properties altered. In agreement with this also, the general picture of the disease in the dog from which this virus was taken was not fully normal. The records of our observations report motor agitation and clonic convulsions. Thus the disease represented as it were an intermediate form between the two varieties of rabies—"street" and "fixed."

These experiments also established that the undamaged arachnoid membrane is an obstacle for the penetration of the virus. If, on the injection of virus into our compartment, the arachnoid membrane proved to be damaged, then no prolongation of incubation took place and the dogs became ill, as usual, on the sixth day. From this it is clear that for infection the virus must move from the place of its introduction, penetrate into the cerebro-spinal fluid and together with the latter reach the point where it can enter the brain. This point is probably situated, not on the outer surface of the cerebral hemispheres, but at their base, where the larger blood vessels penetrate from the surface into the substance of the brain, pushing out before them the arachnoid and pia. This is also the manner of formation around the blood vessels of the adventitious spaces, referred to above, which are accessible to the cerebro-spinal fluid.

Summing up all these data, the conclusion can be arrived at that the circulation of the cerebro-spinal fluid in the brain and the submembranous spaces of the latter plays a part in the development of rabies. It would, however, be premature to form a view of the pathogenesis of the process on this basis alone.

I shall not dwell on this subject now. In dealing with other material it will be necessary to return to it more than once. The basic object of this chapter is to show that the cerebro-spinal fluid and the conditions of its circulation can play a part in the development of certain pathological processes in the brain, including tetanus and rabies. For a conception of this aspect of the subject, contemporary physiology does not have at its disposal an adequate amount of exact data. Hence we were confronted with the necessity of undertaking a series of special researches into the question of the circulation of cerebro-spinal fluid in the brain and the submembranous spaces of the latter.

THE CIRCULATION OF CEREBRO-SPINAL FLUID IN THE BRAIN, THE SUBMEMBRANOUS SPACES AND THE NERVES

CHAPTER VIII

THE CONNECTION OF THE SUBMEMBRANOUS SPACES OF THE BRAIN WITH THE LYMPHATIC SYSTEM

THE question of the formation of cerebro-spinal fluid, its circulation and its secretion from the medullary region, is one of the most difficult in the whole of physiology. In spite of a large number of researches, initiated by Schwalbe as far back as 1869, and continued in the classical investigations of Key and Retzius, even the morphological aspect is far from having been cleared up. Thus the role of the Pacchioni granulations, the existence and structure of perivascular, pericellular and adventitious spaces, the circulation in them, the sources and mechanism of formation of cerebro-spinal fluid, the passage of the latter from the subarachnoid space into the circulatory and especially the lymphatic system—all these are questions which still present problems for the investigator even today and are a long way from having been solved.

It is considered that the subarachnoid space is a collector in which cerebro-spinal fluid accumulates from various medullary regions and from which its secretion begins. It does not, however, possess direct, anatomically defined connections either with the circulatory or with the lymphatic system of the body. On the contrary, within the spinal cord and brain it is continued in the form of special canals running alongside the blood vessels and surrounding them. These canals are termed adventitious sheaths and in the embryonic stage, during the growth of the blood vessels into the substance of the brain, they develop from mesenchyma surrounding the nerve tube (Robin-Virchow spaces). During this process, the blood vessels become, as it were, clothed by the cerebral membranes, pushing them before them. The pia and arachnoid membranes do not completely fuse with one another and form crevice-like canals which are accessible to the cerebro-spinal fluid. Owing to this, the outer wall of these crevices, immediately adjacent to the brain substance, forms a continuation of the pia mater, while their inner wall, lying against the blood vessel, is a continuation of the subarachnoid membrane (Cushing). In the brain substance, the cells of these membranes are replaced by neuroglia; hence the adventitious spaces come into intimate communication with the nerve elements within the brain. Besides these canals leading into the depths of the brain substance, communications of the subarachnoid space with the cerebral ventricles (the foramina of Magendie and Luschka[1]) are to be observed in the posterior cerebral velum.

According to the opinion held by many writers, the movement of cerebro-spinal fluid within the brain substance takes place in the direction towards the subarachnoid space and not in the reverse direction. This was the conclusion arrived at even by the first investigators of the question—Schwalbe, Key and Retzius—who considered the subarachnoid space as the beginning of the secretory system from the medullary region. Recently, the same view has been defended by other authors as well. According to the data obtained by Stern, substances introduced into the cerebral ventricles, or into the brain itself, immediately find their way from there into the fluid of the subarachnoid space, moreover, substances introduced into the subarachnoid space appear in the blood more quickly than after introduction into the system of the cerebral ventricles.

Numerous experiments in regard to this question were performed by the American anatomist Weed, and his school. Weed employed a special method of vital injection into the subarachnoid space and established that not only the fluid of the cerebral ventricles, but also the fluid of the adventitious (perivascular) spaces, moves in the direction of the subarachnoid space. Later, Weed showed that substances when introduced into the subarachnoid space, could penetrate into the adventitious spaces, i.e., within the brain, only under artificial and very considerably increased pressure (50-100 mm. of Hg.). This pressure could entirely change the direction of flow of the cerebro-spinal fluid. But when the injection is carried out under the normal, low pressure (5-10 mm. of Hg.), even if prolonged, the substances introduced do not penetrate within the adventitious sheaths nor, consequently, within the brain. The subarachnoid space is therefore not only topographically external in respect to the brain.

The secretion from here proceeds in two directions, into the venous and lymphatic channels. There are grounds for supposing that secretion into the circulatory system takes place also through the subarachnoid space (Schwalbe, Key, Retzius, Weed and Cushing), and directly into the small veins inside the medullary substance (Sepp).

Sepp disagrees entirely with the views cited above on the subarachnoid space as the starting point of the secretory system of the brain. Putting together the views and experiments of various investigators, he comes to the conclusion that the opinions held on this question are contradictory. This author develops his theory of the secretion, based on study of the structure of the brain vessels

---

[1] These openings are absent in young animals, and sometimes even in adults. In general they can be found only by removing the *plexus chorioideus.*

and the laws of hydro-dynamics. Not only Sepp, but some others as well, deny that the subarachnoid space with its Pacchioni granulations plays any role as a secretory organ (Mott, Papilian and Jippa).

Key and Retzius, on the basis of their experiments, considered that the cerebro-spinal fluid, besides the paths mentioned, is also forced into the peri-neural spaces of all the nerve trunks. From these it passes into the connective tissue surrounding them and further enters the real lymphatic vessels of the general lymphatic system of the body. Justifiable objection was raised against these experiments by Testut, who pointed out that in the posthumous injections carried out by these authors a high pressure was developed in the sub-membranous spaces of the brain such as never occurs under normal conditions. It must be remarked also that in the experiments of Key and Retzius, even under these exceptional conditions, the injection mass by no means moved along the nerve spaces of all the cranial nerves (*n.n. olfactorius, opticus, acusticus, facialis*). In the nerves of the spinal cord, it could usually be seen only as far as the nearest intervertebral ganglion. But this is a place where the membranes do not yet compactly surround the nerve trunk, forming, as it were, lateral outgrowths of the common sac.

Recently, many new investigations of this question have been carried out. They include the work of the above-mentioned American investigator, Weed, who also regards the perineural spaces as the normal paths of outflow from the subarachnoid space. Weed uses a technique of his own for studying the paths of secretion from the subarachnoid space and the circulation in general of cerebro-spinal fluid. I shall permit myself to describe this method in some detail, since a clear conception of it is of essential importance for a correct estimate of the results obtained.

First of all, Weed refrained from any injection into dead bodies and from the use of insoluble injection substances. He also refrained from any artificial, excessive increase of pressure during the injections. As the injection mass, he used a 1 per cent isotonic solution of ferrous ammonium citrate and potassium ferrocyanide. He carried out the injections on live animals in which, after laminectomy, he exposed and cut transversely the spinal cord, together with the membranes, at a particular height of the spinal cord. Previous to this, outside the membranous sac, the nearest nerves of the spinal cord were tied by a ligature and sectioned. The dura mater is drawn away upwards along the medulla and turned back in the form of a cuff. The portion of the spinal column thereby exposed is cut out transversely, and the cuff formed from the dura mater is let down. Into the space formed in this way between the ends of the medulla which has been cut across and the membranes, Weed inserts a cannula through which the injection of his solution is carried out during several hours under a pressure of 100-102 mm. of water.

After death, the animal is dissected and placed for 24 hours in strong formalin made slightly acid with HCl, by the action of which Prussian blue is precipitated from the salts. The distribution of the small particles of Prussian blue in the medulla and the surrounding parts is investigated macroscopically and microscopically. Weed supposes that, under these experimental conditions, the injected liquid added to cerebro-spinal fluid circulates along the natural paths of the latter. Hence, the presence of Prussian blue at any spot is taken as evidence of the normal functional connection of this spot with the submembranous spaces of the medulla.

Using this method, Weed discovered Prussian blue throughout the extent of the subarachnoid space, including the Pacchioni granulations, in the venous sinuses, in the veins of the cranial bones, in the medullary membranes, in the cellular tissue and lymphatic glands of the neck and in others situated close to the spinal column, and, in addition, in the perineural spaces of all spino-cranial nerves and in the mucous membrane of the nasal cavity. As already pointed out above, with a pressure of injected liquid amounting to 5-10 mm. of Hg, he did not succeed in finding Prussian blue in the cerebral ventricles and adventitious spaces. On the basis of these data, Weed supposes that the flow of cerebro-spinal fluid within the medullary substance takes place in the direction towards the subarachnoid space. From here secretion takes place into the circulatory system through the Pacchioni granulations and into the lymphatic system through the perineural spaces of the spino-cranial nerves.

At the beginning, when we started work on the study of the secretion from the submembranous spaces of the medulla, we made use of the method proposed by Weed (experiments of my collaborator M. S. Spirov [1]). He carried out his investigations both on live animals and dead bodies (human embryos of various ages). In these experiments, besides injection of the medulla and membranes, he found also that the salts impregnated the cranial bones, the bones and ligaments of the vertebral column and the cellular tissue surrounding the big blood vessels and nerves of the neck. In addition, particles of Prussian blue were found in the lumina and walls of blood vessels in remote regions of the body, in the paraganglia, kidneys, ureters, etc. This aroused the suspicion that the above-mentioned solution of double salts has the power of diffusely penetrating tissues around the place of injection. In particular, there was marked evidence of this in the work on dead material. Transverse section of the spinal cord also makes it possible for the liquid introduced to penetrate into the blood vessels opened by the incision. On one occasion, Spirov observed that mercury

[1] M. S. Spirov. *Russk. Arkh. Anat., Hist. i Emb.*, Vol. 6, No. 2, 1927.

used as the injection mass had passed into the veins of the vertebral column and even into veins situated beyond its borders.

Hence the data obtained by use of this method cannot be regarded as all of equal value. If, under the conditions described above the injected substance is not discovered in the adventitious spaces, this actually demonstrates that its penetration within the medulla is hindered. As regards the view that the peri-neural spaces of spinal and cranial nerves are the normal paths of outflow of cerebro-spinal fluid, this cannot be considered sufficiently convincing. *In this respect the question still remains open.* Many authors have observed the pene-tration of injection masses, introduced into the subarachnoid space, as far as the lymphatic glands immediately adjacent to the spinal column (Schwalbe, Key and Retzius, Iosifov, Weed and others). Radetzky describes lymphatic vessels running from the perineural parts of the parietal glands, but he does not establish the existence through them of a direct connection of the submem-branous spaces with the lymphatic glands. Magnus and his school, by moisten-ing the medullary membranes with hydrogen peroxide solution, showed the presence here of lymphatic vessels, but like others he could not trace their fur-ther course. In any case, the outcome of the whole is that up to the present time definitely demarcated and organised pathways connecting the submembran-ous spaces of the medulla with the blood and lymphatic systems of the body have not been found.

Our interest being aroused in these questions, we began a series of investi-gations, first of all concentrating attention on the paths of outflow into the lymphatic system, since both the morphology and physiology of these paths have been little investigated. In so doing we had also to make an appropriate alteration in the technique.

CHAPTER IX

OUR INVESTIGATIONS ON THE CONNECTION OF THE SUBMEMBRANOUS SPACES WITH THE LYMPHATIC SYSTEM

THE brain and spinal cord have a common subarachnoid space. A number of data, some of which have been cited above, give us reason to believe that in the higher animals the secretion in the cerebral region is more highly organised than in the spinal region.

Lewandowsky, in an acute experiment with animals, severed the cerebrum from the spinal cord, cutting through their membranes, and observed that after this operation the passage into the blood of substances introduced into the sub-arachnoid space of the spinal cord is very greatly hindered. From this it can be postulated that as a rule the spinal cord partly makes use of secretory apparatuses situated in the cerebral region. In many respects it was important to separate the subarachnoid space *during a chronic, and not an acute* experiment and thus to compel the spinal cord to adapt itself to using only its own secretory apparatus.

I succeeded in solving this task by applying the following simple principle: any foreign body placed in a serous cavity becomes "grafted" onto its walls. The subarachnoid space possesses this property of serous cavities. If we give the form of a ring to some foreign body and place it in the neighbourhood of the boundary between the *medulla oblongata* and the spinal cord, placing it around the latter, then the membranes (*pia, arachnoidea et dura*) grow round it, fixing it firmly in its place. After overcoming a number of technical difficulties, we were able to fulfil this task. The details of the method are given in an article by my collaborator I. A. Pigalev.[1] I shall only point out that the chief difficulties encountered by us were in the two following respects. The first is bleeding. We chose for operations on the dog the region of the second cervical vertebra, in order to isolate as far as possible the whole membranous sac of the spinal cord. In sawing through the posterior wall of this vertebra it was easy to injure the vertebral vessels (*arteria et vena vertebrales*). Owing to various anatomical and technical causes, the bleeding is so difficult to stop that its appearance is almost always a true indication of an unsuccessful oper-

[1] I. A. Pigalev. *Zeitschr. f. d. ges. exp. Med.*, Vol. 61, No. 1-2, 1928.

ation. We learned to avoid this complication by sawing the arc of the second vertebra obliquely and subsequently gradually removing the lateral wall of the vertebral canal by means of Lewer forceps.

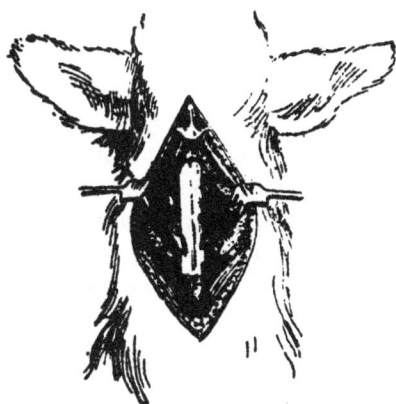

Fig. 4

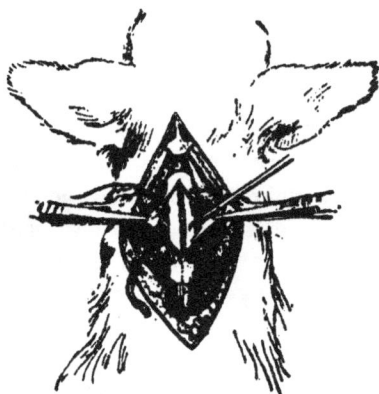

Fig. 5

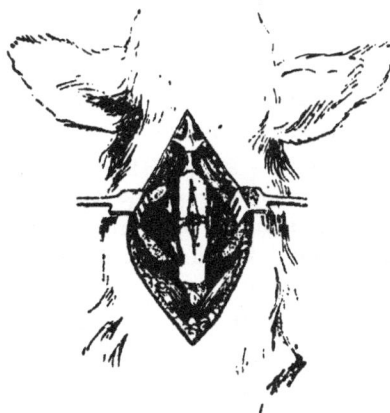

Fig. 6

Figs. 4, 5, 6. Three Moments in the Operation of Inserting a Ring of Muscle Tissue Around the Spinal Cord.

The second complication is the insertion of the ring around the spinal cord. This point does not present any technical difficulties. Nevertheless, owing to violence or haste, the animal suddenly dies after making two or three "terminal" breathing movements, which is due, of course, to the extreme closeness of the *medulla oblongata*. In order to avoid this it is necessary to introduce the ring without lifting the medulla from its seat.

At the beginning of the work, even those cases which were satisfactorily dealt with on the operating table produced complications in the form of subsequent spastic phenomena in the region of the trunk and extremities. Such dogs proved to be unsuitable for some of the later experiments, *e.g.*, for the work with rabies virus or tetanus toxin. Then we substituted a thin strip of muscle (a much softer material) in place of the silk thread used at the beginning. In addition, we began to place it round the medulla in the most delicate fashion possible. Very soon we had dogs which even within a few days completely recovered and subsequently differed in no way from normal. In a number of cases we actually achieved by this means the disconnection, not only of the subarachnoid, but also of the subdural space of the cranial and spinal regions, for the callosity penetrated to the outside from the arachnoid membrane, fusing the latter with the dura mater. By introducing a coloured injection mass into the subarachnoid space of the spinal cord under various pressures, we were able to convince ourselves of its complete isolation.

Our experiments were begun on such animals. We calculated that the spinal cord, deprived of the possibility of using the secretory apparatus of the cerebral medulla, *would in compensation extend its normal secretory paths* and thus make them more accessible for study.

In making the injections, we also refrained from transverse section of the spinal cord and the formation of a cuff from the dura mater. We carried out laminectomy of the last lumbar vertebra and of part of the posterior wall of the sacrum, laying bare the caudal extremity of the membranous sac. On cutting open the membranes we introduced a cannula into the subarachnoid space below the spinal cord, binding it to the membranes by a ligature. As the injection mass, we used India ink, suitably prepared and freed from coarser particles by sedimentation.

The first researches on this subject are due to my collaborator G. F. Ivanov,[1] in whose paper the reader can find both technical details of the method used and references to the literature.

At the outset, we carried out several experiments with fresh carcases of normal dogs. The injection lasted 1-2-3 days under the pressure of a water column of 30-50 cm. Under these conditions, with a dog of average weight, 25-30 c.c. of the ink suspension enters the subarachnoid space during the course of 24 hours. After the injection, the material was dissected and underwent both macroscopical and microscopical study.

Following this, some acute experiments were made with introduction of the ink into the subarachnoid space of living dogs. Finally, a large number of

[1] G. F. Ivanov. *Arkh. Biol. Nauk,* Vol. 27, No. 4-5, 1927; *Zeitschr. f. d. ges. exp. Med.,* Vol. 58, No. 1-2, 1927.

experiments were carried out using fresh carcases of animals in which the sub-membranous spaces had been previously isolated by means of the ring described above.

The results obtained by these methods were completely identical, the only difference being in the intensity; hence I will include them all in a general review.

In the first place, attention was attracted to the fact, already known, that a considerable part of the ink is retained by the arachnoid membrane. The quantity of ink taken up by the cells of the arachnoidea is many times greater than the quantity held on the surface of the spinal cord. It was noticeable that in experiments where the injection tube accidentally penetrated into the sub-dural instead of the subarachnoid space, the ink *merely lay on the surface* of the arachnoidea in the form of a thin crust which could be easily removed and did not penetrate into it. This shows that in relation to foreign particles in suspension, *the behaviour of the cells of the arachnoidea, on the side of the medulla, is sharply differentiated from the behaviour of those cells of the arachnoidea that form the subdural surface.*

This fact is pointed out first of all; in general, however, the retention of foreign particles by the mesothelial cells of the arachnoidea has long been known (Schwalbe). On these grounds, the arachnoidea is considered as largely impenetrable to suspensions introduced into the subarachnoid space. An exception is formed by those parts of it that have a special structure and are situated at definite points in the region of the cerebral medulla (Pacchioni granulations) and spinal cord (Elmann). But what is interesting to note is that in our experiments the lymphatic vessels of the exterior parts of the dura mater of the spinal cord were coloured precisely in those cases when the ink was *introduced subarachnoidally and not subdurally.* In the latter case, as already mentioned, the ink merely adhered to the arachnoidea. In exactly the same fashion, it merely adhered to the dura mater, being very easily removable from the internal surface of the latter and being hardly taken up at all by the endothelial cells. *Consequently the injection of the ink into the lymphatic system of the dura mater is achieved much better from the space whose walls are considered impermeable to the ink.* This phenomenon is only comprehensible on the assumption of special pathways connecting the subarachnoid space with the lymphatic network of the dura mater. The use of a lens to examine the dura mater, which had been washed in water and clarified, revealed the existence in it of a large network of vessels connected by numerous anastomoses. The next place where the ink is discovered easily and in large quantity, both macro- and microscopically, is the lymphatic glands and, in particular, the deep glands lying close to the dorsal wall of the trunk (mesenterial, intercostal and deep cervical glands). The glands are often simply choked with ink. Thus, in some cases the particles of ink or dye can be traced as far as the inguinal lymphatic glands and also the glands of the mesentery of the intestines, on the one hand, and as far as the *ductus thoracicus* on the other.

The latter was observed in just those cases where the injection had been performed on dogs previously operated on by the above-described method. As we anticipated, under these conditions the spinal cord does actually extend its outgoing pathways in compensation. On injection of ink into the fresh carcases of such dogs, the accumulation in the above-mentioned parts of the lymphatic system takes place rapidly and completely. On injection of carcases of normal dogs, we rarely observed ink particles in the lymphatic glands of the mesentery of the intestines and then only in very small quantity. Here however, the impregnation of these structures sometimes produced an intensely black colour. Moreover, we had six experiments where, in spite of placing the ring, complete separation of the membranous sac into its cerebral and spinal portions had not occurred, and precisely in these cases we were able to discover ink particles only in the glands of the dorsal wall of the body.

It must be added to what has been said that the possibility of the ink particles finding their way into remote lymphatic structures through the circulatory system of the body was excluded by a number of experiments made with preliminary ligature of the *aorta, venæ cavæ* and *ductus thoracicus.*

The second circumstance, inclining us to adopt the view of the existence of a direct, anatomically defined, connection between the submembranous cerebral spaces and the lymphatic system of the body, is that on several occasions we observed lymphatic vessels partially injected with ink in the mesentery of the intestines, in the entrances to the spleen and in the parenchyma of the pancreas. On one occasion we obtained an injection of the whole lymphatic network in the caudal regions of the pancreas (experiments of my collaborator V. S. Galkin).

As regards other organs situated on the dorsal wall of the body, the ink was frequently discovered in the suprarenal bodies and also in the substance of the *lig. longitudinale posterius* on the *corpora vertebrarum.*

We observed penetration of the ink under the nerve sheaths only along the course of the optical, auditory, olfactory and facial nerves. During the first period of the work, we did not succeed in discovering intermediary pathways organised in the form of lymphatic vessels between the dura mater and the deep lymphatic glands in closest proximity to it. But subsequently (experiments of my collaborators G. F. Ivanov and K. V. Romodanovsky[1])

---

[1] G. F. Ivanov and K. V. Romodanovsky. *Zeitschr. f. d. ges. exp. Med.,* Vol. 58, No. 3-5, 1927; *Russk. Arkh. Anat., Hist. i Embr.,* Vol. 6, No. 2, 1927.

when Gerota dye was used for injection, we were able to observe that even within 5 minutes from the beginning of injection the deep retro-peritoneal lymphatic glands became visibly dyed blue. The dye was also discovered in some of the afferent lymphatic vessels at some distance from the lymphatic glands.

On immediate injection of ink into the lymphatic glands of the dorsal wall of the trunk, K. V. Romodanovsky sometimes succeeded in obtaining an injection of the vessels leading in the reverse direction from here to the medullary canal. But this injection, also, was only partial.

These data were obtained not only with dead bodies but also with live dogs, in which the ink was introduced under the same conditions during narcosis.

The object of the next research was to establish more exactly the pathways connecting the subarachnoid space with the nearest lymphatic structures at the periphery (mesenterial, cervical, bronchial and inguinal glands). This work could only be carried out by perfecting the method used and all our efforts were concentrated on this task.

My collaborators K. V. Romodanovsky and G. F. Ivanov succeeded in discovering a number of new conditions which considerably improved the results of injection. They turned their attention to the fact that on prolonged injection, the water is rapidly sucked up while the ink remains, filling the subarachnoid space in the form of a compact crust and producing an obstacle to its subsequent passage out of the subarachnoid space.

Experiments made to do away with this phenomenon demonstrated that it depends on the concentration of the solution used in preparing the ink emulsion. If the emulsion is made with distilled water, then the water is rapidly sucked up and the ink becomes thick, hardening in the form of small crusts. But if Ringer's solution is used instead of water there is considerably less thickening of the ink. If, however, Ringer's solution is employed at double strength, then hardly any thickening of the ink takes place and it remains liquid. Such a suspension produces the best injection.

Using this injection mass, we succeeded to a considerable extent in joining up the separate links of the lymphatic chain, and in filling in the gaps between them.

Even during the first period of the work, we had observed the penetration of the ink from the subarachnoid space into the lymphatic spaces and the network of lymphatic capillaries of the dura mater. Under the new conditions, it was already possible to observe the fine lymphatic vessels running to various places from the external surface of the dura mater. They are situated in the cellular tissue of the epidural space of the spinal cord. Particular interest is presented by those which occupy a definitely fixed place. These vessels have their inception on the external surface of the dura mater *in the place where the* lig. denticulata *approach it.*

Subsequently we succeeded in observing that the *lig. denticulatum* actually plays some special role in the process of taking up foreign particles from the submembranous space of the medulla. Thus, in the course of another investigation, my collaborator N. N. Nikitin introduced a 1 per cent solution of trypan blue into one of the cerebral hemispheres of a live dog. The dye was injected to the amount of 1-3 drops through a small trepanned opening, just sufficient to insert the needle into the brain. In so doing, part of the dye flows back through the wound canal and spreads over the surface of the corresponding hemisphere. In order to avoid this, some experiments were performed on dogs, in which a ring of cotton thread, soaked in celluloid, was previously introduced under the dura mater (the method described previously). The injection of the dye was carried out in the thickness of the hemisphere in such a way that the needle penetrated into the interior inside the ring, through the isolated compartment. In those cases where fusion of the ring with the adjacent tissues was complete, the dye did not penetrate generally into the subdural space, and its surplus was retained in the compartment. It is obviously impossible to avoid the dye flowing along the subarachnoid space, since the latter is not flat but descends into the depths of all the sulci.

The dogs tolerate such injections badly. They become limp and usually die within 20-30 hours. On dissection, the dye is discovered in the cisterns and sulci of the brain throughout the extent of the hemisphere taken for the experiment. All these paths are coloured intensely, and the more deeply the closer they are to the place of injection. The corresponding parts of the opposite, healthy hemisphere also contain the dye, but to a much lesser extent. In the region of the spinal cord, the *arachnoidea* is slightly dyed a bluish colour, but usually only in the cervical region. Lower down, the intensity of the colouring rapidly diminishes and from the thoracic region to the caudal extremity the cord and its membranes remain uncoloured. As regards the *lig. denticulatum,* it is found to be coloured *throughout its extent to the end of the spinal cord* and stands out sharply on the white background in the form of a symmetrical, intensely blue strip. It is curious that there is hardly any diminution of the colouring observed on passing downwards from the cerebral end. The degree of colouring, also, on both sides of the body does not depend on which side, right or left, the dye was introduced into the hemisphere. Both of the *lig. denticulata* are usually coloured to the same extent.

The *lig. denticulatum* represents a product of the *arachnoidea.* The latter, throughout its extent, has the capacity of taking up from the cerebro-spinal fluid various foreign bodies suspended in this fluid. This capacity as we have seen, is displayed especially energetically by those of its elements which are turned towards the subarachnoid (arachnoid) space. It is found, however, that even here some of the parts entering into the composition of the *lig. denticulatum*, are distinguished by the degree of their participation in the general process.

In the experiments described, the following was also observed: the *lig. denticulatum*, as is known, is attached by its separate teeth to the inner surface of the dura in the intervals between the places of emergence of the nerve roots. On examination of the points of their attachment we observed on several occasions that in their neighbourhood the dura mater had also been dyed a bluish colour. Hence, we have here not only retention of the dye by elements of the *lig. denticulatum*, but also its transference to the region of the dura mater. If we recall that it was *in this place, but on the external surface of the dura, that we found fine lymphatic trunks,* then the combination of all the phenomena into a single general process becomes obvious.

In cases where the peripheral lymphatic glands are thoroughly injected, the dye can also be discovered in the *ductus thoracicus*. In carcases of animals which, after successful injection, have been washed in running water for several days, considerable decolorisation of the tissues took place. We also observed here fine lymphatic vessels in the mesentery and in the entrances of the spleen that had been coloured by the dye. In some cases, injection of the *thymus* and of the lymphatic vessels approaching it was observed.

As regards injection of the perineural spaces and the spaces of the spinal and cranial nerves, the new technique also gave good results. In the cranial nerves, the distribution of ink under the sheaths (throughout their extent) was only observed in the case of the optical, auditory and olfactory nerves. The ink reached the ends of the *fila olfactoria*, filled the lymphatic network of the nasal mucous membrane, passed to the surface of the latter and exuded from the nostrils. This phenomenon has already been noted by some observers in animal carcases. Key and Retzius, Weed, Baum and Trautmann have described special hollows and stomata on the surface of the mucous membrane of the nasal cavity through which secretion of the injected liquid from the lymphatic network takes place.

Of the other cranial nerves, we found ink under the membranes of the *n. facialis* in its course towards the *ganglion geniculi*. But even with the new methods adopted *we did not succeed in observing penetration of the ink from the subarachnoid space under the sheaths of other nerves farther than to the intervertebral ganglion.* Usually, the ink did not even spread as far as this, but reached only half the distance between the medulla and the intervertebral ganglion. Only when high pressure was applied and ruptures were observed with leakage of ink, did the latter sometimes go outside the limits of the intervertebral ganglion. Thus, on the basis of our experiments, we cannot consider the perineural spaces of the majority of the cranial and all spinal nerves to be the constant and normal paths of outflow from the medullary region and its submembranous spaces.

Later on, in the experiments of my collaborator P. N. Ulyanov,[1] we solved yet another problem. Up to this time, in injecting ink into the subarachnoid space *of a living dog*, we usually employed repeated introduction of the suspension, in a quantity of 4.0-6.0 c.c. We acted in this way both in suboccipital injections and when introducing the ink into the caudal region of the membranous sac. At the beginning of our work, when we used liquid ink, as sold commercially, the animals developed convulsions and frequently died. This compelled us to look for a means of making the ink innocuous, and we achieved this by replacing the commercial liquid by dry India ink, which we triturated in Ringer's solution. This gave us a really harmless preparation which the dog tolerated not only without convulsions, but without any visible signs of disturbance. P. N. Ulyanov injected the ink prepared in this way suboccipitally into one dog eight times in the course of 30 days. At the end of this period, the total quantity of the ink suspension injected amounted to 43.0 c.c. The injections were stopped because at the end it was not possible to obtain any cerebrospinal fluid on making a puncture. The membranous sac was empty and there was no assurance that the ink injected would find its way where required. On dissection, the ink was discovered in the immediate and remote lymphatic glands, which proved to be strongly enlarged and dyed an intense black colour. Moreover, particles of the ink could be seen under the sheaths of many blood vessels and nerves outside the limits of the spinal canal. No cerebro-spinal fluid was found in the subarachnoid space. This case provides evidence of the exceptional adaptability of the submembranous spaces of the medulla in bearing away foreign suspended particles which have penetrated into them. In proportion as the cerebro-spinal fluid disappeared, passive conveyance with the flow was rendered more and more difficult and was replaced by active removal of the ink by phagocytic elements. This explains the occurrence of ink particles in the form of separate spots in the cell tissue of all organs in the vicinity (in the blood vessels, nerves and bones). The dog was killed on the fourth day after the last injection. It is natural that although the immediate and remote lymphatic glands were filled with ink, the latter was not discovered in the lymphatic vessels connecting these glands. In another, acute ex-

1 P. N. Ulyanov. *Arkh. Biol. Nauk*, Vol. 29, No. 2, 1929; *Zeitschr. f. d. ges. exp. Med.*, Vol. 65, No. 5-6, 1929.

periment lasting with interruptions for 13 hours, Dr. Ulyanov injected into the dog under narcosis (using a constant pressure of 30 cm. of water) 60.0 c.c. of "hypertonic" ink suspension. In this case, the lymphatic glands of the dorsal wall of the body were also enlarged 2 or 3 times as compared with normal. But the lymphatic vessels were also strongly injected and (for instance, in the neck) they could be easily distinguished in the region of the chief neurovascular bundle.

Subsequently we succeeeded in introducing still further improvements into the technique of injecting the lymphatic system from the subarachnoid space.

In studying the genesis of epileptic seizures, we were interested in the question of the state of the secretion from the submembranous spaces of the medulla during the time of the seizure (experiments of my collaborator K. A. Efimov [1]).

With this object, we carried out our usual subarachnoid injection into a dog with commercial, liquid, undialysed ink (it is impossible to dialyse the commercial ink, for on so doing it coagulates and is precipitated as a whole). As already mentioned, this preparation by itself produces convulsions in dogs often ending in death. The control dog received the same quantity of a suspension, prepared by triturating a stick of India ink in Ringer's solution. Such a preparation does not produce convulsions and in general is endured very well. The ink was injected into the control dog at the same time as into the experimental animal, and also suboccipitally. At the moment of death of the experimental animal, the control was killed by chloroform and both were dissected.

It was found that during the epileptic attack, secretion from the submembranous spaces into the lymphatic system sharply increased. After two hours of the epileptic state, a large quantity of ink has already been carried beyond the limits of the medulla and penetrates not only into the immediate but also into the more remote lymphatic glands. Especially interesting was the fact that in the live dog, shortly after the onset of convulsions, the ink begins to appear on the surface of the mucous membrane of the nasal cavity and even exudes from the nostrils. The experiment described removes any doubts whether we are confronted with normally existing secretory pathways. On dissection, the mucous membrane of the nasal cavity was found to be dyed locally an intense black colour. Microscopical examination, carried out by G. F. Ivanov, showed the presence of the ink within the lymphatic vessels, forming a dense network in the mucous membrane. In the control dog, after the same period, it was only with difficulty that one could trace the commencement of the passage of

[1] K. A. Efimov. *Zhurn. Exp. Biol. i Med.*, No. 27, 1928; *Zeitschr. f. d. ges. exp. Med.*, Vol. 62, No. 5-6, 1928.

the ink out of the medullary region and its deposition in the nearest lymphatic glands.

These experiments of K. A. Efimov were continued by G. F. Ivanov [1] who came to the conclusion that for injecting the lymphatic system from the subarachnoid space during life, there could hardly be any better method than that of combining injection with the artificial production of the epileptic state in the animal. Especially successful in this case is the injection of the lymphatic system of the nasal mucous membrane and also the lymphatic vessels of the neck, connecting this membrane with the deep-lying cervical lymphatic glands. (Plate 2.)

In addition, one can observe a further series of phenomena, which are otherwise absent; namely, the ink penetrates into the cerebral ventricles and cerebro-spinal canal, into the adventitious spaces of the medullary blood vessels, inside the *septum arachnoidale anterius et posterius*, into the perineural and endoneural spaces of the cerebro-spinal ganglia and of the nerves beyond the ganglia, and also into the perineural spaces of the *cauda equina*. These phenomena are connected with the considerable increase of internal pressure occurring during the epileptic seizure.

Recently Dr. V. A. Chudnosovyetov (Kazan) performed a series of experiments on the same question of the connection of the lymphatic system of the nasal cavity with the subarachnoid space. As regards the method used, he started out from our data, but also introduced some additions. Thus, in order to obtain a more detailed knowledge of the character of the vascular network in the nasal cavity, which becomes filled with ink from the subarachnoid space, he made use of double injection. This enabled him to observe simultaneously the two vascular networks in the nasal cavity—the blood-vessels and the lymphatic vessels. The experiments were carried out on live animals and on fresh bodies. The results are in complete agreement with our observations.

The second improvement introduced by us in the injection technique consists in repeated blood-letting. In the experiment, a dog that has previously (12-15 days beforehand) been operated on, with insertion of a "ring" close to the junction of the *medulla oblongata* and spinal cord, is brought on to the operating table (the experiments were carried out by my collaborator I. A. Pigalev [2]). Under general narcosis, laminectomy is carried out in the region of the sacrum. The cannula is inserted into the end of the membranous sac, below the end of the spinal cord, and joined by a rubber tube to the funnel filled with ink. The pressure amounts to 30-40 cm. of water. Then slight blood-

[1] G. F. Ivanov. *Russk. Arkh. Anat., Hist. ; Emb.*, Vol. 8, No. 2, 1929; *Zeitschr. f. d. ges. exp. Med.*, Vol. 64, No. 3-4, 1929.
[2] I. A. Pigalev. *Zeitschr. f. d. ges. exp. Med.*, Vol. 66, No. 3-4, 1922.

letting is carried out repeatedly. As a result, increased suction of liquids into the lymphatic system, such as is well known on loss of blood, begins. After the death of the dog, injection is continued for 16-20 hours. Under these conditions we succeeded in injecting ink into the lymphatic glands of the mesentery as far as the intestine itself. The injection of the glands where the small intestine passes into the large intestine is especially well seen. It is also possible to observe fine lymphatic vessels, partly filled with ink, in the mesentery of other organs.

In the succeeding experiments (experiments of my collaborator V. S. Galkin [1]), we turned our attention to the significance of the place of injection for the results obtained. It is a fact that, even in the most successful cases, injection of the lymphatic system carried out from the subarachnoid space is never complete. The lymphatic network of the nasal cavity and the cervical glands connected with it are sometimes well filled. In other cases we observe the same thing also in regard to the abdominal organs. The injection into the lymphatic system of the thoracic cavity (glands, vessels) is always weak. We did manage to observe colour here in the glands, but we never found any in the vessels. A review of the material very quickly convinced us that the injection of the lymphatic structures of the body from the subarachnoid space takes place the more easily, the closer they are situated to the place of injection. It is most probable that during the injections the pressure in the subarachnoid space falls fairly rapidly, and is greater at the beginning of the path than at the end. We confirmed this by the following experiment. The fresh body of a dog was laid out horizontally. The dura mater in the cervical, thoracic and lumbar regions was laid bare and, along with the arachnoid, opened by small cuts. Through these cuts, special cannulæ made by my collaborator N. A. Astapov were introduced into the subarachnoid space and connected with vertical glass tubes. The injection was carried out with liquid ink through a fourth cannula inserted into the caudal end of the membranous sac. The pressure was 30-50 cm. of water. In the experiment, it was found that the level of liquid was approximately alike in the two tubes nearest the place of injection but was noticeably lower in the third, distant one. The height of the columns in all three tubes was equalised only after several hours, when the paths of outflow from the subarachnoid space were already choked with ink and movement of the liquid had ceased.

In accordance with these facts, we altered our technique to some extent. In the previous experiments we had introduced ink either suboccipitally (in live dogs) or into the caudal region of the membranous sac (in living and dead dogs). We now decided to carry out injection at various heights of the spinal

1 V. S. Galkin. *Zeitschr. f. d. ges. exp. Med.*, Vol. 74, No. 3-4, 1930.

cord, making use of Astapov's cannulæ or a special, very small Delitsyn cannula designed for injection of the interfascial spaces. A series of experiments were carried out (by V. S. Galkin) which definitely confirmed the importance of the place of injection and enabled us to observe somewhat more than before. The experiments were made on normal dogs and on dogs in which there had been preliminary separation of the subarachnoid space by means of the ring operation.

With injections in the region of the middle of the neck in the fresh bodies of normal dogs, we observed ink not only in the lymphatic network of the nasal cavity but also in the lymphatic network of the frontal sinuses. At the same time we obtained very good injection of the lymphatic glands and cervical vessels.

One observation deserves special mention. The ink penetrated right and left in the deep-lying, pharyngal lymphatic glands and partially coloured them. One lymphatic vessel, which mounted upwards behind the sublingual nerve to the mucous membrane of the nasal pharynx, entered the upper pole of the left glands. Throughout its course the vessel was excellently injected. At the lateral border of the same (left) pharyngal gland there entered three lymphatic trunks, also excellently injected. For some part of their course, these trunks ran almost parallel. The uppermost of them went from the base of the cranium along the inner carotid artery. The two others came down from the region of the transverse processes of the third and fourth cervical vertebræ. Of the vessels running to the right pharyngal gland, only the two upper ones were injected, one from the region of the pharynx, the other along the course of the carotid artery. (Plate 3.) The segmentary disposition of the lymphatic trunks approaching the pharyngal gland may be evidence that this gland itself is also of segmentary origin and in its embryology represents a conglomerate of separate glands which have undergone secondary fusion. Its dimensions and elongated oval form is also indirect testimony to this.

In later experiments of this series, we finally succeeded in producing a good injection of the lymphatic system of the thoracic cavity. In these cases, the injection was carried out from the cervical region of the subarachnoid space in fresh bodies of dogs which had previously been operated on with insertion of a ring.

The following is taken from one of the records: "The ink was deposited in the lymphatic glands lying in a chain along both sides of the trachea and its bifurcation, colouring these glands an intense black colour and filling the fine lymphatic vessels which unite the glands with one another. At the same time, in the abdominal cavity, only one of the retro-peritoneal lumbar glands on each side was injected. The glands and lymphatic vessels of the neck were entirely free from ink." (Fig. 7.)

Generally speaking, *the injection of the lymphatic apparatus of the neck from the subarachnoid space is directly dependent on the injection of the lymphatic network of the nose.* We had noticed this already in the first period of

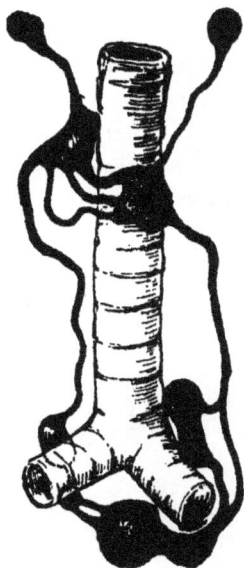

Fig. 7. Injection of the Lymphatic
System of the Mediastinum of a Dog
from the Cervical Part of the
Subarachnoid Space

the work. There is no doubt that the ink can also penetrate into the cervical lymphatic glands through the segmentary vessels, as was proved by our records and drawings. But this is not the main route. In all forms of closure of the nasal outflow, the lymphatic apparatus of the neck almost always remains free from ink.

It also became clear during the work that, for good injection of the lymphatic system of the organs of the abdominal cavity, the cannula must be inserted in the caudal region of the membranous sac. Injection from the region of the cervical and thoracic portions of the spinal cord enables the ink to reach only the first group of abdominal glands, situated on the dorsal wall of the trunk.

It seems to me that the facts adduced prove beyond question that there is a direct, anatomically defined connection between the subarachnoid space and the lymphatic system of the body. This exists both through the lymphatic network of the nasal cavity and through the special, possibly segmentary, lymphatic trunks.

The *fila olfactoria* must be included among the paths of outflow along the perineural spaces of the nerve trunks. Possibly, one should also include here certain other cranial nerves. We do not deny that under special conditions, for instance with high pressure in the submembranous spaces, other cranial and spinal nerves may also participate in this process. The spaces of nerve trunks do not have valves, and the movement of fluid in them can take place in both directions. But, judging from our material and also from the consideration of the material of other writers, *we cannot regard these spaces as constant pathways of outflow from the medullary region.*

CHAPTER X

THE MOVEMENT OF CEREBRO-SPINAL FLUID WITHIN THE MEDULLA AND SUBMEMBRANOUS SPACES

In regard to the question of the circulation of cerebro-spinal fluid within the medulla and submembranous spaces, the researches of numerous workers have established a number of authoritative facts (Key and Retzius, Cushing, Coeub, Weed, Mott, Baum, Papilian and Stanesku Jippa, Stern, etc.). Nevertheless, in this question, also, there is much that is far from clear. During our work we succeeded in making some observations which supplement those already known.

It was mentioned above that on suboccipital injection of India ink into living animals it is always present in the cerebral region, *being found mainly*

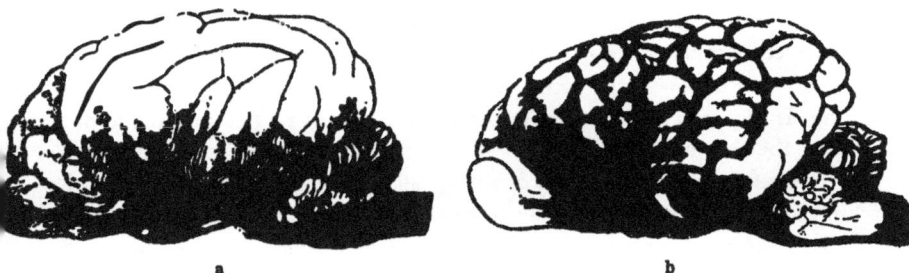

a   b

Fig. 8. Distribution of India Ink in the Subarachnoid Space of the Canine Cerebrum.
a) Vital injection. b) Post mortem injection

in the sulci and cisterns at its base. On posthumous injection, the distribution of ink in the cerebral region is much more uniform, and it can be observed everywhere at the bottom of the sulci on the surface of the hemispheres. These data were confirmed subsequently more than once by observations of my collaborators Drs. P. N. Ulyanov and V. S. Galkin. In the course of them it was found that the amount of ink filling the subarachnoid space during life depends directly on the quantity of ink used. If there is little ink, it almost always accumulates at the base of the cerebrum.

From this it can be concluded that under *normal conditions of circulation the chief direction of the flow of cerebral fluid in the submembranous spaces of the cerebrum is towards the base of the latter.* After death, when circulation of cerebro-spinal fluid has ceased, the ink, under artificial pressure, passively and therefore uniformly fills the cisterns of the subarachnoid space. This is also observed during life if the pressure exceeds a certain value, beyond which the normally existing conditions are distorted.

One of the conditions determining the circulation of fluid in the subarachnoid space of the canine cerebrum is its outflow. At the outer surface of the cerebrum the outflow takes place through the Pacchioni granulations, and at the base through the perineural spaces around the *fila olfactoria*. These spaces, it was demonstrated, represent a more powerful route and therefore exercise an influence over a greater area.

In order to obtain a more concrete idea of the degree of strength of the nasal path of outflow, we carried out the following experiments. (Experiments of my collaborator V. S. Galkin.[1])

We have already seen that the division of the subarachnoid space into its cerebral and spinal portions during chronic experiments has as its consequence a compensatory extension of the connections of the spinal cord with the lymphatic system of the body. At any rate, under these conditions the passage of the injected substance into the lymphatic system is markedly improved. Subsequently we obtained the same improvement by employing repeated bloodletting. In this way a definite indicator was established for judging the dynamic state of the channel interesting us. It remained to make clear what would be the consequences for the region of the spinal cord if the nasal path of outflow from the subarachnoid space were to be closed.

The method employed by us for this purpose was described in the first part of this book in the chapter on the nervous mechanism of epileptic seizures. It consists in the operative separation of the dura mater from the *lamina cribrosa*. In so doing, all the *fila olfactoria* are ruptured. The openings of the *lamina cribrosa* subsequently become closed by connective tissue. At the end of two or three weeks after the operation, the dogs underwent the injection experiment, carried out in the usual way, *i.e.*, beginning on the living dog under narcosis and ending on the dead body.

As a result, it was discovered that the mere obliteration of the nasal path of outflow of the cerebro-spinal fluid has the same consequences on its circulation in the region of the spinal cord as is produced by the isolation of the whole cerebral part of the subarachnoid space. Under these conditions, an injection carried out from the caudal end of the membranous sac provided an exceptionally complete picture of the passage of ink into the corresponding parts of the abdominal cavity. In particular, we observed several times the colouring of the

[1] V. S. Galkin. *Zeitschr. f. d. ges. exp. Med.*, Vol. 72, Nos. 1, 2, 1930.

whole chain of glands of the mesentery up to the intestine, and also injection of the lymphatic system of the pancreas.

These experiments furnished further confirmation of the existence of a direct connection between the lymphatic apparatus of the neck and the corresponding network of the nasal cavity. If the ink did not penetrate into the latter, then it was not to be discovered in the glands of the cervical region. In one case, the closure of the nasal path of outflow was incomplete. The ink passed into the nasal cavity and was then immediately found in the lymphatic glands of the neck.

In another series of experiments, a comparison was drawn with those experiments where the passage of the injected substance into the lymphatic system was improved by repeated blood-letting. Here also, it was found that the result of closing the nasal path of outflow was not only not worse, but even better than this experimental device. We draw the conclusion from this that *the outflow of cerebro-spinal fluid through the lymphatic network of the nasal cavity is considerable.* We recall that the passage of cerebro-spinal fluid into the venous sinuses in the region of the Pacchioni granulations follows the type of filtration through animal membranes. Here there is a mechanical barrier to the path of outflow. As a result, the flow of fluid in the cerebral part of the subarachnoid space can take several directions, but *the strongest of them is found to be that which leads to the base of the brain.* In cases where foreign suspended particles occur in small quantity in the subarachnoid space, they are passively carried with this flow and are partially retained in the corresponding sulci and cisterns. It is highly probable also that this mechanism is one of the causes producing so-called basal meningitis.

The subarachnoid space is common to the cerebral and spinal medulla. If in the normal dog the flow of cerebro-spinal fluid in the cerebral region has a more or less constant direction, then this cannot fail to be reflected also in the spinal part of the membranous sac. Appropriate experiments of ours have confirmed this (experiments of my collaborator G. F. Ivanov [1]).

As already pointed out, on suboccipital injection of ink, it can always be found subsequently in the sulci and cisterns at the base of the cerebrum. On the side of the spinal cord the ink does not spread far. This is shown particularly clearly if the ink is introduced in small quantity and the subarachnoid space is not freed previously from the cerebro-spinal fluid held there. When the fluid flows out in a quantity exceeding the volume of the suspension introduced, then the latter penetrates also into the region of the spinal cord. However, *even under these conditions,* it rarely descends lower than the thoracic part of the

---

[1] G. F. Ivanov. *Arkh. Biol. Nauk,* Vol. 27, No. 4-5, 1927; *Zeitschr. f. d. ges. exp. Med.,* Vol. 58, Nos. 1, 2, 1927.

membranous sac and practically never reaches its caudal end. If the ink is introduced into the caudal part, then, independently of the amount taken, *it always spreads in the direction of the cerebrum and can be discovered in the cisterns at the base of the brain.* The same data were obtained by my other collaborator, I. A. Pigalev, in experiments on rabbits with suboccipital injection of tar emulsion.

All this is evidence that along a considerable part of the subarachnoid space the cerebro-spinal fluid has a progressive movement in the cranial direction. It is difficult to determine the velocity of this movement. According to some data obtained in experiments by my collaborator P. N. Ulyanov, in narcotised animals, the ink from the caudal end of the membranous sac reaches the head only after several hours. The actual velocity in natural conditions is greater, especially in the normal moving animal. Moreover, on its way, the ink is vigorously taken up by the cells of the arachnoidea and hence its movement is not free. Finally, it must be borne in mind that the cerebro-spinal fluid flows in the submembranous spaces not in one direction, but in several.

Desiring to obtain a dynamic picture of this process at various levels of the spinal cord, we performed the following experiment on several occassions (experiments of my collaborator V. S. Galkin[1]). By the aid of the "ring" described above, the subarachnoid space in a dog was divided into three regions, upper, middle and lower. After the usual period, the animal underwent the injection experiment, which was carried out separately in each of these regions. It was found that from the upper and lower regions, good injection of the lymphatic system of the corresponding regions towards the periphery was always obtained. The injection from the middle section, however, yielded almost no results. Practically the same thing, with employment of a somewhat different method, was observed also by my other collaborator, P. N. Ulyanov.

The conclusion must be drawn from this that the intensity of outflow of cerebro-spinal fluid into the lymphatic system is not the same at different levels of the subarachnoid space. *At the cranial and caudal end of the membranous sac, it is greater than in the middle.* From the point of view of the history of development, the secretory apparatus in the caudal part of the membranous sacs is the older. In lower animals, apparently, it plays the chief role. Recently, V. M. Karasik has shown that, on hæmorrhage in the region of the central nervous system in frogs, the products of disintegration of the extravasated blood are conducted away precisely in the caudal part of the membranous sac, through the perineural spaces of the nerves of the hind extremities.

Such were the data obtained by us in regard to the circulation of cerebro-spinal fluid in the submembranous spaces of the central nervous system.

[1] V. S. Galkin. *Zeitschr. f. d. ges. exp. Med.*, Vol. 74, Nos. 3, 4, 1930.

We also made some observations on the subject of the circulation of fluid within the medulla itself. Some of these related to the central canal of the spinal cord, others to the medullary substance.

The following experiments (made by my collaborator P. N. Ulyanov [1]) were performed to clear up the question of the movement of fluid in the central canal. Under general narcosis, the carotid and vertebral arteries of a dog were ligatured on both sides in the lower part of the neck. This was followed by a broad trepanning, laying bare both hemispheres of the brain. Decerebration by Sherrington's method was rapidly carried out with a blunt instrument (spatula). The brain was divided at the level of the posterior quadrigeminal bodies exactly at the place where the *brachia conjunctiva* come together. The entire cerebrum in front of this place was removed. Bleeding at the bottom of the middle cranial pit from the caritid arteries ruptured in removing the cerebrum is sometimes rather persistent, in spite of the preliminary ligature of the vessels in the neck. It can best be stopped by strewing dry plaster of Paris at the bottom of the cranial cavity and stirring the resulting mixture with the finger. It is easy to ligature the *art. basilaris* in the furrow of the *pons*.

The head of the dog is fixed so as to be at the same level as the spine. If now the cerebellum is cautiously raised, then the anterior cerebral velum is ruptured and the cavity of the fourth ventricle opened. Into this we introduced 1-2 drops of "dialysed" ink by means of a fine pipette. The dog was artificially kept warm and was periodically given cardiacs. Under these conditions, the experiments can be continued for many hours. From time to time, the introduction of ink into the cavity of the fourth ventricle is repeated in the same way as before. After the death of the dog, the spinal column is fixed and subjected to microscopical examination.

It was found that ink particles are to be discovered along the whole course of the central canal. In its caudal part there is even more than in the middle, since on reaching the end of the canal the particles of ink are held back and accumulate here as in a filter.

In this form, the experiment was also carried out several times on dogs that had undergone a preliminary operation with insertion of a "ring" at the boundary between the *medulla oblongata* and spinal cord. Owing to the pressure of the callosity on the neighbouring tissues, some difficulty was created for the penetration of the ink along the central canal. However, here also we found ink particles along its length, although in lesser quantity.

It was shown above that the cerebro-spinal fluid within the subarachnoid

[1] P. N. Ulyanov. *Arkh. Biol. Nauk*, Vol. 31, No. 5, 1931; *Zeitschr. f. d. ges. exp. Med.*, Vol. 78, Nos. 5, 6, 1931.

space moves towards the cranial end of the membranous sac. The facts just described justify us in assuming that the *liquid within the central canal, on the other hand, has a progressive movement in the caudal direction.*

Recently, P. Remlinger and J. Bailly have carried out a number of experiments on the pathogenesis of rabies. Besides answering the basic question, on account of which they were performed, it seems to me that these experiments give a basis for judging the direction of flow of the cerebro-spinal fluid in the cerebral substance itself.

The authors inoculated rabies toxin into the cortex and then periodically investigated the virus content of various parts of the brain. It was found that during the initial period the virus disappears from the place of inoculation and only reappears there after eight days, and then in a quantity less considerable than in the nuclei of the nerves innervating the salivary glands. The authors draw the conclusion from this that the nerve nuclei, especially those of the salivary glands possess specific sensitivity to virus.

I think that another explanation is possible here. The virus only disappears temporarily from the point of inoculation. It is not destroyed. Consequently, it is only swept out of the region of injection. On being transferred into other parts of the brain, it multiplies on the way by geometrical progression. The quantity of it in the brain stem, as is well known, is always relatively more than in other places. If the flow of fluid within the cerebrum is directed to its base, *i.e.*, to the mid- and hind-brain, then it would be natural for the minute particles of virus to be carried here in the first instance. As a result of tremendous multiplication, the virus secondarily fills or, according to the accepted expression, "invades" the nervous system. Then it reappears at the place of inoculation, but now not only here but also in the peripheral nerve trunks. This gives no reason to assume that the virus has an especial affinity to the nuclei of the salivary glands. The only fact in favour of this view is the constant presence of virus in the saliva in the street form of rabies; but it must not be forgotten that this is almost the shortest path along the nerve trunk to a gland with external secretion; in the second place, the salivary glands produce a very large quantity of secretion in the course of 24 hours, at the same time expelling the virus from its boundaries. The latter circumstance is of extreme practical significance and hence special attention is concentrated on it. Much less attention has been given to other glands. In this regard, we have only isolated reports of individual observers who from time to time have discovered virus in the pancreas and lachrymal glands (Bombici, Cherevkov, and others). Puntoni even found it at times in the gastric juice.

It seemed to me that the presence of the virus in other glands of external secretion should be just as constant as in the salivary glands. In particular, this should hold good for the lachrymal glands which have such a short nerve path to the brain. I commissioned my collaborator Dr. A. M. Cheshkov[1] with the investigation of this subject. The data of the analysis carried out by him can be summarised as follows:

1) Determination of the content of street virus in the lachrymal glands of dogs.

2) Determination of the content of fixed virus in the lachrymal glands of rabbits.

3) Study of lachrymal glands in human material.

For the first series of experiments, the lachrymal glands of a dog that was dying or had just died from the street form of rabies were extracted under sterile conditions. An emulsion prepared from this gland was inoculated sub-arachnoidally into another dog. When this dog became ill and died, the corresponding gland material was taken from it and the experiment repeated under the same conditions. Besides this, microscopical examination of the brain was always carried out after death of the animal, together with biological tests on rabbits.

Out of ten dogs operated on in this way, nine died from the street form of rabies. That is to say, in 90 per cent of cases, street virus was found in the lachrymal glands of the diseased dog.

Out of ten rabbits inoculated with *virus fixe*, the latter was found in the lachrymal glands in four cases. The result was verified by biological test, consisting of two transfers.

A curious detail was observed here. On transfer, the incubation period in two cases was prolonged from the usual four days to six days, in one case to seven and in one to as much as eight days. In the secondary transfer it diminished again in all the rabbits to the usual four days. Thus, fixed virus, after remaining for some time in the lachrymal gland of the rabbit, already begins to change its biological properties.

In human material, taken from the bodies of persons who had died from hydrophobia, the corresponding test was carried out three times. In all three cases a positive result was obtained.

We are justified in drawing the conclusion from these experiments that the presence of rabies virus in the lachrymal glands of the animal was not an exception. Specially important here was the discovery of fixed virus (in four animals out of ten), since it is usually considered that *fixed virus is absent even from the salivary glands of the rabbit.*

These data enable us to form the opinion that in the case of the salivary glands also, the reason for the penetration of street virus is not that it is in

[1] A. M. Cheshkov. *Zeitschr. f. d. ges. exp. Med.*, Vol. 78, Nos. 1, 2, 1931.

some way attracted to the nerve centres of these organs. It is not a question of separate centres, but of the whole brain-stem, to which the virus can be carried passively, *e.g.*, by the flow of cerebro-spinal fluid. On multiplying, it secondarily passes from here into various other nerve regions.

We described above the data of Weed's experiments, establishing that the pathway from the subarachnoid space into the interior of the brain is hindered. In our experiments on live dogs we observed that ink penetrates along this path only under conditions of considerably increased intra-cranial pressure, *e.g.*, during convulsions. Hence the flow of liquid in the subarachnoid space normally takes place in the direction of the submembranous spaces. *The adventitious spaces of the cerebral vessels are the sole, more or less definite, structure capable of serving for this purpose.* They are undoubtedly accessible to the cerebro-spinal fluid, and a large proportion of them open precisely on the base of the brain.

Summarising the results of our work, it must be considered that the material described confirms the role played by the subarachnoid space in the process of secretion from the brain and spinal cord. However, we would not deny that, under certain conditions, cerebro-spinal fluid could also enter the brain through the adventitious spaces of the blood vessels. Both processes may even take place simultaneously. We saw, for instance, in our experiments that this happens during an epileptic attack. It is probable that it occurs also under the other physiological conditions, and this is confirmed, moreover, by experiments with rabies virus (*virus fixe*). It was shown above that the uninjured medullary membranes are an obstacle to the penetration of the virus into the brain. Below, we shall see that the nerve sheaths also are impenetrable to the virus. Consequently, the virus in the subarachnoid space *finds some pathway into the brain besides the surface of the brain itself or the surface of its nerve roots.* The only case when dogs sometimes (very rarely) do not fall ill is when the virus is carried in very small amounts into this space; in that case, the virus is eliminated from the subarachnoid space before it has had time to penetrate into the brain. In an immense majority of cases, however, the disease does develop. Consequently the question is not one of the possibility of the penetration of cerebro-spinal fluid from the subarachnoid space into the interior of the brain, but only of hindrances to this penetration. These hindrances can be created by the flow of fluid in the reverse direction in the adventitious spaces. It is permissible to think that not only exceptional conditions, such as epileptic attacks, but also intensified muscular work and alterations in depth and rhythm of breathing, are capable of altering temporarily the velocity, and sometimes also the direction, of flow of cerebro-spinal fluid within the adventitious spaces.

CHAPTER XI

ON THE PENETRATION OF VARIOUS SUBSTANCES INTO THE NERVE TRUNK AND THEIR MOVEMENT ALONG IT

THE study of the circulation of cerebro-spinal fluid cannot be restricted to the topographical limits of the medulla and its submembranous spaces. Such an attitude would be obviously inadequate, if only because there are no real limits either to the medulla or its membranes. Nerve trunks pass out in the region of each segment of it, and the membranes pass out with them. The spaces within the nerve trunks are thus connected with all parts of the submembranous spaces.

It was mentioned above that neither the old data, nor those recently obtained, permit us to regard the nerve spaces within the trunks of the majority of nerves as constant paths of outflow for cerebro-spinal fluid. However, in experiments where the normal relations are disturbed, for instance in cases of prolonged increase of intra-cranial pressure, the nerve spaces did assume this function. The conclusion must be drawn from this that *decreasing the pressure, permanently or temporarily, will have the opposite consequences*; the fluid contained in spaces of the nerve trunk should now pass from there into the medullary region.

The existence of such a path would represent a threat to the constancy of composition of cerebro-spinal fluid, maintained by a number of different devices, including the barrier: substances unable to pass through the barrier from the blood would be able to reach the medulla by a detour through the spaces of the nerve trunk.

The segmentary structure of the central nervous system and the number of nerve trunks provide the pre-conditions in this case for considerable variations in the composition of the cerebro-spinal fluid. *But, as we know, there are no such variations.* This is a contradiction which cannot be left without examination.

The question as a whole is made up of two parts.

The first problem is to make clear whether the lymph in the spaces within the nerve trunks can actually move towards the centre, and what forces control this process.

The second problem is to establish why foreign substances occurring in the blood do not penetrate into the cerebro-spinal fluid along with the lymph of the nerve trunks.

These two problems are closely connected with one another and were worked upon simultaneously.

A number of data led us to the conclusion that the process of formation of nerve lymph is marked by the same specific features as the formation of cerebro-spinal fluid. But it is very difficult to determine the composition of nerve lymph by direct chemical analysis; attempts to collect it without violence are bound to fail, while every artificial means gives a falsified product. Only an indirect way remains.

Attention is first of all attracted here to the old clinical observations that testify to the exceptional morphological and functional stability of nerve trunks in cases where inflammatory and even necrotic processes take place in neighbouring regions. Not infrequently it can be seen that nerve trunks, although surrounded for a considerable part of their course by pus, or dead and disintegrating tissue, nevertheless preserve not only their external appearance, but also the full measure of their functions.

At the end of the last century, interest was aroused in the question of the distribution of live viruses and toxins, on their introduction into a nerve trunk. One must mention here the work of Guillan, Homen and Laitinen, Orr and Rows, and others. Among Russian scientists, Rakhmanov studied the penetration into nerves of various chemical and microbe poisons, and also of certain dyes. All writers mention local changes in the vicinity of the nerve trauma, and progressive degenerative phenomena right up to the point of entrance of the nerve roots into the spinal cord. Inflammatory phenomena were also found, with formation of infiltrates around the endoneural vessels.

It has been frequently noted that undamaged sheaths represent an obstacle to the penetration of many substances from outside into the undamaged nerve trunk. These obstacles, however, are not absolute. It is well known that the application, for example, of chloroform or solutions of cocaine to the surface of the nerve trunk results in loss of excitability and complete interruption of conductivity along it.

Experimental data obtained in my laboratory have shown that for a number of substances, not only entrance, but exit through the undamaged sheaths of the nerve trunk is hindered (experiments of my collaborator P. N. Ulyanov [1]). These experiments were as follows:

The chief branch of the sciatic nerve—*n. tibialis*—was exposed under narcosis by a cut in the hollow under the knee joint of a dog. By means of a fine injection needle, 1.0-2.0 c.c. of a 2 per cent potassium iodide solution

[1] P. N. Ulyanov. *Zeitschr. f. d. ges. exp. Med.*, Vol. 64, Nos. 5, 6, 1929.

was slowly introduced into the nerve. Local swelling of the nerve followed. This gradually diminished as a result of the movement of the solution under the sheaths into adjacent parts. Following this, the same sciatic nerve was exposed by a special cut in the region of the hip-joint. The nerve was lifted up very cautiously, without damaging the small nerve branches and surrounding tissues, and a small flat watch-glass was placed under it. The nerve above the watch-glass was covered by a piece of cotton-wool moistened with warm physiological solution. During the following hours, the cotton-wool was taken up several times and tested for iodine content. The result was negative. In those cases where the nerve sheaths, in the portion of the nerve above the watch-glass, were cut, and the nerve bundles slightly moved, iodine was easily found within a short time in the cotton-wool placed on the nerve. These facts show that some substances, introduced into the nerve trunk are capable of being retained a long time within its sheaths, and are also conveyed along it. There is no doubt that the movement here was stimulated by local increase of pressure, produced by the injection, since the experiment showed that it took place in both directions. The difference in the extent of the movement above or below depends in part on the direction of the injection, *i.e.*, in practice, on the direction in which the point of the needle is inserted. If the injection of potassium iodide solution is carried out slowly, selecting for this purpose a portion of the sciatic nerve closer to the pelvic region, then iodine can sometimes be found also in the cerebro-spinal fluid. Experiments with a similar technique were performed by Dr. Ulyanov on some nerve trunks of the vascular system. He inserted fine needles into the sheaths of vascular bundles situated close to the spinal column and he carried out the injection under definite pressure. After a certain time, the substance introduced (dyes, potassium iodide) could be found in the cerebro-spinal fluid and even within the medulla, along the course of its blood vessels. It was necessary, however, in these experiments, to use a rather large volume of substance (above 10.0 c.c. in the case of dogs), since the sheaths of the vessels have a very fragile structure. On the injection, the fluid here very easily flows along the basic trunk and its branches, penetrating along the latter into the corresponding organs, including the central nervous system.

Thus, the penetration into the medulla of substances introduced into the spaces of nerve trunks or the sheaths of vessels does not encounter any special obstacle. This is not only the case for substances with a special affinity or "tropism" to the nervous system. We observed it also in experiments with indifferent substances. Hence, *the conditions underlying the process under consideration are of a general character.* However much they may have been exaggerated in our experiments, only the quantitative side of the matter is open to question.

More complicated is the question of the mechanism of the penetration of foreign substances into nerves.

In spite of the considerable number of researches which have been devoted to this subject, the matter is far from clear. It is usually approached from the point of view of tropism, *i.e.*, specificity. It is, of course, difficult to estimate phenomena when they are approached as regularities of a special order; hence, the matter has in the main been restricted to registering them. We know, for example, that tetanus toxin moves along the nerve trunk, but we know *neither the mode of its entrance into the trunk nor the forces determining its movement*. Looking through the relevant literature, it is easy to convince oneself that the first question has found its solution only in the word "affinity," while the second *has not even been raised*. Up to now, the task of the investigator has been mainly to elucidate the morphological substratum of the process, *viz.*, to find out whether the perineural and endoneural nerve spaces serve as paths for the movement of neuro-tropic toxins and viruses, or whether the axis cylinders also play a part in this process. Both views have their adherents, and it is very likely that both are correct. This series of researches began with experiments and observations on rabies (Pasteur, Roux, Chamberlain, Babes, Centanni), but the greater part of it was made with tetanus toxin (Gumprecht, Marie and Morax, Meyer and Ransom, Tizzoni and Cattani, Wassermann and Takaki, Brunner and Bruschetini, Aschof and Robertson, and recently Gottlieb and Freund, Teale and Embleton, etc.).

The dynamic side of the phenomenon and its mechanism has hardly been touched upon in the researches enumerated.

In commencing work in this sphere, we set ourselves three tasks:

1. To make clear whether chemical or biological affinity ("tropism") is an indispensable condition for the entry of a particular substance into the nerve trunk, or whether this is possible also for indifferent substances.

2. To determine where exactly in the nerve trunk this passage takes place.

3. To determine what forces guide the further movement of a substance that has already entered the nerve trunk.

The solution of these three problems is to be found in the following experiments of my collaborator P. N. Ulyanov.[1]

In a dog under narcosis, we injected simultaneously into the substance of the *muscular triceps suræ* of both right and left legs similar amounts of an aqueous solution (and partly suspension) of carmine. To make sure of the symmetry and equality of the injections, the muscles were exposed by a cut in the skin, which was sewn up immediately after introducing the dye. Fol-

[1] P. N. Ulyanov. *Zeitschr. f. d. ges. exp. Med.*, Vol. 64, Nos. 5, 6, 1929.

lowing this, we caused the above-mentioned muscle on one side to work for some hours. This was done by rhythmic stimulation of it through the skin by means of current from an induction coil. The muscles on the other side were left at rest. Narcosis was maintained until the end of the experiment, following which the animal was killed with chloroform and dissected.

It was found that on the side left at rest the dye had moved only an insignificant extent from the place of injection and had been imbibed by the tissues in the immediate neighbourhood. Even at the level of the hollow under the knee-joint, the cellular tissue and vascular walls hardly contained any dye, while the nerve trunks were uncoloured. On the side where the muscles had been at work, the nerves were dyed over a much longer distance, up to the middle of the femur, or even higher. On one occasion we observed that not only was the entire sciatic nerve dyed, but also the corresponding nerve roots. Dye was even present in the adjacent parts of the medullary membranes. Subsequently, similar observations were made with other substances. I shall omit an account of these experiments because they gave approximately the same result, without introducing any essential additions.

In this way it was found that on the creation of special conditions many substances are able to penetrate within the nerve trunk from surrounding tissues. In our experiments, we altered the osmotic processes in the tissues by introducing solutions and suspensions of foreign substances into them. A common trauma was inflicted on the tissue elements, *i.e.*, the process was studied in an artificial environment. However, there is a reason why we are able, not only to discuss the results obtained, but also to put them directly alongside those previously known.

The reason is this. In the experiments with tetanus toxin that provided the basic material for our conclusions on the subject under discussion, *exactly the same conditions prevailed.* The experiment begins with the injection of toxin into healthy tissues. The toxin preparations usually employed leave no doubt that, besides specific effect, there occurs here also common trauma of the surrounding parts, produced by the complex mixture of various chemical substances completely foreign to the organism. The resulting non-specific consequences of a physico-chemical character develop in the tissues immediately after the injection, while the specific results are delayed for many hours and even days. Consequently, *the conditions in which laboratory tetanus was studied are also artificial, and their artificiality is of the same order as in our experiments.*

Thus, the first of the problems set by us was decided. The second, *viz.*, the question of the place where the process of penetration into the nerve trunk takes place most easily, was elucidated by the same experiments. In order that the agent introduced should appear in the nerve spaces, it was found most convenient to introduce it into the substance of the tissues. It is clear that with this method of introduction the agent is introduced into the terminal branchings, perhaps even the nerve endings. Axis cylinders, gradually becoming divested of sheaths, enter into close contact with tissue elements and, together with the latter, are subjected to the action of various nocuous influences. In regard to muscle, for instance, it is known that there is here even a direct passage of the sheath of a motor nerve fibre into the sarcolemma of the cell.

The third problem was solved in the following way. Every introduction of foreign substances into the tissue gives rise to osmotic processes. Through the cell membrane, some substances leave the cell, others enter it. The pressure developing in this process can be the primary stimulus for the movement of the substance along the nerve. Muscle contractions create an additional factor, since the work of the muscles is one of the chief conditions for the movement of lymph, not only in the muscles themselves, but as expressed also in other parts of the body, including the subcutaneous cellular tissue.

The data given above allow us now to add here also the lymph circulation in the nerve trunk spaces. This was confirmed by the following series of experiments by my collaborator A. S. Vishnevsky.[1]

In two dogs of like weight and growth, he laid bare one of the sciatic nerves by an incision and injected a drop of methylene blue into it. The minimum quantity of substance must be used, for on increase of pressure at the place of injection the dye visibly spreads on both sides until the pressure is equalised. Moreover, a portion of the dye can issue through the puncture and colour the cellular tissue, which obscures the result. On sewing up the wound, one of the dogs was placed in a chamber with such a low ceiling that the dog remained for the most part lying down. The other dog was harnessed to a small cart loaded with a stone. It was made to draw this cart for some hours, and this was repeated several times. Subsequently, both dogs were killed by bleeding.

It was found that the dye moved along the nerve in a centripetal direction more rapidly in the dog which carried the load. The result of the experiment was the more pronounced, *the nearer the nerve portion taken was to the muscle*. From this it is clear that muscular work not only facilitates the entry of substances into the spaces of the nerve trunk, but also *is the force driving these substances farther*.

As is known, there are no lymphatic vessels within the nerve trunks under the perineuria and endoneuria; they occur only in the fatty cellular tissue of

[1] A. S. Vishnevsky. *Arkh. Biol. Nauk*, Vol. 28, No. 2, 1928; *Zeitschr. f. d. ges. exp. Med.*, Vol. 61, Nos. 1, 2, 1928.

the epineuria. It is possible that a part of the nerve lymph finds its way by this path into the general lymphatic channel. But the intra-trunk spaces are not morphologically defined—they consist of continuous communications along the whole course to the central nervous system and its submembranous spaces. By increasing the pressure at the commencement of the path, *i.e.*, in the muscle, we obtain an accelerated movement of lymph within the nerve trunk. It is clear that the same result should be obtained if we succeed in lowering the pressure at the other end of the path. This was confirmed by the further experiments of A. S. Vishnevsky.[1]

In two dogs of like weight and growth, the sciatic nerve in the pelvic region was exposed under narcosis as before. A drop of methylene blue solution was injected into it.

After injecting the dye, the skin wound was sewn up and one of the dogs underwent maximum extraction of the cerebro-spinal fluid. The other remained as a control. After some hours the dogs were killed by blood-letting. The epidermal stitches were undone and the nerve again exposed. Measurement was made of the extent of the dyed portion centrally from the place of injection.

It was discovered that, during the same period, the nerve was dyed for a greater distance in the dog from which the cerebro-spinal fluid had been extracted than in the control. To obtain a distinct result, it is necessary to select for injection a portion of the nerve *as near to the medulla as possible.*

In other experiments of A. S. Vishnevsky, we injected into the dogs a greater volume of methylene blue solution, not, however, into the nerves, but into the long spinal muscles at the vertebral column itself. Following this, the cerebro-spinal fluid was withdrawn. After some hours, the dogs were killed and dissected. Here we also obtained coloration of the nerve roots and even of adjacent parts of the spinal cord. It must be mentioned, however, that in the spinal cord the dye is never uniformly distributed. Only that part of the medulla is dyed which lies *below the place of entry of the nerve roots.* The rest of their vicinity remained white.

Since the publication of our experiments, they have been repeated in various places. The results obtained coincide in general with those observed by us. Horsber and Whitman, who injected toxins and dyes into nerves, have established even exceptionally short periods for this movement. Kenji Fujibayashi regards this pathway as the shortest and most accessible passage to the central nervous system. Kiroshi Ogata describes the chemical characteristics of substances which are most easily able to penetrate in this direction along the spaces of the nerve trunk.

[1] A. S. Vishnevsky. *Ibid.*

Thus, various substances that are injected or independently find their way into a nerve, subsequently enter the constant flow of its lymph. The nerve spaces have no valves to regulate the direction of movement of the fluids they contain. Hence the movement can take place equally in either direction. Where the subarachnoid pressure is higher than that of the part of the nerve beyond the membranous sac, the movement will be centrifugal; under the reverse conditions it will be centripetal. In the latter case, the fluids of the nerve trunk are able to penetrate into the medullary region under all its membranes, *i.e.*, to make their appearance both within the medullary trunk and outside it in the subdural and subarachnoid spaces. As a rule, centripetal movement is apparently of more constant occurrence than centrifugal, at any rate for the majority of spinal nerves. As we have seen, the velocity of this movement can be increased by a number of natural causes or artificial measures.

In our experiments, movement along the nerve was secured for indifferent substances. The movement of substances possessing chemical or biological affinity to the nerve tissue can also take place in another way. It follows from this, that in this process one must *strictly distinguish between two mechanisms —active and passive. The movement of toxins and some other substances takes place as a result of their affinity to nerve tissue; it is an active movement and must inevitably be connected with the nerve structure itself. Movement along the nerve spaces is always passive.* On penetrating into the spaces, foreign substances, both indifferent and specific, are carried farther owing to the movement of the nerve lymph itself. Thus, *specific substances have a double path for their distribution.*

These conclusions, in their turn, give rise to a number of others.

1. We saw that the lymph of the nerve trunks is able to pass into the region of the central nervous system. Consequently, *in enumerating the various sources for the formation of the cerebro-spinal fluid, both within and without the medullary substance, one must also include the lymph of the nerve trunks.*

2. It is obvious that the tissue fluid of the nerve trunks is not ordinary lymph; otherwise all substances circulating in the general lymphatic channels would penetrate into the region of the central nervous system. It is not possible to say what quantity of nerve lymph actually reaches the medulla and what quantity leaves the nerve en route. If the nerve lymph did not differ in composition from ordinary lymph, then, in view of the number of nerve segments, there would be a danger of continual or periodic variations in the composition of cerebro-spinal fluid. Such variations do not exist. This implies a special permeability of the vessels and membranes in the region of the nerve

trunks at the periphery, in other words *a separate peripheral nerve barrier* closely allied to the central one in its properties.

3. On gross changes of the physiological conditions, *e.g.*, on direct introduction of some foreign substance into the muscle, the normal resistance of the peripheral nerve barrier is destroyed. This occurs, not so much along the course of the already completely defined nerve trunk, as in the region of the terminal branchings or even the nerve endings. This provides an explanation of certain facts, well known in the laboratory and clinic. Thus, we know that the effect of intra-muscular injections of specific sera considerably exceeds the effect of subcutaneous injections. The difference here is too great to be ascribed to the rapidity of absorption alone. From this point of view, it is comprehensible that many neuro-pathologists still prefer cutaneal application of mercury in the treatment of specific diseases of the nervous system, and some syphilidologists apply intra-muscular injections of mercury and salvarsan. Finally, the mechanism of so-called para-vertebral anæsthesia, in which the anæsthetising substance is introduced into muscles situated directly at the *proc. transversæ* of the vertebræ, may perhaps also be explained by the same facts.

4. The last conclusion relates to fatigue. Under normal conditions of muscular work, the circulation in the muscles is adapted to the new circumstances, so that products of combustion do not accumulate in the working muscles. When, however, the work is excessive or very prolonged, a number of consequences develop, included under the general term fatigue. The state of fatigue includes not only muscular phenomena, but also changes in the nervous system. In estimating the genesis of these phenomena, one must perhaps also take into account the mechanism which has been the subject of investigation in this chapter.

It remains to describe one further group of facts. This concerns the question of axis cylinders. Do they play any part in the process we are investigating, or is the matter restricted solely to the perineural and endoneural spaces?

A positive solution of this problem is based on indirect data, mainly on the fact that tetanus toxin enters into chemical combination with nerve tissue. This is partly confirmed also by histo-pathological observations (the relevant literature has been mentioned above). There are no facts permitting an estimate of the phenomenon under direct experimental conditions. There is no doubt that it is very difficult or even impossible to make a direct experiment in this case. Hence, everything that the experimental form of work is capable of giving deserves attention here.

Two factors must be taken into account in organising such work

In the first place, the substance taken for experiment must penetrate from the periphery into the medulla actually along the nerve trunk and not through the blood.

In the second place, the subsequent presence of this substance in the medulla must not be open to doubt.

Rabies virus is a "substance" such as is required. Under natural conditions this virus, as is known, passes into the medulla along the nerve. The mechanism of the movement is still unclear, as was recently emphasised by such a specialist in rabies as Kraus. The virus moves not only centripetally but also centrifugally (E. Roux and others, most recently—Nicolau). It is possible that the live virus spreads actively through, or "invades," the entire central and peripheral nervous system. This, however, does not interfere with our experiment, since only the movement of the virus in the direction of the medulla is important for the development of the disease. Both the active and the passive factor can play a part in this movement. The latter can, of course, be registered by means of our technique.

Experiments were carried out on dogs (experiments of my collaborators W. H. Gantt and A. V. Ponomarev [1]). *Virus fixe* was used for infection.

Virus fixe was introduced in the muscles of dogs in the form of a 10 per cent emulsion, which had been freed from granular fragments by various means and had the appearance of a slightly opalescent solution. The injection was carried out in a number of places, in order to bring the virus into contact with as large a quantity of nerve elements in the muscles as possible. The amount of emulsion used was 30.0 c.c. The injection was performed into the deep-lying muscles of the spine and neck in the neighbourhood of the vertebral column. As always, the dogs for the experiment were selected in pairs. From one of the dogs, extraction of cerebro-spinal fluid was subsequently undertaken. No fluid was extracted from the other (control) dog. The extraction of fluid from the first dog was repeated on the same and on the following day.

As a result, the dogs that had undergone extraction of cerebro-spinal fluid developed rabies in a considerable percentage of cases. Not one of the control dogs became ill.

We were not satisfied with the method of these experiments since it did not exclude the possibility of the virus penetrating into the medulla from the blood. Therefore the following series of experiments was carried out with injection of fixed virus directly into a nerve, after which extraction of cerebro-spinal fluid was undertaken. The animals experimented on were also dogs.

At the beginning, we introduced the virus into the substance of the sciatic

[1] W. H. Gantt and A. V. Ponomarev. *Arkh. Biol. Nauk,* Vol. 29, No. 3, 1929. *Zeitschr. f. d. ges. exp. Med.,* Vol. 66, Nos. 5, 6, 1929.

nerve on one side and did not obtain the anticipated effect. The animals did not become ill. The experiments were made with all virus stocks in the possession of the Institute of Experimental Medicine. We had only one case of illness in more than fifteen animals. Then we began to introduce the virus into both sciatic nerves, also accompanying this operation by withdrawal of cerebro-spinal fluid. The dogs did not become ill. It must be considered that *virus fixe*, when introduced into the nerve trunk from muscles, is able to move a greater distance, while the same virus, when introduced directly into the nerve trunk, somehow loses this capacity.

We attempted to solve the riddle of these phenomena by means of experiments that have recently been performed by A. S. Vishnevsky and P. N. Ulyanov. The former injected a drop of dye under the sheath of the nerve trunk. The latter introduced the dye into the substance of the muscle, and subsequently for several hours stimulated the muscle by an electric current, causing rhythmical contraction. In this case the dye moved considerably further along the nerve than in the experiments of A. S. Vishnevsky, and sometimes even reached the spinal cord. In addition, we had at that time already made experiments on the question of the mechanism of development of "trophic ulcers." These experiments are described below. To obtain trophic disturbances, we introduced various irritating substances (pus, mustard gas, formalin, croton oil, etc.) into the sciatic nerve of dogs. In these experiments, the injection was made in the substance of the undamaged nerve trunk, under its sheaths. Other nerves were cut transversely and the irritating agent introduced from the surface of the cut between the fibres of the central end. *In cases where the irritant was applied to the surface of the severed nerve, "trophic" disturbances developed more rapidly and were considerably more intense.* We explained this as due to the fact that a double trauma of the nerve trunk took place here and that, moreover, an additional path was opened up to the nerve cell, not only through the nerve spaces but also through the axis cylinders, which are inaccessible for direct injections.

An opportunity presented itself for testing this by experiments with *virus fixe*. We began by injecting the virus in the same quantity and at the same place of the sciatic nerve as before. The virus was injected only on one side; but following its introduction, the nerve was severed with a sharp knife through the middle of the part swollen by the injection. After this, the cerebro-spinal fluid was extracted, but also only once. *In spite of the fact that the greater part of the virus flowed back into the wound from the severed nerve, almost all the dogs developed rabies.* The number of animals developing the disease with this method of infection almost equalled the number of those becoming ill as a result of direct injection into the medulla. It would seem that when the nerve trunk is severed after the injection, the chances of the virus penetrating into the medulla, especially through the nerve spaces, must be considerably decreased: in the first place, the local pressure, artificially raised by the injection, immediately falls; in the second place, almost everything introduced under the sheath of the nerve flows out again. Yet the result was the reverse. It is clear that the nerve spaces play no part here. *The only remaining structures are the axis cylinders.*

THE ROLE OF THE NERVOUS SYSTEM IN THE PATHO-GENESIS OF CERTAIN INFECTIOUS DISEASES

CHAPTER XII

THE ROLE OF THE NERVOUS SYSTEM IN THE PATHO-GENESIS OF CERTAIN INFECTIOUS DISEASES

THE data obtained by us in the course of our study of the circulation in the medulla, its submembranous spaces and spinal nerves, gave rise to a number of new working hypotheses for investigating the role of the nervous system in pathological processes.

In the first place it was necessary to continue observations on the action of various substances penetrating independently, or artificially introduced, into the region of the central nervous system. Here special attention is attracted by the groups of so-called specific substances, *i.e.*, viruses, toxins and their anti-bodies. Having established previously the role of cerebro-spinal fluid in the pathogenesis of rabies, we could not but ask ourselves why there exists no passive immunisation and specific treatment of this disease. The question is not new. It has already been raised repeatedly, but its solution has been sought either "in a test-tube" or in connection with the circulatory system.

Towards the end of the last century, a number of writers almost simultaneously made an observation which has subsequently become part of the theory of so-called "meningeal permeability" (*"permeabilité méningée"*). This theory had its basis in the fact that the chemical composition of cerebro-spinal fluid differs more strongly from that of blood than that of transudates, and, consequently, that cerebro-spinal fluid is not an ordinary transudate. Subsequently, it was found that in various pathological processes, for instance in acute, and also tuberculous meningitis, the composition of the cerebro-spinal fluid is altered (Widal, Sicard and Lesné). Widal and Sicard (1897) also showed that many substances (methylene blue, potassium iodide, etc.), when introduced artificially into the blood of an animal, or independently finding their way into the blood (specific agglutinins), do not pass thence into the cerebro-spinal fluid and cannot be discovered in the latter. In 1898, in a work on "cerebral tetanus," E. Roux and Borrel pointed out that immunity to tetanus toxin is not absolute. If the toxin is introduced in the medulla of an immunised animal, the latter develops tetanus, in spite of abundance of anti-toxin in the blood. In this way it was established for the first time that tetanus anti-toxin, occurring in the blood, does not exhibit its action in the medulla.

These observations were subsequently applied also to diphtheria. Ransom, Kafka, Karlson, Hektoen, Becht, Gröer, Gärtner, Redlich, Pötzl, Hess, Lemaire, Debré, Goldmann, Wittgenstein, Krebs and others, have already demonstrated by special experiments that specific anti-bodies of sera, including anti-toxin, penetrate into the cerebro-spinal fluid only in minute traces. It gradually became evident that a great number of other colloids and crystalline substances encounter hindrances to their penetration from the blood into the medullary region. Very soon investigators began to connect the above-mentioned phenomenon not only with "meningeal permeability" but with the permeability of the walls of medullary vessels in general. Stern and Gautier proposed a new name for this phenomenon: "the hæmato-encephalitic barrier." Further investigations have already shown that not only the vessels of the medulla and its membranes possess a special selective permeability, but that in other organs also the vessels are not uniformly accessible to various substances circulating in the blood. Widal and Sicard must be regarded as the writers who laid the foundations of this theory, but its significance for immunology was first of all shown in the above-mentioned experiments of Roux and Borrel. At the present time there already exists an enormous literature on this subject, both clinical and experimental. Those interested can find references in Kafka's book (*Die Zerebrospinalflüssigkeit*), and also in the books of Gellhorn and Walter.

I shall not dwell on this any longer, since we are only interested in the fact, firmly established long ago, that, *as a rule, anti-bodies of specific sera either do not pass at all from the blood into the medulla, or penetrate into the latter only in very small quantity*—for instance, when their concentration in the blood reaches a high level.

In the so-called specific diseases of the central nervous system this circumstance has repeatedly evoked attempts to produce injection of serum directly into the region of the central nervous system. Thus, Roux and Borrel, in cases of spontaneous tetanus in man, proposed subarachnoid introduction of anti-toxin. Kocher recommended introducing it even into the cerebral ventricles. However, even this means has rarely proved efficaceous.

Still less is obtained by the application of antirabic serum in rabies. It has never been observed to produce a specific effect *in cases of intra-cerebral infection* of animals. Thus, Kraus and Marie, in spite of many years' work, could not note any effect of it on the organism. The same is reported by Keller, Clairmont, Murillo, Miessner, Kapfberger, and others. Reports of positive results from the application of antirabic serum are isolated and have not been subsequently confirmed. As early as 1835, Tizzoni and Centanni described some experiments in which antirabic serum prepared by them exhibited a prophylactic action, provided the infection was subcutaneous.

In 1913, Pfeiler obtained positive results by subdural introduction of antirabic serum in sheep which had been infected *through the anterior chamber of the eye*. Fermi also observed the specific action of his serum on animals. But he inoculated them only with his virus (*"virus Fermi"*) and only subcutaneously. Kraus and Fukuhara tested these experiments under the same conditions and with the same virus, but obtained a negative result. To sum up, the question of the prophylactic and curative action of antirabic serum in all methods of infection has received a negative decision. In the book, *Lyssa bei Mensch und Tier*, a joint work of three great specialists—Kraus, Gerlach and Schweinburg—this view is expressed in the most categorical fashion.

It follows that a positive effect of the application of antirabic serum is at any rate a very rare exception. On the contrary, there are a large number of reports providing evidence that antirabic serum exhibits specific properties only *"in vitro,"* i.e., by direct mixture with virus.

Such was the position of the question when we commenced work on it.

We could not explain the contradictions between the experiments carried out *in vitro* and *in vivo* as being due to the low rabicidal properties of the serum. Some investigators (Tizzoni and Centanni) used sera, the rabicidal power of which was exhibited *"in vitro"* in a dilution of 1 : 25,000. A fraction of a gram of such a serum would be sufficient to neutralise the virus throughout the entire brain of a man. This brought us to the conclusion that in all conditions of introduction of the serum *in vivo*, the rabicidal substances do not encounter the virus. If the serum is introduced into the blood—it is prevented by the "barrier." On subarachnoid injection, the serum gets into a space from which access into the medulla is hindered, and, on the contrary, it is easily removed from the medullary region.

The matter can only be made fully clear by means of experiments which take the above-mentioned conditions into account.

With this aim in view, we decided to utilise certain data provided by the observations on circulation described above, *i.e.*, we decided to study the problem, *not from the limited standpoint of the specific reactions in rabies alone, but with the purpose of determining the general conditions for the appearance of different substances in the medulla and its submembranous spaces.*

This made it possible to apply to other processes the data obtained from studying one process. Naturally, the volume of the work was thereby increased; this, in its turn, permitted us to observe a number of phenomena that did not stand in direct relation to our original problem.

RABIES

As a starting point, we made use of the data obtained in studying the action of the products of disintegration of nerve tissue. We have seen that the effect of their action was sharply intensified when a large quantity of cerebrospinal fluid was withdrawn before the subarachnoid injection. New experiments on these lines with antirabic serum were made on dogs (experiments of my collaborators A. V. Ponomarev and A. M. Cheshkov [1]).

The number of animals used was sixteen. The infection was always subarachnoid or subdural. The serum was also introduced subarachnoidally—in some cases before infection, in other cases after it, with an interval of 6-20 hours on either side. For injection, Leningrad stock of *virus fixe* was used in a dilution of 1/100 or 1/500 (unfiltered emulsion), in an amount of 0.4-0.5 c.c. Before introduction of the serum, the maximum quantity of cerebrospinal fluid was extracted from the dogs. Sometimes a second injection of 3.0-5.0 c.c. of serum was made. Each experiment was accompanied by a control.

Almost all the experimental dogs remained healthy. Only one became ill, and in its case the incubation period was prolonged to twelve days. All the control animals, infected simultaneously with the same dose of virus, became ill and died within the ordinary period.

These data provide reason for thinking that with subarachnoid introduction *both the virus and the serum enter the medulla by the same paths.* Hence, on the establishment of conditions favourable to the penetration from the subarachnoid space into the medulla, the serum was able to exhibit its specific action even when several hours elapsed between infection and injection of the serum. *The serum, as it were, overtook the virus on the paths of distribution of the latter.*

The experiments described established also that there is no difference between the action of serum *in vitro* and *in vivo.* The lack of effect in applying this serum in the organism thus depends to a considerable extent on the fact that it does not encounter the virus. At any rate, creating conditions for this encounter guarantees the exhibition of the reaction.

Those of our experiments in which the time of application of the serum was delayed for 20 or more hours after the time of infection ended in failure. From the account given below it will be evident that *these failures are not to be explained only by the mechanical conditions of circulation,* although these conditions undoubtedly can play a certain part in this respect.

[1] A. V. Ponomarev and A. M. Cheshkov. *Comptes rend. de la Société de Biologie,* S. du 2 Juillet, 1927, Vol. 97, p. 376.

A useful effect is only achieved as long as the virus has not passed beyond a certain range, which is accessible from the subarachnoid space. We saw that not all substances introduced into this space enter the medulla by diffusion. For many of them, and especially for the virus, a locus of entry must be assumed, and it is only along this path that the anti-bodies of the serum can come into contact with the virus in sufficient quantity.

In order that rabicidal substances should penetrate into the medulla *from the blood*, the integrity of the above-mentioned "barrier" must be destroyed. There are a number of artificial devices that have been used for increasing the permeability of the medullary vessels. These devices include:

1) Superheating the body and, in particular, the medulla (diathermy).

2) X-rays.

3) Ligature of the urethra (N. K. Rosenberg).

4) Introducing various substances into the blood, *e.g.*, diptheria toxin, tuberculin, etc. (Stern, Baatard).

5) Injection of hypertonic salt solution into the blood.

6) Lowering the subarachnoid pressure by withdrawal of cerebro-spinal fluid, and other means.

Some of the above methods are employed also in the clinic in cases where it is desired that a particular remedy, normally not passing the "barrier," should reach the medulla. For many experimental purposes, however, and particularly for the solution of the problem facing us, some of these methods were inapplicable, since they resulted very rapidly in the death of the animal (ligature of the urethra), others were too weak (superheating, introduction of hypertonic solutions), and did not yield any result in our hands. The means listed above may perhaps be suitable for studying the physiological phenomenon itself—the permeability of the wall of the medullary vessels. *But in experiments with the introduction of antirabic serum into the blood of animals infected intra-cerebrally, we did not obtain any effect from their use.* Only on introducing antirabic serum into the blood and following this by maximum extraction of cerebro-spinal fluid, did we sometimes observe a *retardation* in the development of rabies. The incubation period was somewhat prolonged but even in these cases we never saved the animal from rabies, even if the intra-cerebral infection took place before or immediately after the extraction of cerebro-spinal fluid. However, it was on this method that our attention became focused.

Of all these methods, it is the oldest. At any rate, even those who first investigated the question of the permeability of the medullary vessels (Sicard, N. K. Rosenberg, etc.) describe in detail how the extraction of cerebro-spinal fluid must be carried out to prevent substances occurring in the blood from getting into the fluid.

The essential advantage of this method is that: 1) nothing is introduced into the organism from without, and 2) the result appears almost from the moment of application. The only defect of this means for our purpose lies in its weakness. It was necessary to strengthen its action.

In the course of another investigation, I had occasion to make an observation which enabled me to achieve the necessary increase in permeability of the medullary vessels. In making various operations on the cranium and brain of dogs, I noted that if the maximum quantity of cerebro-spinal fluid was withdrawn immediately before trepanning, there was no bleeding from the bones, or the bleeding was insignificant. This fact proved to be constant and was made the subject of special study, which I entrusted to my collaborator Dr. A. S. Vishnevsky.[1]

The experiments were performed as follows. While the dog was under narcosis, trepanning was performed above the *sinus sagittalis* or above one of the big bony veins of the skull. Heavy bleeding occurred. Immediately, the cerebro-spinal fluid was extracted by suboccipital puncture. From the very beginning of the extraction, the bleeding almost suddenly ceased. It was sufficient to re-introduce the fluid for the bleeding to be renewed. If the bleeding proceeded from the exposed *sinus sagittalis* then, in proportion as the fluid was withdrawn, the wall of the sinus collapsed; it no longer protruded above the dura mater but caved inwards, forming a small groove. We now use this means in all cases of more or less serious trepanning of the canine cranium.

If the cerebro-spinal fluid is extracted from a dog, re-introduced and then extracted again, the fluid will no longer be colourless. On repeating this procedure, it gradually takes on a yellowish, and later, a red colour. If the action is continued, using the whole available quantity of cerebro-spinal fluid, then, not only the fluid of the subarachnoid space, but also the fluid of the ventricles becomes coloured, and acute hæmorrhage occurs in the cerebral substance itself.

We have termed this procedure "pumping" (in French, *"pompage"*). For brevity, I shall use this term in what follows.

We decided to apply the method of "pumping" for enabling anti-rabic serum to penetrate from the blood into the brain (experiments of my collaborators A. V. Ponomarev and A. M. Cheshkov [2]).

---

[1] A. S. Vishnevsky. *Zhurn. Exp. Biol. i Med.*, No. 12, 1926-27; *Arch. f. kl. Chir.*, Vol. 146, No. 2-3, 1927.

[2] A. V. Ponomarev and A. M. Cheshkov. *Comptes rend. de la Soc. de Biol.*, S. Ju 2 Juillet, 1927, Vol. 97, p. 376.

These experiments were performed in the following way. We introduced antirabic serum into the auricular vein of two rabbits of like weight. Following this, cerebro-spinal fluid was extracted from one of them by suboccipital puncture, and then immediately re-introduced and extracted afresh. In some cases the procedure stopped here; sometimes, however, it was repeated once or twice more. At the end, we usually did not re-introduce the extracted fluid. The infection of the rabbits was always carried out intra-cerebrally, the material used being 1 per cent emulsion of *virus fixe*. At the beginning we had at our disposal only serum of weak titre; hence the infection was carried out two or three hours before, or within two to three hours after, the introduction of the serum. The control rabbits, in which the same quantity of serum was injected into the blood, but without reinforcement, were infected at the same time and in the same way.

With very few exceptions, the experimental rabbits remained healthy. The control animals became ill and all of them died.

Such experiments were carried out by us in large numbers with uniform results. After antirabic serum of a high titre (S. Fein) had been prepared in the Institute of Experimental Medicine, it was possible to increase the interval between the introduction of the serum and the moment of infection to a considerable period (up to 20 hours). Subsequently, a certain number of such experiments were performed on dogs with the same results.

In estimating the results obtained, it is necessary to take note of the fact that this was *the first occasion* in the whole history of the study of the conditions of passive immunisation in rabies *that antirabic serum constantly exhibited its specific action in the organism, even in cases of intra-cerebral infection of the animal.*

Later on, we tested the destruction of the "barrier" by pumping, not only in regard to specific anti-bodies, but also in regard to virus.

Hitherto, the question of the possibility of rabies infection through the blood has not been finally decided. The majority of writers deny this possibility (Pasteur, Marie, Kraus, Nocard, Babes, Bombici, etc.). Helman even considers that the virus is destroyed in the blood. According to the experimental data of Cherevkov, the virus when introduced into the blood, disappears from it within a few minutes, but it can be found in many tissues and organs.

Our experiments along this line were performed as follows (experiments of B. M. Yovelev [1]). A 25 per cent emulsion of rabised brain was prepared, filtered through gauze and centrifuged for some time to remove the larger particles. Of the centrifuged liquid, 3.0 c.c. were very gradually introduced

[1] B. M. Yovelev. *Arkh. Biol. Nauk*, Vol. 30, No. 4, 1930; *Zeitschr. f. d. ges. exp. Med.*, Vol. 74, No. 1-2, 1930.

into the auricular vein of rabbits. Following this, some of the rabbits underwent simple extraction of the cerebro-spinal fluid; to others, the above-described
method of "pumping" was applied. Then the rabbits received a further 5.0
c.c. of the same emulsion. The control rabbits only received introduction of
emulsion into the blood, in the same quantity, and also on two occasions.

Only one of five rabbits undergoing simple extraction of cerebro-spinal
fluid became ill. In the other series, where "pumping" was carried out, four
rabbits out of five became ill. All five control animals remained healthy.

These experiments demonstrated very clearly that "pumping" is a real
means for increasing the permeability of medullary vessels even for particles of
organised matter (including filtrable virus), and in the strength of its
action considerably exceeds the extraction of cerebro-spinal fluid. Moreover,
the experiment confirms that rabies infection through the blood meets with
hindrance under normal conditions. The animals did not become ill even
when the virus introduced exceeded greatly the quantities possible in the spontaneous form of infection.

Recently, Schweinburg also carried out a series of experiments on guinea-
pigs in order to test the intravenous route of infection of rabies. Using a large
volume of virus, he obtained the disease in 50 per cent of cases. On this basis,
he considers that the negative result in our experiments depended, not on the
degree of permeability of the medullary vessels to the virus, but on the employment of liquid emulsion in small doses.

I think that there is a misunderstanding here. We divided the quantity of
emulsion used into two portions precisely because the introduction of the whole
amount at once was accompanied by serious symptoms (panting, convulsions).
Under such conditions, many of the rabbits died in a short time with symptoms
of pulmonary embolism.

The fact that in the experiments described, not one of the control rabbits
became ill, while almost all (four out of five) of those subjected to "pumping"
became ill, leaves no doubt that this process is influenced by the degree of permeability of the medullary vessels. On the contrary, Schweinburg's conclusions
are more open to objection. With the injection of large volumes of foreign
liquid into the circulatory system, the guinea-pigs have to deal not only with
the specific virus contained in the liquid, but also *with the fact of the injection
itself*. The composition of the blood is here sharply (even if temporarily) altered, and this must inevitably lead to an abnormal state of the vascular walls.
Such conditions of infection with virus through the blood never occur normally and *must be likened to the embolic* form of infection, *i.e.*, to immediate
introduction of the virus into the brain. But even under these conditions only
50 per cent of Schweinburg's animals became ill. If his experiments had been

performed under our conditions of technique, *i.e.*, with a still greater injury to the vascular walls, he would have obtained not 50 but a full 100 per cent.

DIPHTHERIA

The above-described method of mechanical destruction of the "barrier" has no special application limited to rabies. Consequently, it was of interest to study its influence on the course of all those pathological processes in the treatment of which specific anti-bodies, in particular anti-toxins, are employed.

Our first experiments were made with diphtheria toxin, the connection of which with the medulla has been pointed out in a number of clinical and histo-pathological observations (Monti, Baginsky, Arnheim, Kleinschmidt). In diphtheria, nervous symptoms so frequently come into the forefront that it has given rise to the proposal (Francioni and Bingle) to inject diphtheria anti-toxin into patients intra-lumbarly, which was successfully done by Bingle in severe cases. His proposal received almost no support. It is probable that this is to be explained by the fact that in cases of medium severity, even simple injection of the serum under the skin—and especially into the blood and muscles—produces a good effect. If, however, this means gives no result, it is already too late and the anti-toxin becomes useless whatever the manner of its introduction.

In our experiments, performed by my collaborator A. V. Ponomarev,[1] we made use of the data of Dönitz and Berghaus concerning the quantitative and temporal relations between toxin and anti-toxin permitting the latter to exhibit its specific effect in the organism. Dönitz showed that if 15 MLD of diphtheria toxin is introduced into the blood of a rabbit weighing 1.8-2.0 kg., and then within 60 minutes afterwards this is followed by 1850 units of anti-toxin, the rabbit cannot be saved and dies approximately on the third day. We performed preliminary experiments which confirmed this.

For each of our experiments, rabbits were selected in pairs. Within 60 minutes after the introduction into a vein of 15 MLD of diphtheria toxin, the rabbits were given, also intravenally, 1850 IU. After 5-10 minutes, "pumping" was carried out on one animal of each pair. This operation was performed under ether narcosis. To equalise the conditions of the experiment, all the control rabbits also underwent ether narcosis, but no "pumping" was carried out on them.

The original experiment was made with eighteen pairs of rabbits. All the eighteen control animals became ill and died in the usual course. Five of the experimental animals did not become ill at all; eleven outlived their controls

[1] A. V. Ponomarev. *Arkh. Biol. Nauk*, Vol. 28, No. 4, 1928; *Zeitschr. f. d. ges. exp. Med.*, Vol. 64, Nos. 1, 2, 1928; *Compt. Rend., de la Soc. de Biol.*, Vol. 97, 1927.

by 3-5 days, and only two died at the same time as their controls. Then we changed the conditions of the experiment and began to introduce the anti-toxin, not 60, but 45 minutes after the toxin. The rest of the procedure remained as before. Under these conditions, it was now the rule for the experimental animals to survive, while the controls died after living only a little longer than in the experiments of the first series.

The facts given above establish without a shadow of doubt that in diphtheria intoxication the nervous system is not drawn into the pathological process to the same extent as other organs and systems of the body. *Its disease is the fundamental condition determining death.* In our experiments, only those animals survived in whose organism conditions had been created for better penetration of the anti-toxin from the blood into the brain. If the anti-toxin reached the region of the central nervous system in time, anxiety about other organs was removed and recovery ensured. The same amount of anti-toxin in the blood, the heart, the suprarenals, etc., proved useless as long as the central nervous system remained outside the sphere of the specific reactions.

We convinced ourselves that the anti-toxin actually enters the brain after "pumping" by special experiments on dogs, the cerebro-spinal fluid of which neutralised the toxin both *in vitro* and *in vivo*. Here, a further point was made clear: after "pumping," especially if it is repeated, the quantity of anti-toxin in the cerebro-spinal fluid gradually increases and attains a maximum, not in the hours immediately following, but on the second or third day.

Later, the anti-toxin content of the cerebro-spinal fluid falls, but in some cases anti-toxin can be found until the seventh or even tenth day.

TETANUS

Our experiments with tetanus toxin were performed approximately according to the same plan. I shall not describe them in detail, mentioning only that corresponding results were also obtained here, though not to the extent that might have been anticipated. The experimental animals on the average outlived their controls by a short period, but finally they also died. The suspicion was inevitably aroused that the useful effect here was connected more with the procedure of "pumping" *per se*, than with the specific antibodies themselves.

DYSENTERY

Experiments with dysentery toxin were performed on rabbits. As the investigations of Kraus and Dörr have shown, these animals are very sensitive to dysentery toxin. The pathological results of dysentery intoxication find expression in the rabbit not only in the region of the intestinal tract, but also in the nervous system, in the form of convulsions and paralysis (Heller, Dörr).

The technique of our experiments (experiments of my collaborator A. V. Ponomarev[1]) was the same as in those with diphtheria toxin. Only the amounts of reacting substance and the times employed were changed. The result was that the rabbits subjected to "pumping" either did not become ill or outlived their controls. The same result was obtained when the rabbits were not subjected to "pumping" but the serum was divided into two parts, one-third being introduced subarachnoidally, and the other two-thirds into the blood. The control rabbit received the whole amount of serum into the blood only. In some cases we had recourse to repeated introduction of serum in various doses in experimental and control rabbits.

The data obtained by application of anti-dysentery serum to animals already diseased proved of interest. After diarrhœa had occurred, and especially on the first appearance of the paralytic symptoms, we introduced the serum into the experimental rabbit both through the blood and subarachnoidally, while in the control rabbit it was introduced only through the blood.

In a number of cases *we obtained a good curative effect* in the experimental animals. In four cases we obtained recovery in animals in a state of prostration, without even strength enough to stand on their feet. With the same doses of anti-toxin, we *did not succeed* in saving diseased animals if the serum was introduced only into the blood.

SCARLATINA

Many infectional processes cannot be reproduced in animals. Consequently we had to turn to clinical material.

At the present time, treatment with anti-toxin serum is frequently employed in scarlatina. When we began our work (1926), there was almost no concentrated anti-scarlatina serum, and the normal dose for severe cases in adults was 100.0-200.0 c.c—otherwise no effect was obtained. The data given by us above provide reason for thinking that by the use of so large a volume of serum a certain proportion of the anti-bodies penetrate from the blood into the medullary region, and that it is this that forms the indispensable condition for any curative effect. But in that case we ought to be able to obtain the effect by subarachnoid injection even with very small doses of the serum.

I made this proposal to Professor G. A. Ivashentsov, the head of the Botkin Infectious Diseases Hospital in Leningrad. A number of such experiments were performed under his control, in this hospital, by Drs. H. G. Kotov

[1] A. V. Ponomarev. *Loc. cit.*, p. 139.

and B. N. Kotlyarenko.[1] Unconcentrated anti-toxin serum to an amount of 4.0-10.0 c.c. was injected into scarlatina patients only subarachnoidally by means of a lumbar puncture. In all these cases the serum was not introduced into the blood or muscles.

By the summer of 1927, 57 observations had been made: 27 cases were the toxic form of disease (categories II, III and IV according to Mozer), 13 were toxic-septic (categories II and III) and 17 were septic-toxic (categories III and IV).

Among the cases treated by subarachnoid injection of serum, *there were no light forms.* They included only patients whose condition in general called for treatment by serum. The prognosis in the case of these patients can be judged from the following statistics.

Our observations were made in the winter of 1926-27 when the scarlatina epidemic was at its height. In 1926, there were 3,296 cases being treated in the Botkin Hospital, in 1927 there were 3,367 scarlatina cases. The general mortality from scarlatina in 1926 was 4.8 per cent, while in 1927 it was 4.2 per cent. The majority of cases were light forms. Only those patients were treated with serum who were actually in need of it, either from the form or the severity of the case. The mortality here, in spite of serum treatment, was 20 per cent. Thus, during the period when our 57 patients were in the hospital, 107 patients received anti-toxin serum by intra-muscular injection and 21 of them died.

For intra-muscular injection, 100.0-200.0 c.c. of serum were used, while for the intra-lumbar injection we took 4.0-10.0 c.c. (about 6.0 c.c. on the average). Parallel observations were carried out with both methods.

Of the 57 persons treated by intra-lumbar injection of serum, 6 died (10.5 per cent); of these, 5 cases belonged to category IV of Mozer, for which Mozer himself reckons a mortality of 99.8 per cent, regarding this form as the preliminary to agony.

In one case of intra-lumbar use of the serum, no direct effect upon the symptoms was obtained. It is noteworthy that a second introduction of serum in large quantity into the muscles, carried out on this patient on the following day, also had no direct curative effect (the patient all the same recovered).

In the remaining cases, *the direct effect upon the symptoms was produced in the same period and in the same form as by the use of other methods of introducing anti-toxin.* The impression was created that with this means an effect was obtained even more quickly and decisively.

---

[1] N. G. Kotov and B. N. Kotlyarenko. *Zhurn. Micr. Pat. i Inf. Bol.,* Vol. 6, No. 2, 1928; *Verhandl. d. deutsch-russisch Scharlach Kongresses vom 11.-14. Juni 1928 in Königsberg.*

This direct effect was expressed primarily in the abolition of "intoxication symptoms" (clouding of consciousness, delirium, convulsions, general excitation or depression, retention of urine, diarrhœa, vomiting, cardio-vascular symptoms, etc.).

At the same time, *the roseolous rash disappeared or faded considerably*. Of the petechial rash, there remained only the petechia themselves on a pale background. The disappearance of the rash took place in all cases independently of the severity of the disease.

At the same time, *the redness and swelling in the throat also decreased or passed off*. A complete parallelism was observed in the process of disappearance of rash and sore throat. The intoxication symptoms, the rash and sore throat, once they had disappeared, did not return.

The temperature fell in 50 cases out of the 57. In this regard, the authors say in their paper: "Subdural introduction of serum . . . gives a definite, rapid and, in cases without complications, final critical fall of temperature."

The earlier the application of serum treatment, the better was the effect. For obtaining the effect from the serum, preliminary extraction of large amounts of cerebro-spinal fluid proved unnecessary.

Subsequent data concerned scarlatina nephritis. Of the above-mentioned 107 scarlatina patients treated with intra-muscular serum injections, 18 died during the first days of the illness. Among the remaining 89 patients, 22 cases of pronounced nephritis were subsequently observed (25 per cent), of which 3 ended fatally. Among our patients, however, numbering 51 persons, who recovered after intra-lumbar injection of serum, nephritis in the proper sense of the word was not observed in a single case. Short-lived albuminuria (1-3 days) was noted only in 3 cases, and in 2 other cases albuminuria (without admixture of blood, without diarrhœa, and with normal temperature) lasted about 2 weeks.

It is necessary to take note also of the development of the meningeal reaction on intra-lumbar injection of serum. In this respect, all the patients were divided into two groups. One group consisted of patients in whom injection had been made with serum prepared with the addition of a trace of carbolic acid as a preservative. This group included 27 persons. In 5 of them there were no symptoms of "meningism"; in 4, these symptoms were rather pronounced, and in 18, light.

The second group, consisting of 30 persons, had been given serum preserved by the addition of chloroform. Among them meningeal symptoms were not observed in a single case. This must obviously be ascribed to the action of the chloroform; when some patients were injected intra-lumbarly with serum containing neither carbolic acid nor chloroform they developed symptoms of meningism.

Later, a number of new observations were made on intra-lumbar injection of serum in scarlatina cases, with approximately the same result.

In drawing conclusions from the data given above, it must be remarked that in a number of cases subarachnoid injection alone of small quantities of anti-toxin serum gave a full therapeutic effect expressed in fall of temperature, disappearance of rash and sore throat, and marked improvement of the general state. *This effect could not be obtained from the same quantity of serum by injecting it by the intravenous, intra-muscular or subcutaneous route.*

Shortly after the publication of these facts, corresponding experiments were made by Dr. N. I. Morozkin in Smolensk at the Infectious Diseases Clinic of Professor M. I. Pevzner (*Vrachebnaya Gazeta*, 1930, No. 3).

The material comprised 50 cases. As regards age, they were mainly children from six months to twelve years. Half the total number of these patients had the severe septic form of scarlatina with early complications (purulent adenitis, otitis, mastoiditis). The remaining half of the cases were referred by the writer to the category of toxic scarlatina of average severity (up to 40° temperature, pronounced intoxication, abundant rash, membranous exudation without necrosis). In this group of patients, intra-lumbar introduction of serum "invariably produced a rapid effect," with doses of anti-toxin several times smaller than employed in intra-muscular injections. In the septic form of scarlatina, intra-lumbar introduction of serum gave only temporary lowering of temperature and transient decrease of intoxication. The writer comes to the conclusion that even small doses of anti-toxin, if introduced intra-lumbarly, have a good therapeutic effect in cases of toxic scarlatina. The question of treatment of severe septic scarlatina by this means is not decided. The author considers that a defect of this method for therapeutic purposes lies in the meningeal symptoms, which in two of his cases were accompanied by bladder disturbances that were not quickly eliminated. The writer gives preference to the method of intra-muscular injection of serum, since this does not produce the above-mentioned complications.

I do not consider myself competent to decide this question. Moreover, this was not the object of our experiments. Their aim was the study of the pathogenesis of the toxic form of scarlatina, and in this respect the result obtained has undoubted interest. On intra-lumbar injection of anti-toxin *in quantities that were inactive by any other method of introduction*, it was not only "nervous symptoms" that disappeared, and not only the "general state" that was improved. Changes took place in a number of other *local processes, such as rash and sore throat, and, perhaps, nephritis was prevented.* The amount of serum employed by us proved ineffective when introduced directly through the blood into the diseased organs themselves, but from the medullary region they put an end to all the pathological processes in those organs.

This is undoubtedly a problem which can only be solved by studying the origin and nature of these specific "local" processes.

<h3 style="text-align:center">MEASLES</h3>

The external symptoms of disease in measles are very similar to those of scarlatina, *viz.*, sharp onset, first signs of local infection in the mouth and throat, rash, and high temperature.

At the present time, prophylactic use of serum of convalescents from measles has become rather popular generally. For this purpose, the serum is employed in small doses that give no directly visible curative effect. The latter can also be obtained by increasing the dose.

It is impossible for a number of reasons to test the resemblance in pathogenesis of measles and scarlatina on considerable clinical material. In the first place, the patients comparatively rarely require specific treatment and consequently the experiment has only its own justification. In the second place, it is very difficult to select material which would make it possible to regard the experimental results as convincing, since the course of the illness itself often varies. However, we succeeded in obtaining some cases which were of considerable value as proofs (cases of Drs. N. G. Kotov and B. N. Kotlyarenko).

These were cases of infection within the hospital; three children of approximately the same age happened to be exposed to infection simultaneously. They were kept under observation. In all of them, at the same time, "Koplik spots" appeared on the mucous membrane of the cheek. Each of them received an injection of 8.0 c.c. of serum from measles convalescents, in two cases in the blood, in the other subarachnoidally by means of a lumbar puncture. For the latter injection, a case was chosen in which the "Koplik spots" were exhibited in a very marked form. The first two children became ill on the following day and subsequently passed through the usual history of the disease in average severity. The child in whom serum had been injected subarachnoidally did not develop the illness. All that happened was that five days afterwards the temperature rose slightly ($37.4°$) and a slight and non-typical rash appeared (serum symptoms?). Within 24 hours, the rash disappeared and the temperature returned to normal.

These cases can be summed up in the following way. In the blood system of two of the patients, there was introduced a quantity of serum which proved inadequate for producing an effect. This is clear from the fact that there was no alteration of the development and course of the illness in these patients.

In the third patient, the same, *i.e.*, also an inadequate, quantity of serum was introduced subarachnoidally. Here, the illness did not follow, or at any rate, it was delayed for five days.

What then are measles and scarlatina, if blockade of the nervous system alone held back or extinguished all the symptoms of these diseases?

It is clear that here, just as in scarlatina, the "local" symptoms (rash, sore throat, Koplik spots) *cannot be regarded as independent*, and are by no means evidence of an actual affection of the peripheral tissues by a specific irritating agent which has produced the disease itself. We obtained an opportunity of convincing ourselves of this by yet another example.

The serum of a measles convalescent (10.0 c.c.) was introduced subarachnoidally during the first period of the illness into a patient with already pronounced rash and high temperature (39.8°). Within twelve hours, the temperature fell critically and the rash disappeared. But the case is not interesting on this account. On the very first day of the illness, symptoms of pneumonia were noticed, with a focus in one of the lungs (early "measles pneumonia"). The dissipation of the pneumonia focus occurred simultaneously with the disappearance of the other symptoms of the disease, and within even a few days this focus could no longer be diagnosed.

When all the symptoms of the disease fall out one after another, the disease itself comes to an end. If this process takes place owing to reactions of the nervous system, then it must logically be said that the nervous system *was not only drawn into the disease, but itself organised the external manifestations of the disease.* All the rest was only the consequence of this action.

CHAPTER XIII
GENERAL REVIEW

In our further work we tested under the same conditions a number of other specific sera. These included polyvalent sera—streptococcus, staphylococcus, cholera and typhoid sera. A few observations were carried out on human beings, but the vast majority of the experiments were on animals. We did not observe any clear advantages in the action of these sera, whether by subarachnoid injection or by the method of "pumping." The effect was either absent or accidental. The general impression from this series of experiments was negative rather than positive. This is comprehensible. Subarachnoid injections or "pumping" produce, by themselves, a trauma of the nervous system. If these means are not followed by a reaction specifically useful *ad hoc,* they inevitably make the position worse. All the sera enumerated above, it is known, give no marked effect even when employed in the usual form. Contemporary medical practice hardly takes them into account. If the laboratories, nevertheless, continue to prepare them, it is chiefly for scientific purposes.

It is customary to consider that the absence of specific action depends here on accidental causes, on the type of animal, on the properties of the anti-body taken, on the form of immunisation, etc.; it is still hoped, that in the course of time, changes in the manner of preparation of these sera (*i.e.,* more perfect methods) will settle the problem in a positive sense.

We, however, doubt this. We have seen that the exhibition of specific action of sera in the organism is connected with something more than the mere presence of definite properties belonging to these sera. *The fundamental issue here concerns the properties of the reacting object* and the character of those processes which are exhibited in the form of disease. I shall permit myself to dwell a little on this subject.

Does the specific character of the action of sera depend on whether we are dealing with an "anti-toxin" or a "bactericidal" serum?

It does not. This was already demonstrated above in the case of antirabic serum. Its specific properties were previously only accessible to study *in vitro.* We are now able to observe them *in vivo.*

The second question is: Do the "bactericidal" sera enumerated actually possess specific properties?

Yes, they do, for *in vitro* they exhibit a series of specific reactions with appropriate anti-bodies. Moreover, the manner of their preparation is not in any way different in principle from the manner of preparation of anti-toxin sera. The difference is not essential, it relates solely to the methods of obtaining the antigen, and the time, quantity and place of its injection.

Finally—and this is the chief question—are there any peculiarities in the character of the action of anti-toxin sera?

There are none. Their specific properties are undoubtedly also only exhibited *in vitro*. To observe them in the organism, it is necessary to take very exact account of the time. The diphtheria clinic demonstrates the violent increase in the percentage of failures with anti-toxin treatment with every day's delay in its employment. Laboratory experiment testifies to the same thing even more categorically. Here, it is already not days of delay but hours and even minutes that play a role. Almost the same thing can be said of laboratory experiments with tetanus. The appearance of the initial local symptoms is usually a sign of fatal danger, whatever the manner and whatever the extent of subsequent serum treatment.

The reader will remember that we observed the same thing in our experience with rabies.

It is clear that there are no reasons why anti-toxin sera should differ in this respect from bactericidal sera. It is also clear that the *conception of infectional and toxic processes as processes which are specific from start to finish is incorrect. In all these cases, the specific agent only starts the process. The subsequent development of the latter is governed by other conditions which the specific serum is not able to abolish.*

It will now not appear surprising that intra-lumbar introduction of anti-toxin (as indeed every other form of its introduction) has not decided the question of the treatment of septic scarlatina. *The latter is a supplementary process arising on the basis of scarlatina.* As in diphtheria, the transition to this new form of disease may occur very rapidly, almost simultaneously with the toxic symptoms. It follows from this that the absence of curative effect of many sera *is no evidence that they are weak or destitute of specific properties.*

Passing to consideration of the genesis of individual symptoms of the infection process, we shall have to admit that at least some of them *are secondary*. This is the case for the rash of measles and scarlatina, and also for sore throat. It is natural that the question of local changes in diphtheria should also have arisen.

In the development of diphtheria, the leading part played by the nervous system also stood out very distinctly. Using one and the same quantity of anti-toxin, only those animals survived in whose organism conditions were created for the anti-toxin to reach the medulla. Data, testifying to the capacity of diphtheria toxin to unite with various tissues, are therefore mainly of theoretical interest.

C. Levaditi and St. Muttermilch placed pieces of organs (heart, kidney, spleen, bone marrow) for short periods in a solution of diphtheria toxin and observed retardation in the growth of tissue culture. This retardation was easily neutralised by anti-toxin. In 1928, Dr. I. M. Gakh repeated these experiments with the same result. However, when he began to take for tissue cultures, pieces of organs of animals that had died from diphtheria intoxication, then the cultures grew excellently in spite of the fact that the doses of toxin were, in general, enormous (200 MLD). The author gives no explanation of this phenomenon. However, we are justified in drawing from it the conclusion, at least, that in the conditions of the living organism, diphtheria toxin, even in large doses, does not cause irreparable disturbance in the tissues mentioned.

The matter is quite otherwise with the nervous system. We described above the experiments of Roux and Borrel, which established that immunised animals die from tetanus if the toxin is introduced into the brain. Planer and Potpeschnig repeated these experiments with a similar result, taking diphtheria toxin instead of tetanus toxin. We, in our turn, performed a series of experiments along these lines with diphtheria toxin (experiments of my collaborators N. N. Nikitin and A. V. Ponomarev[1]).

Rabbits and guinea-pigs were used as the experimental animals. In rabbits the anti-toxin was introduced into the blood in large quantities (500-1000 IU). This was followed shortly afterwards by subarachnoid injection of diphtheria toxin in doses of 10 or 5 MLD. All the rabbits died, very few of them surviving for more than 24 hours. A still more convincing result, however, was obtained in a second series of experiments. In these, we not only introduced the same quantity of anti-toxin into the blood as in the first series, but accompanied it by "pumping." Only after this came subarachnoid injection of toxin. All the rabbits, of course, considerably outlived the rabbits of the first series, and many of them even survived. When we passed from doses of 5 MLD to 2 MLD, then survival of the rabbits subjected to "pumping" became the general rule. However, at a later period (from the twelfth to the twentieth day or later, many of these animals also died, showing

[1] N. N. Nikitin and A. V. Ponomarev. *Arkh. Biol. Nauk*, Vol. 30, No. 1, 1930; *Zeitschr. f. d. ges. exp. Med.*, Vol. 70, No. 3-4, 1930.

symptoms of emaciation, increasing weakness and paralysis). The diphtheria toxin, having been given the possibility of encountering at the same time both the anti-toxin and the nerve tissues, partially reacted with the latter, and even found time to produce irreparable alterations in it. *Even if the toxin was subsequently entirely neutralised, this did not restore the structure and function of the nerve cell.*

The experiments on guinea-pigs were performed under analogous conditions. As in the case of rabbits, we introduced large doses of the anti-toxin into the blood and only a little toxin subarachnoidally. Like the rabbits, they all inevitably died.

One curious phenomenon was noticed during this series of experiments. It is well known that in guinea-pigs affections of the suprarenal glands are considered to be a typical sign of death from diphtheria intoxication. They can be observed in other animals also, but in a less marked degree. *We discovered these changes in our guinea-pigs on dissection.* They may have been somewhat less marked than in cases of intoxication through the blood; but they were, nevertheless, clearly defined, even on macroscopical examination. The same applies also to the heart muscle and ganglia.

It is worth while devoting some attention to these facts. Under our conditions of experiment, every molecule of toxin that passed out of the medullary region into the blood was immediately neutralised here, since the anti-toxin had been introduced previously to the toxin. *The toxin reached the heart or suprarenal glands only in this inactive form.* When, under the same conditions, we introduced the toxin not subarachnoidally but into the blood, even very large quantities had generally no consequences. In other words, in our experiments the impulse to alterations in the heart and in the medullary substance of the suprarenal glands came from the nervous system, for it is only on the nervous system that the diptheria toxin could act. *In other words, these peripheral affections in diphtheria are secondary.* Their cause is not the toxin but the new relations now established between the tissues and the injured nerve centres.

Consequently it was found that in diphtheria, as in scarlatina and measles, *certain of the "local" processes are of a peculiar nature and call for special consideration.*

Now if the disappearance or prevention of local symptoms depends solely on the immunisation of the nervous system it must be admitted that the local reactions of immunity may also proceed in neither the place nor the manner usually accepted. This in its turn gives rise to the question of the nature of "general" disturbances.

To finish the examination of the materials in this chapter, it remains to give an estimate of the technical means employed by us, which we have called "pumping."

In the experiments described here, our object was to bring about a rapid change in the permeability of the medullary vessels for the conveyance of specific anti-bodies into the medulla.

In addition, however, to the products required by us, the way was opened to all other substances present in the blood. For a certain period the permeability of the medullary vessels is altered in general. This is a fact which must certainly be taken into account.

This is not all. It has already been pointed out, in dealing with the material relating to convulsive phenomena, that even simple withdrawal of the cerebro-spinal fluid can alter the usual form of reaction to a particular irritating agent. The effect of "pumping" is bound to be even stronger. *If only from the point of view of its mechanical effect, it must be regarded as a specific form of brain massage.*

We are very well aware of the fact that the nervous system *exhibits its functions in the organism only by producing changes in other organs.* In this respect, it always inevitably acts in a dual fashion. If changes take place within the nervous system one can be assured that they will also find their expression at the periphery. The normal cycle of reactions is altered if the normal state of the nerve is destroyed. We have convinced ourselves of this on many occasions. Below will be found a series of examples of the same character.

My collaborators Drs. A. M. and M. L. Petrunkin [1] performed a series of experiments with salts of magnesium and bromine, which on introduction into the blood of rabbits, intra-muscularly or even into the stomach (bromine), produce narcosis in these animals.

The first part of the work was devoted to working out the experimental conditions, *i.e.,* the conditions in regard to times and doses. The latter depends to a considerable extent on the size of the animal. We finally adopted the following form, whereby the experiments yielded clear results.

The animals were selected in pairs. Their weight was 1.6-1.8 kg. The experiment began by one of the animals undergoing "pumping" under ether narcosis, while the other, to equalise the conditions, was given only narcosis. After 40-60 minutes, there was injected intra-muscularly (into the femoral and gluteal muscles) 8.0-10.0 c.c. of a 10 per cent solution of $MgCl_2$.

Even after a very short time, a difference could be noted. In the course of the following 3-10 minutes, the normal rabbit became limp, lay down and went to sleep. Narcosis speedily developed. In the rabbit subjected to "pump-

[1] A. M. and M. L. Petrunkin. *Arkh. Biol. Nauk,* Vol. 29, No. 1, 1929; *Zeitschr. f. d. ges. exp. Med.,* Vol. 68, Nos. 5, 6, 1929.

ing," not only was there no narcosis, but even sleepiness was not always observed. While the control animals were already lying immovable and did not react to external stimuli, the rabbits subjected to "pumping" were still running about the table all the time, sniffing at their sleeping companions and even nibbling at turnips offered to them. After some time, they also became limp, sat without moving and bristled up, *but they reacted to contact and did not lie on their sides.* Very soon they completely recovered. When on two occasions we injected 18.0 c.c. of $MgCl_2$ solution, instead of 10.0 c.c., into the rabbits, the animals subjected to "pumping" also went to sleep, but only after 20 minutes from the time of injection, and they woke up within an hour. The controls slept within 3 minutes after the injection, and died after 25 minutes.

To obtain a clear result, it is necessary that the magnesium should be introduced, *not immediately after "pumping,"* but after 40-60 minutes. Hence, what is important here is *not so much the destruction of the normal permeability of the medullary vessels, as the process which develops in the nervous system as a result of our interference.* It is only after a certain period of time that it reaches the necessary level, and it then exercises a clearly marked influence on the course of other reactions.

In addition, it is of course impossible to doubt that the process termed narcosis proceeds fundamentally within the central nervous system. After "pumping," magnesium entered the nervous system in a greater quantity than without this operation; in spite of this, narcosis was either lacking or much more weakly expressed than in the controls.

From this the conclusion must inevitably be drawn that the character of the action of a particular substance does not depend only on its special properties, quantity or mode of application. In making an estimate of the complicated effect, *it is necessary in each separate case to take into account all the conditions of combination or non-combination of the substance taken with the substratum, and also the continually varying reciprocal relations of the separate parts of the reacting substratum.*

In analogous experiments with bromine, we introduced this substance into the stomach. The narcotic effect of bromine on rabbits begins to appear only after some hours. Consequently we introduced it, not 40-60 minutes after "pumping," but immediately after it. As a result of "pumping," the rabbits went to sleep within 4-5 hours and narcosis persisted 1-2 days. In the normal rabbits, sleep appeared only after 15-20 hours, and narcosis lasted altogether a few hours. There were cases when complete narcosis did not develop at all in the normal rabbits. *Consequently, in the experiments with bromine, the result was the opposite of that obtained in experiments with magnesium.*

In attempting to explain this fact, the following supposition was made. Magnesium is a cation. According to Loeb's rule, it should unite with the carboxyl group of the protein molecule in an alkaline medium. Acidifying the medulla ought to diminish the combination of magnesium with proteins and thus weaken its pharmacological (narcotic) action.

Bromine, on the other hand, is an anion. By the same rule, its combination with protein will take place in an acid medium by means of the free amine group present under these conditions.

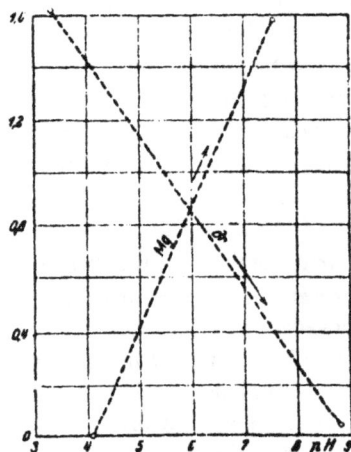

Fig. 9. Diagram Showing the Influence of the Acidity of the Medium on the Combination of Magnesium and Bromine with Gelatine

These considerations led to a new group of experiments which were similar in every way to those described above, with the exception that "pumping" was replaced by the introduction of acid or alkali into the blood. For acidification a 1/10 N solution of HCl was used, for alkalisation, a 2½ per cent solution of Na_2CO_3.

Under these conditions, magnesial narcosis does not develop in the "acidified" rabbits, but the "alkalised" animals quickly go to sleep and remain in narcosis for a long time. This is the more noteworthy in that, on introduction of alkali alone without magnesium, the rabbits remain lively and even become restless, while the introduction of acid produces depression.

The experiments with bromine were organised on the same lines. 20 c.c of a 35 per cent solution of sodium bromide was introduced by means of a tube into the stomach of the rabbits, shortly after one of the pair had received an injection of acid in the blood, and the other of alkali. The "acid" rabbits quickly became limp. After 3-5 hours they were already in a state of narcosis which lasted for 1-2 days and frequently ended in death. Under otherwise similar conditions, in the rabbits in which alkali had been injected, not only did narcosis not develop but even sleep was not always observed. After 24 hours, when the "acid" rabbits were under narcosis, their "alkaline" companions could be considered almost normal.

When A. M. and M. L. Petrunkin transferred these same experiments into the purely chemical sphere, the following result was obtained. Bromine and magnesium unite with gelatine, and also with the proteins of the human brain, in exact accordance with Loeb's rule. That is to say, *as the medium becomes more alkaline, the magnesium is bound by them in greater quantity. On the contrary, with bromine the same reaction proceeds in proportion to the acidification.* This is made clear by the diagram on page 153. (Fig. 9.)

This shows that *"pumping" leads not only to a change in the state of permeability of the walls of the medullary vessels.* The specific form of irritation of the nervous system obtained in this way is expressed, evidently, by the destruction of the normal course of many other processes in the organism, including possibly its acid-alkali equilibrium.

One further detail must be mentioned here. The experiments of Lumière have shown that variations of pH in the blood, produced by addition of acid or alkali to the blood of guinea-pigs, last for a very short time and disappear within 1-2 hours. In our cases, this period was sufficient not only for temporary but also for final changes in the course of the processes interesting us. It follows from this that *the course and outcome of some biological reactions are determined from the very first moment of action of the irritating agent on the object concerned.*

I shall describe one further group of materials in order to characterise the nature of "pumping" *as a means that results in not one but many different consequences.* This material concerns some observations on epidemic cerebro-spinal meningitis. They were obtained as early as 1926 and were the logical consequence of our experiments on rabies, diphtheria, scarlatina, etc.

The indications for the appropriate experiments seemed obvious for there could be no doubt that the antigen is located in the region of the central nervous system. One must consider that the auto-immunisation commences at the same time as the process itself. After 2-3 weeks, auto-immunisation should be considerable. However, we know that by this time the disease not only has not subsided, but is rather at the climax of its development. If now the access to the brain of specific anti-bodies occurring in the blood can be strengthened, the recovery must thereby be accelerated.

"Pumping" appeared to be the appropriate means for realising this aim, since after the first two weeks the thick pus filling the subarachnoid space usually becomes more fluid and watery, and is easily withdrawn through the needle.

An obstacle to the performance of the experiment can only be encountered in another respect.

It was in experiments with meningitis that we first decided to apply "pumping" to human beings. It is natural that the conditions necessary here should be somewhat different from those in experiments on animals, where we used the entire quantity of fluid that could be extracted and it was sufficient to repeat the procedure two or three times in order to obtain a useful effect without harmful consequences. In man, however, the quantity of cerebro-spinal fluid is very large; it increases with age, attaining 150-200 c.c. To use even one-third or one-quarter of this quantity for "pumping" may prove harmful. Consequently, we decided to use an injector with a volume of only 10.0-15.0 c.c., repeating the extraction and re-introduction of the fluid 10-15 times. In this form, "pumping" was admissible for human beings also, especially in meningitis; the quantity of fluid in this disease is usually so much enlarged that this alone often makes daily punctures a necessity.

Further, clinical surgery is acquainted with, and has employed a form of lumbar anæsthesia, due to Bier, in which the anæsthetising substance (cocaine) is introduced and withdrawn several times. This method was proposed by the French surgeon Le Filliatre for mixing the cocaine solution with cerebro-spinal fluid. The object in this case was to spread anæsthesia to parts of the central nervous system situated above the lumbar region of the spinal cord. The author did not mention any deleterious consequences from the use of this technique.

Our experiments on the application of "pumping" in epidemic meningitis were carried out in 1925-26 in the Filatov Hospital in Leningrad, in collaboration with Dr. Y. K. Panferov. The patients were seven children. They had already been repeatedly subjected during a considerable period to lumbar punctures in order to lower the intra-cranial pressure. No perceptible improvement had been noted. Then the lumbar puncture was combined with "pumping." The fluid was extracted and re-introduced 5-8 times and finally poured away; the syringe was then replaced on the needle and the whole procedure repeated 5-10 times more. At the end, the liquid was allowed to flow freely from the needle in the same quantity as had previously been let out from the patient by simple puncture. This procedure was repeated in the next few days. Five of the children recovered without defects, the favourable turning point of the disease more or less clearly coinciding with the time of application of "pumping." The sixth patient also recovered, but the recovery could not be connected with our procedure. The seventh patient died some days after the first employment of "pumping." We could not escape from the idea of a possible connection between this death and the use of our procedure, and no further experiments with cerebro-spinal meningitis were undertaken.

Two years later, Dr. S. N. Markov (of Ufa) employed "pumping" in a case of adult meningitis with good results. In 1930, these experiments were repeated by Dr. M. B. Litvin (at Mogilev on the Dnieper). His material included both simple and complicated cases. Besides "pumping," the author employed also other methods of treatment (repeated serum injection, proteinotherapy, "autoliquortherapy," etc.).

On the strength of his material, he comes to the conclusion that "the general effect of pumping in cerebro-spinal meningitis is equivalent to the effect of the usual lumbar puncture." The author does not connect the recovery of his patients with the procedure indicated.

Looking through the short extracts from his protocols, we see that in almost all of them "pumping" was employed only once. We employed it repeatedly, with intervals of 1-2-3 days, combining it with the regular puncture. The data in our possession provide evidence that in this form the procedure has had an undoubted influence on the course of some cases of cerebro-spinal meningitis. The same must be said also of one of Dr. S. N. Markov's cases.

He began the treatment of his patient by repeated lumbar punctures. They were not successful. After the first "pumping," however, the temperature at once dropped by 2.5°C. and the general condition sharply improved. In the days immediately following, a new rise of temperature was observed, but after "pumping" it dropped to normal on the same day. The procedure was repeated twice more with the same effect, after which the temperature did not rise again and the patient recovered.

It is interesting to note that exactly the same was observed in one of our cases. On the day of the first "pumping," the temperature fell to normal, and remained so on the following day. The next day, the temperature rose and the general condition changed accordingly. A repetition of "pumping" did away with all these phenomena, again for two days. The general picture was renewed twice more, after which there was no further relapse and the patient recovered.

These and similar observations convinced us that in some cases of cerebro-spinal meningitis, "pumping" undoubtedly has a favourable effect on the course of the disease. It would seem that the result obtained ought to confirm us of the correctness of the assumptions made earlier. However, comparison with a number of other facts *cast doubt on whether we were dealing here with specific reactions.*

In point of fact, if the antigen is present in the brain, then why is it essential for producing anti-bodies that it should leave the brain and penetrate into other organs through the blood? Immunity could be developed also on the spot. If we do not find this, for example, in rabies, it is only because the process of progressive affection of the nervous system develops here in violent fashion. Nevertheless, it is possible to obtain a certain degree of active immunity of the central nervous system even towards rabies (as we found several times as far back as 1926 in the experiments of my collaborator A. V. Ponomarev[1]). Brain inoculated with rabies was treated with cerebro-spinal fluid in a thermostat, filtered through a filter candle and the filtrate repeatedly injected into rabbits subarachnoidally. In the succeeding infection, these animals were noticeably more stable than their controls.

Things should be even better with meningococcus. It is undoubtedly a weak stimulant. The disease persists for weeks and frequently not only ends in recovery, but even in recovery *ad integrum.*

Attention should also be paid to the rhythmical character of the improvements and succeeding outbursts of the disease, frequently observed in cerebro-spinal meningitis. If the improvement takes place under the influence of a specific factor, what determines the relapse?

From this point of view, it is also impossible to explain the fact of the protractedness of the disease. The laboratory method of active immunisation produces the required effect in a much shorter period than 1½-2 months. Yet we know that cerebro-spinal meningitis sometimes lasts even longer than this.

Perhaps, however, the nervous system is incapable of active immunisation, or this process is retarded in it?

Looking through the literature, it is easy to convince oneself that this question has been investigated, but with very contradictory results. The question has been examined in relation to various anti-bodies—hæmolysins, agglutinins and anti-toxins. Neufeld did not find hæmolysins in the cerebro-spinal fluid of rabbits treated with subarachnoid injections of sheep erythrocytes. Muttermilch, under the same experimental conditions, discovered them both in the blood and in the cerebro-spinal fluid, but their strength was approximately 100 times higher in the blood. Illert, Grabow and Plaut discovered,

[1] Speransky. *Ann. de l'Inst. Pasteur,* Vol. 41, 1927.

also in rabbits, that under appropriate conditions hæmolysins and agglutinins make their appearance in the cerebro-spinal fluid by local formation and not by passing out of the blood. The quantity of these substances in the blood, however, was 10-80 times greater than in the fluid. Marie immunised animals by injecting tetanus toxin into them intra-cerebrally in minimal doses, but he did not obtain the desired effect. Muttermilch and Salomon repeated these experiments, substituting anatoxin for the toxin. Animals treated by this means withstood intra-cerebral injection of fatal doses of tetanus toxin. Descombey, under the same experimental conditions, obtained a contrary result, and on these grounds denies the difference between subcutaneous and intra-cerebral methods of immunising animals with tetanus toxin.

To clear up the question finally, we decided to perform a series of experiments with diphtheria anatoxin (experiments of my collaborators N. N. Nikitin and A. V. Ponomarev[1]).

The animals used in the experiments were rabbits and dogs. The latter, on account of their size, are more suitable, and in their case the technique is simplified. In addition, the quantity of cerebro-spinal fluid in the dog is much greater than in the rabbit. Hence, with subarachnoid injections of the same dose of anatoxin, its composition will change relatively less. This, in its turn, diminishes the general nerve trauma and the local shock thereby involved to those elements which have to be drawn into the process under examination.

Vaccination in the rabbits was carried out subarachnoidally and intra-cerebrally, in the dogs only by the subarachnoid route. The control animals in both groups were vaccinated subcutaneously. The anatoxin injections were repeated several times at weekly intervals. After the lapse of various periods since the last inoculation (from eight days upwards) the animals were given intra-cerebral injections of diphtheria toxin. *The rabbits received 10, the dogs 100 or 250 fatal doses intra-cerebrally.*

All the experimental animals remained healthy, not only during the days immediately following, but also during the whole subsequent period. *All* the controls died within periods of 10-48 hours.

Long before the test with the toxin, the cerebro-spinal fluid and serum of the dogs had already been tested for anti-toxin content. It was found that the titre of the fluid was only twice as low as that of the blood. This gives every justification for considering that the anti-toxin in the cerebral region of our dogs was of local origin and had not penetrated there from the blood as a result of meningeal irritation. We injected anti-diphtheria serum subarachnoidally into other dogs, and after various periods determined its amount

[1] N. N. Nikitin and A. V. Ponomarev. *Arkh. Biol. Nauk*, Vol. 30, No. 1, 1930; *Zeitschr. f. d. ges. exp. Med.*, Vol. 70, Nos. 3, 4, 1930.

in the cerebro-spinal fluid; already within one or two days the anti-toxin could not be found there. Yet meningeal stimulation from serum is not a whit less than from anatoxin. Taking into account the quantities of the one and the other, one must consider that the irritation produced by serum is even greater. Our animals, however, *a month after the final vaccination withstood the intra-cerebral introduction of 250 fatal doses of diphtheria toxin easily and without showing any symptoms.*

On comparing these data with those given above, it is clear that the production of anti-toxins proceeds more successfully in the region of the central nervous system than the production of other anti-bodies, *e.g.*, hæmolysins or agglutinins. This is explained by the fact of the special sensitiveness of nerve elements to toxins; toxins and toxoids are stronger irritating agents than erythrocytes and bacteria, the more so as the erythrocytes and bacteria must first be disintegrated, and this disintegration takes time.

Among incidental observations made by us in the course of the above-described experiments, it is worth noting that *the strength of the anti-toxin in the serum of dogs inoculated subarachnoidally was always higher than in that of dogs inoculated subcutaneously.* Consequently the additional irritation of the nerve elements by a specific antigen led to a more vigorous production of anti-bodies in other parts of the organism as well.

The data obtained show also that *active local immunisation of the central nervous system is not only possible but is the most hopeful form of immunity.* Its development begins from the first days of the action of the antigen, and even within a fairly short time can be determined by suitable biological tests.

This once again confronted us with the question whether recovery from cerebro-spinal meningitis is actually connected with specific reactions between the antigen and anti-bodies, and whether it has been objectively and incontrovertibly proved that the meningococcus is the cause of the disease from beginning to end.

We have no objective proofs of this, and still less any that are incontrovertible. The process was and remains problematical. In commencing experiments on "pumping" in patients suffering from epidemic meningitis, we shared the generally accepted point of view and connected the undoubted effect obtained in certain cases with immunity reactions. Subsequent work caused us to alter our original conceptions and made us look for other explanations. The large number of experiments described in the preceding chapters of this book show that both simple extraction of cerebro-spinal fluid and "pumping" exercise a marked influence on the course of many processes. In addition to the reactions of the medullary vessels and membranes, it is necessary to take into account the *irritation which this operation produces in the nervous system.* The degree and direction of biological reactions in various parts of the organism, including the nervous system itself, are altered; this can increase some pathological phenomena and weaken others. Hence, in judging the method of "pumping," we must take into account not only the "barrier," or the permeability of the vascular wall, but also the fact that this procedure is *a specific form of "brain massage."*

A study of the properties of the reacting object and of the character of its reactions is the basic task for elucidating the nature of the phenomena under consideration.

Our experiments in this connection form the subject of the following chapters of this book.

THE CONDITIONS AND FORMS OF DEVELOPMENT OF DYSTROPHIC PROCESSES WITHIN THE NERVOUS SYSTEM

CHAPTER XIV

THE MECHANISM OF SEGMENTARY AFFECTIONS OF THE NERVOUS SYSTEM THROUGH THE NERVE TRUNK

In one of the preceding chapters, devoted to the question of circulation, when analysing a series of data that we had obtained, we divided the movements of various substances along the nerve trunk into two forms—active and passive. The form based on a biochemical reaction between the substance introduced and the nerve tissue we called active. This, in turn, implies that *active movement is always an injury.*

The processes developing as a result of the penetration of foreign substances into nerves proceed, consequently, in at least two ways. On the one hand we have the irritation or rupture of peripheral nerve parts, *subsequently bringing reflex mechanisms into play*; on the other hand, the central nerve cells may be the direct substratum of the *action of the substance used.* Both processes occur simultaneously, being superposed on one another, and create a very complex combination in which it is not easy to distinguish the component elements.

The processes taking place within the nervous system can only be judged by the external reactions reflecting these processes at the periphery. We consider local tetanus of a particular group of muscles as one of the forms of nerve reactions because it can be easily eliminated by severing the appropriate nerve. In exactly the same way, we have seen that sore throat and rash in scarlet fever are liquidated by influences exerted on the nervous system. Since the onset of tetanus is usually connected with the toxin making its appearance in the peripheral nerve regions, it was interesting to test this *as a method of investigating the genesis of other local processes,* using other substances as irritants.

This naturally brought us to the question of trophic ulcers. The formation of ulcers on the cornea of rabbits after stimulating the Gasserian ganglion by an electric current was first observed by Magendie. Samuel—one of the founders of the theory of the trophic function of the nervous system—used chemical irritation of various nerve structures for producing tissue disturbances. We decided to make this the starting point of our work.

Among the local pathological processes arising as a result of illness, or of injury to the nervous system, are included chronic ulcers. In man, they develop most frequently on the lower extremities. Charcot observed long ago that not every injury to a nerve results in dystrophic lesions of the tissues, and that these lesions are connected *not with the cessation of the functioning of the nerve, but with its irritation.* According to the observations of the American surgeons, W. Mitchell, Morehouse and Keen, partial injury to nerves is more dangerous in this respect than complete severance. They pointed out also the role played by infection and inflammation of the lesioned nerves. Thus trophic ulcers, after injury to the sciatic nerve, usually arise in cases which are accompanied by suppuration and where neuritis occurs during healing.

Chronic ulcers of the extremities in dogs were obtained comparatively long ago by Levashev and Lapinsky, and their experiments were later confirmed by others. The principle of the method is the application of some chemical substance to the sciatic nerve (for instance, a thread soaked in sulphuric acid, iodine or croton oil). Some 2-3 months afterwards, ulcers developed in a few of the animals (about 20 per cent) on the side corresponding to the place of injury. A. S. Vishnevsky [1] repeated these experiments, and devoted special attention to the role of suppuration and constant mechanical irritation of the centripetal end of the severed sciatic nerve in dogs. He produced suppuration in the operation wound, and, in addition, stitched the centripetal nerve end to the unparalysed muscles. The contractions of the muscles produced a continual slight trauma of the nerve.

As a result, he succeeded in obtaining chronic ulcers on the corresponding extremities of the dogs in *100 per cent of his experiments.* The ulcers developed within 1½-2 months, independently of the conditions under which the animals were kept, and frequently healed after the removal of the neuroma of the centripetal end of the severed nerve.

Thus, the development of trophic ulcers on the extremities takes place fundamentally after the manner of a reflex. Irritation of the centripetal end of the damaged nerve provides the starting point for the whole process.

A number of other facts, however, provide reason for thinking that *the process is not limited to this.* In the first place, we are not dealing here with a simple reflex. As is well known, the medical treatment of trophic ulcers consists not only in the removal of the neuroma of the spinal nerves, but also in the section of the sympathetic paths; Leriche achieved this by peri-arterial sympathectomy, Razumovsky by alcoholising the vascular sheath, Diez by partial incision of the sympathetic chain, etc.

[1] A. S. Vishnevsky. *Vestn. Khirurg. i Pogr. Obl. [Messenger of Surgery and Related Fields]*, No. 39, 1928.

The second point lies in the relapses. Statistics of all forms of interference by operation show that relapses after curing trophic ulcers occur in the vast majority of cases. The causes producing relapses in some cases are also noteworthy. Thus, A. S. Vishnevsky noticed that in a number of his patients operated on by Molotkov's method, ulcers already healed *easily suffered a relapse when the patients caught grippe*. When the grippe passed away, the ulcer also healed again.

He also directed attention to the indubitable importance of age, both for the formation of trophic ulcers and for their healing.

All this gives rise to the idea that the injury to the nerve creates not only a point of irritation at the periphery but also some kind of pathological focus in the centre. *The elucidation of the conditions for the origin of this focus became the subject of our work.*

The original experiments consisted in the following (experiments of my collaborator A. S. Vishnevsky [1]). The sciatic nerve in the middle part of the thigh of a dog was sectioned under narcosis. A small quantity of mucilaginous purulent secretion taken from a chronic suppurating focus of a human being, was applied to the centripetal end of the nerve and partly rubbed in. The wound was sewn up. Following this the cerebro-spinal fluid was extracted, and this extraction was repeated every 2-5 days (3-5 times in all). No further irritation was inflicted in the region of the operation wound itself.

About 7-12 days later, fluctuating swelling, loss of hair and, finally, ulceration occurred on the corresponding foot-pad, usually at the back of it, and also on the lobe of the heel. The ulceration rapidly enlarged, both peripherally and in depth, involving tendons, joints and bones so that sometimes the process had to be diagnosed not as ulcer but as gangrene. In some dogs this led to the complete separation of the toes and parts of the foot-pad. Sequestration of the bones frequently occurred, not in the joint or in the neighbourhood of the epiphysal end of the bone, but in the middle of the diaphysis of, for instance, the metatarsal bones. All this occurred *in the midst of completely healthy tissues*, unconnected by any inflammatory phenomena with the operation wound. Thus, a process which, in the hands of previous investigators, required a period of 2-3 months, developed under these new conditions much more rapidly and intensely. (Plates 4 and 6.)

But more than this, in all our cases after a certain period (from 5-10 days up to 8 weeks) a similar non-healing ulcer or gangrene appeared *on the symmetrically situated place of the other, healthy, foot*. (Plate 5.) The formation

[1] A. S. Vishnevsky. *Vestn. Khirurg. i Pogr. Obl.*, No. 41, 1928; *Zeitschr. f. d. ges. exp. Med.*, Vol. 63, No. 5-6, 1928.

of symmetrical chronic ulcers at the extremities has long been known in the clinic and is quite familiar. But this fact had not previously been obtained experimentally in conditions ·vhere the nerve on only one side was used for the experiment.

It is important to mention that the possibility of a direct cause for the formation of these ulcerations, *e.g.*, trauma, was excluded. In the majority of cases, the process begins with œdematic swelling in a restricted spot. The skin becomes thin, and a fluctuating focus is observed under it. If this is cut open, a serous bloody fluid flows out; it is evident that the deep-seated tissues are already affected. Hence, dystrophy begins from the underlying parts and only gradually reaches the surface, forming there a non-healing ulcer.

Subsequently it was discovered that infection of the injured nerve is not the sole, or even the chief, factor in the development of symmetrical affections. Instead of mucilaginous purulent secretion, we took bile which was injected into the centripetal end of the severed sciatic nerve. Extraction of the cerebro-spinal fluid was carried out as in the experiments of the first series. The operation was performed under sterile conditions and the wound healed *per primam*. The results here were not different. Others of my collaborators used as irritants various chemical substances (mustard gas, croton oil, acids, alkalis, formalin, phenol, etc.) and fresh emulsions of normal organs, and they observed the same consequences (Pigalev and Kuznetsova, Suslov, Galkin [1]). Consequently, the phenomena described are not connected with myelitis of infectional origin, which, as is known, can sometimes be produced in animals by introducing an agent of infection within the nerve trunk. However, something similar must have taken place here also, for *symmetrical affections of the extremities in dogs can develop only as the result of a symmetrical affection of the nervous system.*

Study of the movement of various substances along the nerve trunk provides a number of facts which suggest the possibility of the direct action of the substance taken on the cells of the central nervous system. But this action alone can hardly explain everything. Also, it is impossible to study this action separately from other factors, because the axis cylinders, *i.e.*, parts of the same central elements, are subjected to irritation from the very moment of penetration of the irritating agent into the nerve; consequently, the irritation begins before the irritant penetrates into the nerve cells. Moreover, in a number of cases the effect of the action of the irritating agent was manifested by destruction of the tissues at a very late stage: in some cases, sym-

[1] I. A. Pigalev and Z. G. Kuznetsova. *Arkh. Biol. Nauk*, Vol. 30, No. 1, 1930; *Zeitschr. f. d. ges. exp. Med.*, Vol. 67, Nos. 1, 2, 1929; G. V. Suslov, *Arkh. Biol. Nauk*, Vol. 32, No. 2, 1932; *Zeitschr. f. d. ges. exp. Med.*, Vol. 83, Nos. 3, 4, 1932.

metrical affections of the soft tissues and bones in the healthy foot of the dog were noted on the fourteenth day from the beginning of the experiment, in other cases only after 2-3 months. After this period, there is not a trace left in the organism of the irritating agent itself, the more so as this agent is applied only once.

In studying the consequences of freezing the cerebral cortex in dogs, we already encountered a similar phenomenon. If the irritation proceeding from the injured portion reached a particular strength, *we were not able to arrest it, even by removing the irritating agent.* In some cases this process takes place rapidly, in others more slowly, but it proceeds approximately on the same lines as those described by us in the case of the affection of the supra-renal glands in diphtheria intoxication, where the corresponding changes developed *when not a single molecule of toxin could enter into direct contact with them.*

Another of my collaborators, P. N. Ulyanov, also made it the aim of his investigations to obtain symmetrical affections on irritation of one side only. But, as the place of application of the irritating agent, he used not the nerve trunk, but the muscles, *i.e.,* the finer nerve branches and nerve endings. Consequently, the conditions here were fairly close to those of our experiments with tetanus toxin.

Dogs were used for the experiment. A 2-5 per cent solution of potassium iodide was applied as the irritating agent.

At the beginning of his work, P. N. Ulyanov compared the rapidity of formation of epidermal rashes and ulcerations obtained by using various forms of iodine intoxication of animals—intravenous, subcutaneous and intra-muscular. It was found that symptoms of iodism, in the form of papulæ, blisters, erosions and genuine ulcers, appeared even more quickly after intra-muscular than after intravenous injections.

Further, they were not merely the result of general poisoning. This was made clear by experiments in which the potassium iodide solution was introduced by the intra-muscular route and, moreover, on one side of the animal's body. In these cases the skin affections were also unsymmetrical. They both appeared earlier and were more intensely expressed on the side of the injection. If the potassium iodide solution was introduced into the muscles of one of the hind extremities, then rash, baldness and eczema developed, first on the same extremity, then in symmetrical places on the opposite leg, and only later on the skin of other parts of the body. Hence, we are confronted here also with a process beginning segmentarily.

In weighing up the results obtained, one must not omit to mention their correspondence with those observed in experiments with tetanus toxin under analogous experimental conditions. The effect is here also expressed primarily on the side of the irritation, the beginning of the generalisation of the process, also, is segmentary tetanus and, finally, tetanus takes hold of the whole muscular system in approximately the same sequence as in the dissemination of the skin affection. If we start out only from the data of the genesis of these processes, then it seems that *there is actually no unbridgeable gulf between certain forms of rash on the skin and tetanus.*

Another form of symmetrical dystrophy resulting from unilateral irritation was obtained by my collaborator Dr. P. V. Manenkov.[1] Fragments of copper wire were introduced into the anterior chamber of one eye of a dog. As a result, an inflammatory process developed in the cornea and iris—sometimes even panophthalmitis.

Beginning with the first day, extraction of the cerebro-spinal fluid was carried out and this was repeated after each 2-3 days. In some cases, disease of the other eye appeared after 5-15 days. The first symptom of this was photophobia, followed by pericorneal hyperæmia, increasing from day to day; this is soon followed by a weak, or sometimes stronger, restricted or diffuse opacity of the cornea. On one occasion we observed that the blood vessels of the borders of the cornea began to grow into it in a thick layer. The other pathological changes included foci of obscuration in the *corpus vitreum* of the "sympathetic" eye. The sterility of these foci was proved bacteriologically at the time of dissection.

It is possible to demonstrate the symmetry of nervous changes on unilateral chemical (infectional) trauma of the nerve trunk, not only in the case of trophic ulcers, but also in the case of other processes. I shall permit myself to cite some examples of this kind from our work. An investigation of the question of nerve regeneration is included here. I entrusted this work to my collaborator A. S. Vishnevsky.[2] The histological part of the investigation was carried out in the laboratory of B. S. Doinikov.

The process of nerve regeneration is made up of two parts: the growth and union of a syncytium of protoplasmic connecting strands and the outgrowth of axis cylinders from the centripetal end of the severed nerve (Cruikschank, Waller, Perroncito, Ramon-Kakhal, Bielschowsky, Heidenhain, Ranson, Krasin, Doinikov).

In studying the circumstances which facilitate or, on the contrary, hinder the normal course of this process, individual investigators have taken account of a number of conditions, such as the size of the defect, the position and de-

[1] P. V. Manenkov. *Arkh. Biol. Nauk*, Vol. 29, No. 1, 1929; *Zeitschr. f. d. ges. exp. Med.*, Vol. 63, Nos. 5, 6, 1928.
[2] A. S. Vishnevsky. *Zeitschr. f. d. ges. exp. Med.*, Vol. 76, Nos. 1, 2, 1931.

gree of separation of the pieces, infection, scars, foreign bodies, etc. The conditions enumerated are all local, and mostly even external. The possibility that the nerve regeneration may be influenced by processes taking place in the complex organism has not attracted the attention it deserves. The question of the role of the nervous system itself in this action has also been left unexamined.

Our investigation consisted of three series of experiments. They were alike in plan, except for the time at which the material was taken for histological treatment. In each experiment, two animals were included—an experimental and a control animal. The operation of exposing and severing the right and left sciatic nerves in the region of the hip joint was carried out under narcosis on both of them simultaneously. In the experimental animal, the left sciatic nerve was immediately sewn up, but into the central end of the right nerve there was introduced some chemical or biological irritant (croton oil, virulent microbes, etc.). The sewing up of the left sciatic nerve was also carried out in the control animal, but no foreign substance was introduced into the central end of the right nerve. At the end of the operation, the cerebro-spinal fluid was extracted from both animals. The extraction of fluid was repeated once or twice more during the next few days. After a certain time, the animals were killed and the portion of the sciatic nerve in the immediate vicinity of the suture was subjected to histological examination. In the first series of experiments, the material was taken for treatment 2-3 days after the operation, in the second series, after 7-8 days, and in the third series, after 6-7 weeks.

The following are the results in the form as recorded by A. S. Vishnevsky.

FIRST SERIES (2-3 DAYS)

In the group of *experimental* animals, *there was no sign of regeneration in the nerve.* The only result is a separation of the fibrils ("effilochements de Cajal") and a few isolated growth bulbs. At the same time, preparations taken from the *control* group show at the place of suture *a clear picture of the inception of a regenerative process.* A very large number of young axons are visible, terminating in growth bulbs, and also the first stages of formation of Perroncito spirals.

SECOND SERIES (7-8 DAYS)

Experimental group. In the region of the nerve suture, one notices the presence of fine axis cylinder fibres, in places woven together in the form of a "felt" (irregular growth following the type of formation of neuromata). The growth bulbs are small and few in number. *Only in some places do the individual fibres cross the line of suture.* In the vast majority of cases, the fibres end centrally, at a considerable distance from the boundary of the scar.

Control group. Very *vigorous regeneration* in the region of the nerve suture. The axis cylinders lie close to one another. Throughout the whole extent they grow out in straight lines. The majority of the axis cylinders already pass beyond the line of suture.

A certain number of axis cylinders are to be noticed growing in the central direction and also furnished with growth bulbs.

THIRD SERIES (6-7 WEEKS)

Experimental group. Along the whole line of suture in the midst of the scar tissue, the fibres cross one another in disorder, forming a "felt." The axis cylinders are thin, with rare and small growth bulbs. *Only isolated fibres pass across the line of suture.* (See Plate 7.)

Control group. The place of the former suture is occupied by a completely restored nerve. There are no longer any elements of regeneration. The young fibres run in rows within the newly formed perineural sheaths. Regeneration of the nerve in the immediate neighbourhood of the peripheral end is complete. (See Plate 8.)

All this was obtained in the normal course of development, amid healthy tissues and under absolutely the same local conditions for both groups of animals. In spite of the fact that the irritating agent was applied in the experimental group to a topographically remote portion, and even on the opposite side of the body, it had the result of almost completely arresting the regeneration of the nerve. The process took a course as if an insurmountable barrier had been artificially created at the place of suture.

In subsequent experiments, it was found that the extraction of the cerebro-spinal fluid, although it plays a part in this process, is not indispensable. Chemical trauma of the nerve trunk gives by itself approximately the same results.

These data establish that remote influences have an effect upon the course of local processes and permit us to estimate in a new way the significance of factors whose action has always been accounted local. In the first place, one must refer here to infection. We have seen that the presence of infection on the opposite side of the body exercises the same influence on the process of regeneration as if the place of the nerve suture itself had been infected. It follows inevitably from this that where suppuration occurs in the region of the operation itself, the process is not limited to the immediate destruction of surrounding tissues. *The disease involves not only the nearest portions of the axis cylinders, but also the corresponding nerve elements as a whole, temporarily or permanently depriving them of the capacity for regeneration.*

The following example, belonging to the same order of phenomena, is concerned with vascular innervation. I shall demonstrate it in two forms. The first is in regard to observations of the so-called Löwen reflex. This name is used in physiology to denote the widening of the blood-vessels of an organ, resulting from stimulation of the central end of a severed receptor nerve, as long as the vaso-motor fibres have been preserved in the other nerves (Löwen, Bradford, Bayliss).

The experiments were carried out in my laboratory by P. S. Kupalov and F. D. Vassilenko.[1] For the experiment they took dogs in which 2 per cent solution of potassium iodide (3.0-5.0 c.c. per kg. weight of the animal) had been introduced 10-15 days beforehand into the muscles of one of the hind extremities. As was pointed out just above, this method was also employed by Ulyanov in studying the process of formation of symmetrical skin diseases.

The conditions of the experiment were as follows. The dog was put under curare and subjected to tracheotomy. Artificial respiration was used, and hot

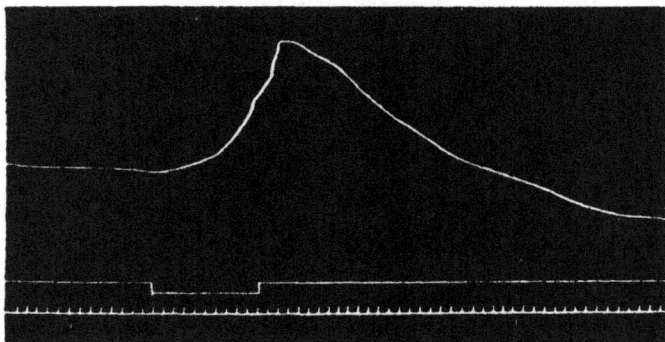

Fig. 10. Löwen Reflex of the Hind Extremity of a Healthy Dog on Irritation of the Centripetal End of *N. Peroneus*. Separation of the Coils, 110 mm.

water bottles applied for warming. In order to exclude the influence of adrenalin, the suprarenals on both sides were removed. After exposure and section of the *n. saphenus* or *n. peroneus*, plethysmographs connected with Marey capsules were attached to the hind extremities.

In all, six dogs were taken for the experiment. In not a single case was the Löwen reflex obtained, whether of the extremity into which the potassium iodide solution had been introduced some days beforehand or of the opposite "healthy" foot. An equal number of normal animals, used as controls, under the same experimental conditions exhibited the Löwen reflex in a normal form, as can be seen from the curves reproduced here. (Figs. 10, 11.)

A second form of experiment, also testifying to the symmetry of vascular changes after nerve trauma on one side, was performed by my collaborator E. P. Zakaraya.[2]

[1] F. D. Vassilenko. *Zeitschr. f. d. ges. exp. Med.*, Vol. 74, No. 5-6, 1930.
[2] E. P. Zakaraya. *Arkh. Biol. Nauk*, Vol. 31, No. 2-3, 1931; *Zeitschr. f. d. ges. exp. Med.*, Vol. 80, Nos. 5, 6, 1932.

The animals used were rabbits. As in a number of other cases, the experiment began with section of one of the sciatic nerves and poisoning of its centripetal end by croton oil.[1] Following this, 20-30 c.c. of a 1 per cent solution of trypan blue were injected into the auricular vein of the animal. Sometimes only one injection was used, sometimes it was repeated on the following day.

Trypan blue is a colloid dye and is not able to penetrate through the "barrier" into the region of the central nervous system. It was of interest to discover whether the properties of the "barrier" were altered in this case, and if so, in precisely what form, *i.e.*, whether along the whole extent of the spinal cord and cerebrum, or only in the region of the corresponding nerve segments.

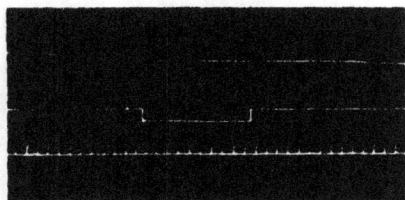

Fig. 11. Absence of Löwen Reflex of the Left Hind Extremity on Irritation of the Centripetal End of *N. Peroneus.* (Two weeks before the experiment, a 2 per cent solution of potassium iodide was injected intra-muscularly in the right hind extremity of the dog.)

The experiment confirmed the latter. It was found that under these conditions trypan blue actually penetrates into the medullary region, dyeing the arachnoid and pia membranes a blue colour, as well as several segments of the medullary substance itself, close to the injured nerve. When the sciatic nerve was taken for the experiment, the greatest quantity of trypan blue penetrated into the caudal region of the spinal cord. From here the intensity of the colouring diminished in the direction of the cerebrum and by the middle of the thoracic portion the spinal cord was unstained.

In other cases the nerves of the brachial plexus were subjected to mechanical and chemical trauma; here the cervical portion of the spinal cord was coloured and also the basal and posterior regions of the cerebrum. The thoracic and lumbar parts of the spinal cord did not contain any colour. It

---

[1] It should be mentioned that rabbits prove to be much more resistant to croton oil than dogs. The latter are very sensitive to the introduction of this substance into the nerve and are easily killed by a dose of 0.2-0.3 c.c., especially if the preparation is fresh. Hence, in experiments on dogs it is better to dispense with injection and confine onself to pricking the centripetal end of the nerve with a needle moistened with the oil.

should be added that the distribution of trypan blue was uniform over the right and left halves of the spinal cord, *i.e.*, the process here also was symmetrical. (See Plate 9.)

Our observations on the development of segmentary nervous affections were not limited to the data described above. But the other facts concerned with this matter served at the same time to elucidate new details in the process under consideration; hence, these supplementary data will be given in the course of the further exposition.

Thus, the first thing that demands special emphasis is the *question of the irritating agent and of irritation in the genesis of segmentary pathological reactions.* It will be necessary to return to this subject more than once, but the material just analysed raises the question in a sufficiently marked form. Chemical or infectional trauma of various nerve structures at the periphery can easily become the starting point of this complex process. *Its development proceeds along two lines.* The sum total is made up of the immediate injury to the nerve elements by the substance itself and of an unusual form of nerve irritation. The latter may not only distort the functioning of the nerve cell, but even destroy it.

In our experiments, under exactly regulated and equalised conditions, the effect was not always equal in degree. The external symptoms of disease *differed from one another, sometimes very sharply, as regards time of appearance and degree of expression, as well as subsequent history.* Between the moment of application of the agent and the changes objectively revealed, *there always elapsed a certain period* of several hours, days or even weeks. During this period, the animal was not different externally from a healthy one. Within its nervous system, however, a hidden process was developing, as is evident from the results of all the experiments. We may supplement these results by one of the observations of my collaborators N. A. Astapov and I. P. Bobkov.[1]

While studying the mechanism of the action of mustard gas and lewisite in circumstances of direct irritation of a nerve trunk, they made the following experiments, among others. The place where the sciatic nerve passes out of the pelvis was exposed by a cut in the gluteal region of a rabbit. The cut was always made at the upper edge of the *m. gluteus*, and the latter was pulled downwards medially by means of a hook. This was done in order to keep the place of operation as far as possible from the region of the perineum and scrotum. Exactly where the sciatic nerve passes out, the *n. pudendus* branches off from it and passes through the *foramen ischiadicum minus* into the *cavum ischiorectale*, running further to the perineum and sexual organs. A platinum

[1] N. A. Astapov and I. P. Bobkov. *Med. Sanit. Vopr. Protivokhim. Zashchit.* [*Medical and Hygienic Questions of Anti-Chemical Defence*], Symposium, No. 1, 1932.

loop with a 2 per cent solution of mustard gas or lewisite in acetone was applied to the fine trunk of the *n. pudendus*. The solution vaporised almost immediately and the wound was tightly sewn up.

It is important to mention that no signs of inflammatory reaction are usually observed at the place of application of these substances in the above-mentioned concentrations, whether immediately afterwards or at a later period. The operation wound always healed *per primam*.

During the following 2-3 days, the rabbit remains healthy. Then a small bluish spot appears on the skin of the corresponding scrotum, at its distal end. The surrounding tissues become swollen. The spot gradually increases in size and the process terminates in dry mortification of the skin of the corresponding scrotum over a greater or lesser extent. At the same time the size of the testicle increases. The testicle and scrotum on the opposite side remain normal. After a few days, the above-described phenomena begin to disappear. *Then swelling of the scrotum on the opposite, "healthy," side makes its appearance.* Here the process does not usually go so far as mortification, and the testicle on this side is affected even later, when the process has already come to an end on the side that had been subjected to irritation.

These experiments vividly demonstrate the development of the process by stages. At the beginning, we have the general latent period, during which the process taking place within the nerve network remains invisible. After the local symptoms have begun, *this latent process continues and periodically sends out proofs of its development to the periphery. Thus, a sequence of latent periods for each stage of the process arises.*

Already at this point, I should like to raise the question: What is the precise difference between the above-described period and the incubation which *is considered a characteristic sign of infectional processes and is regarded by many as the initial stage of "struggle" between micro-organisms and the macro-organism?*

The facts adduced in this chapter demonstrate that certain forms of irritation of peripheral nerve apparatuses can easily be the occasion for the development of a segmentary affection of the nervous system. If the nerve elements have suffered and not recovered, if they have preserved traces of the pathological process formerly taking place here, then measures directed towards removing pathological changes in the tissues at the periphery will not save the situation. If the nerve elements that have suffered are drawn, directly or indirectly, into the orbit of some other nervous process, this inevitably adds something to the pathological irritation already existing.

This makes it comprehensible why relapses are observed in the majority of trophic ulcers when treated in the human clinic by operation of the nerve paths. The statistics with which I am acquainted (Mathey-Cornat, Durente, Shamov, A. S. Vishnevsky, Stradyn, Levenson, etc.) are uniformly discouraging in regard to surgical interference with either the sympathetic or central nerve paths.

The real illness is not the ulcer at the periphery. By severing the paths of the pathological reflex, we do not treat the basic injury, but, like the ostrich, we bury our heads in the sand, *we make the process invisible for us.* While temporarily destroying one of the links, we not only leave the cause of the phenomenon intact, but even strengthen it, since the act of operational interference is itself an additional nerve trauma. And we know that on relapse the process is frequently renewed on a much larger scale. The work of A. S. Vishnevsky, devoted to the treatment of spontaneous gangrene by neurotomy of the spinal nerves, brings forward convincing data testifying to the fact that the useful effect of operations is the more clear and lasting, the less the extent of surgical interference. Repeated neurotomy resulted as a rule in marked aggravation both of the gangrenous symptoms and of the general state of the patient.

CHAPTER XV

THE EXTENSION OF THE DYSTROPHIC PROCESS BEYOND THE LIMITS OF THE SEGMENT

T HIS chapter contains materials obtained by approximately the same experimental methods as those described in the preceding chapter.

We saw that nerve trauma usually leads to unilateral or symmetrical dystrophy and that the difference depends chiefly *on the magnitude of the irritation.* There is reason to think that the same cause can also govern the development of the process outside the limits of the segment primarily affected.

For further analysis of the subject, we pursued our work in various directions. It included also a study of the morphological consequences of nerve trauma. It is not possible to expect very much from this method. Morphological changes in nerve cells are delayed in comparison with functional changes. Structural derangement, when it has become accessible to immediate observation, is usually evidence of a process that has already gone a long way. The attractiveness of this method lies in the fact that it gives a very distinct idea of the changes in the vital properties of the cells. It also permits us to follow, to a certain extent, the sequence in the development of the process.

This work is still far from having reached a conclusion; consequently I shall only describe here materials from some of the researches of my collaborators, where the experiments partly ended in a histological analysis. The latter was conducted under the general guidance of B. S. Doinikov.

Included here are the researches of B. S. Doinikov, E. P. Zakaraya, G. V. Suslov, Y. M. Zhabotinsky, and partly those of I. A. Pigalev, A. S. Vishnevsky, S. I. Lebedinsky, E. A. Uspensky and O. P. Vishnevsky.

The object of the work was histological analysis of various parts of the nervous system at various periods after the application of chemical or infectional nerve trauma at the periphery. A large number of animals were used for the experiments—dogs, cats, rabbits and rats.

In the majority of cases the irritating agent was introduced into a nerve and the operation wound was sewn up. In some cases, the same substances were applied to the skin or injected into the tissues. The animals withstood these operations fairly well in general, although local dystrophic processes developed in them. A certain number of the animals, however, died even within a short period, exhibiting symptoms of general dystrophy. Others lived for a comparatively long time, at any rate the time was sufficient both for observations and for performing new experiments. After, the requisite period, we killed the animals, and the material underwent histological treatment (Nissl, Marchi, Cajal's silver impregnation according to de Castro, Favorsky, etc.).

Study of the objects concerned showed that morphological changes develop in the central nervous system not only after introduction of an irritant directly into the nerve, but also *after its application to the skin or after injections into the tissues.* In all these cases, the changes were *qualitatively alike,* differing only in degree.

It is interesting to note that, on chemical trauma of the nerve trunk, the extent of morphological changes within the central nervous system *did not always correspond to the concentration of the agent used.* Tests were made with varying strengths of solutions of formalin, mustard gas, acids, etc. On analysis of the state of the nerve regions remote from the point of primary irritation, the general impression was obtained that *weak concentrations of one and the same substance produce in those regions the most marked morphological changes.* This once more confirms that in the process under consideration the effect is due not so much to the immediate action of the irritating agent transferred from the place of injection to the proximal nerve regions, as to the state and degree of the irritation itself. The latter presumes the presence of an energetically reacting substratum. With high concentrations of the substance, local destruction of the tissues can be very large; but the irritation of the nerve, arising in the injured region where the tissues are destroyed, may be insignificant.

It was discovered, further, that the injection of the irritating agent into the nerve without severing the latter *produces much smaller consequences* than injection into the centripetal end of the severed nerve, even if the quantity of substance taken was smaller in the second case.

Finally, it was found that there is *no special difference between the chemical and infectional form of nerve irritation* in the general picture of the changes produced.

The nerve trunk. Within the injured nerve trunk, the process is expressed in necrosis, distributed unequally among separate nerve bundles. On injecting a weak solution of formalin (1.5 per cent), part of Schwann's cells and also of the vascular and endoneural elements are preserved. The most marked reactive changes are encountered in the epineuria and perineuria (infiltrations, productive reaction, thickening of the perineurium). Leucocyte infiltration takes place during the first days in the region of the demarcated zone. In the part of the nerve distal from the place of injection there are various degrees of Wallerian degeneration, while in the proximal part there develops an increasing neuritis of various intensities.

The nearer to the medulla the portion of the nerve undergoing trauma, the higher does the neuritis extend, reaching the inter-vertebral ganglia and even the nerve roots. The inflammatory reaction diminishes in proportion to the distance from the place of infection. The same holds good of the degenerative changes of the nerve fibres. Only in a minority of cases does the marked picture of inflammation and degeneration extend for more than 2-3 cm. Above this, one finds endo-arteritis of the nerve vessels, small infiltrations and slight degenerative changes of the parenchyma (with a large number of Elzholz bodies in the nerve fibres).

The inter-vertebral ganglia. In the ganglia corresponding to the injured nerve, there are both inflammatory and parenchymatous changes. The inflammatory reaction makes its appearance after 5-10 days and is localised at the proximal or distal pole of the ganglion (Plate 10.), more rarely in its stroma as well. (Plate 11.) It consists of *a strip of infiltrate, which, as it were, partitions the nerve transversely and enters* the region of the nerve roots. (Plate 12.)

This reaction is interesting also because its development is not confined to the ganglia of the segment affected. It is true at the beginning (5-6 days) it is visible only here; subsequently, however, analogous changes make their appearance *in the ganglia and roots of the opposite, "healthy," side,* and after that in other ganglia as well, sometimes even in all ganglia of the right and left sides of the spinal cord.

The changes in the nerve cells of the inter-vertebral ganglia are exhibited in several different forms:

1. The most frequent form is accumulation of chromatophilous substance in the neighbourhood of the nucleus and scarcity of it at the periphery of the cell. (Plates 11 and 13.)

2. "Primary irritation" of the cell—central chromatolysis with lateral disposition of the nucleus.

3. Diffuse or restricted chromatolysis without marked alteration of the nucleus.

4. "Severe affection" of the nerve cell—hyper-chromatosis of the nucleus and disintegration of the cell body.

It never happens that all the cells of the ganglion are affected in the process; *only a certain proportion of them suffer.*

The spinal cord. In all cases, changes in the spinal cord are more clearly pronounced in the region of the segments corresponding to the place of primary irritation, and also in the neighbouring segments. The intensity of the changes differs in different cases; both inflamatory reactions and proliferation of the glia occur. (Plates 14, 15.) In addition, there are always changes in the parenchyma as well. The latter are usually reversible and not pronounced.

The proliferation of the glia takes place in the border glia cells, especially close to the point of entry of the roots; there is a diffuse growth of the glia into the white and grey matter and around the blood vessels. The glia proliferates also around the nerve cells, both those that have been altered and those that are not visibly affected. (Plate 16.) It is possible to observe here the development of complete and incomplete fringes of glia round the nerve cells or their separate offshoots, the formation of rosettes of glia, *i.e.*, accumulations of glia at the place of the dead nerve cells, and more rarely—phenomena of neuronophagy. During the first 5-8 days, all these forms of reaction are expressed more sharply on the side of the trauma, afterwards they sometimes become symmetrical and even extend beyond the limits of the segment, gradually diminishing in intensity.

The inflammatory reaction is exhibited in the form of swelling and marked colouring of the inside of the vessels, infiltration around them and also at the point of entry of the nerve roots, and infiltration into the pia mater and its recesses, into the white matter, and into the grey matter close to the central canal. It is important to note that precisely in those cases where inflammatory symptoms are especially strongly pronounced at the level of the primarily affected segments, foci of inflammation are almost always scattered also along the cephalic and caudal sections of the spinal cord and cerebrum. These are usually localised round the vessels and at various points of the medullary membranes (*encephalo-myelitis disseminata*).

This is an important fact. A number of communications have recently appeared in Western and American literature indicating the fairly frequent occurrence in rabbits of phenomena of encephalo-myelitis, developing spontaneously and showing no evidence of its presence during life (Bull, Lewy and Tiefenbach, Oliver, McCartney, Balo and Gal, Seifried, Ostertag).

While fully confirming these data, we, nevertheless, cannot regard the encephalo-myelitis in our animals as spontaneous, since its direct connection with the primary nerve trauma was clearly marked. Moreover, we conducted our experiments not only with rabbits, but also with other animals, including dogs. Especially in the last-named, along with gradual development of general dystrophy on the basis of the nerve trauma, morphological degenerative phenomena are always found.

Parenchymatous changes of the spinal cord and cerebrum are exhibited in the form of various types of degeneration of the nerve cells. Most frequently these are reversible changes: diffuse chromatolysis, sometimes with slight hyper-chromatosis of the nucleus, spotted chromatolysis, accumulation of chromatophilous substance in a layer around the nucleus and its scarcity in the peripheral layers. (Plate 16.) "Primary irritation" of the cell rarely occurs, and then only in motor cells of the anterior horns. "Severe affection" of the cell is still more rare. (Plate 17.)

It always happens that only some of the cells are altered. Great interest attaches to preparations where, of two nerve cells lying side by side, *one has suffered so strongly that it must be considered dead, while the other has an absolutely normal appearance.* Such cases are not rare. They demonstrate once again that we are confronted by a complex process which cannot be viewed merely as the result of the immediate influence of the foreign agent on each element in particular. In that case it would be absolutely inexplicable why one cell was killed while a neighbouring cell, situated only a few microns away, did not even suffer. The destruction of the cell becomes comprehensible *provided that it is recognised that its cause is the distortion of the relations between this cell and other nerve elements that have changed their function under the influence of irritation.*

It is characteristic that the reaction of the glia is frequently absent around heavily altered nerve cells and occurs around nearby cells that are normal or have been only slightly altered.

The extent of alteration of the nerve cells is usually greater on the side of application of the irritating agent. In severe cases, this difference disappears. Like the symptoms of inflammation, the parenchymatous changes of the nerve cells are strongly marked in the segments which have primarily suffered, but are also met with far outside the limits of these segments.

It was found that the *morphological and physiological changes develop in equal degree*: the greater the dystrophic processes in the tissues at the periphery, the wider is the region they embrace and the more severe and widespread are the changes within the nervous system.

The role of the *locus of primary irritation* is of interest in this respect.

My collaborator G. V. Suslov began his researches with chemical trauma of the sciatic nerve. Morphological changes within the central nervous system, both in the region of the corresponding segment and outside its limits, were here almost always very marked; so also were the symptoms of symmetrical dystrophy in the tissues of the hind extremities (loss of hair, ulcers, falling off of the claws). Y M. Zhabotinsky began part of his experiments by producing chemical trauma of one or several nerves of the fore extremities. The morphological consequences within the nervous system were in general the same as in Suslov's experiments, but their extent proved to be considerably less. Symmetrical changes in the spinal cord itself and in its inter-vertebral ganglia were sometimes absent or only weakly expressed. At the same time also, it was not possible to note dystrophic symptoms in the tissues of the fore extremities. This, however, did not prevent the subsequent development of general dystrophy which thus set in without a preceding stage of segmentary changes.

There is yet another curious observation to be found in the investigations of Doinikov and Zhabotinsky. When, after chemical trauma of a fore extremity, morphological changes were strongly pronounced in the region of the cervical segments, equally marked changes appeared also in the lumbar section of the spinal cord. *The thoracic segments, however, remained almost unaffected by the process.* Consequently, the process can spread unequally, *leaving untouched extensive nerve tracts.* It is clear that if the whole thing amounted to a mere spreading of the irritating agent itself along the nervous system, nothing of this sort could happen.

However, it does not follow from this that we deny altogether the possibility of direct action of an irritating agent introduced into the nerve trunk on the elements of the central nervous system. We recognise the active role of this mechanism in giving rise to the phenomena under consideration, and we find continual confirmation of it in our researches, particularly in our morphological data. It is sufficient here to refer only to two facts. Both of them were obtained in the experiments of my collaborators Zakaraya and Suslov.

While investigating the consequences of intravenous injection of trypan blue in chemical trauma of the spinal nerve, Zakaraya [1] found that the intensity of coloration of the outer layers of the dura mater was much greater in the experimental group of animals than in the control group. In spite of the fact that only one of the sciatic nerves was subjected to trauma, the intensity of absorption of the dye by the mesothelial elements of the dura mater was sharply intensified *throughout the extent of the spinal cord and even of the cerebrum.* Consequently, the irritation of a spinal nerve by the foreign agent produced an intensification of the absorption of dye over the whole extent of the outermost of the medullary membranes. After this the other foreign agent was held back in the region of this barrier with much greater energy than normally.

The second fact was as follows. It has already been pointed out that one of the reactions to chemical or infectional nerve trauma is infiltration of the inter-vertebral ganglia. The reaction develops, not only in the ganglia corresponding to the injured nerve, but also in the neighbouring ganglia, and even in the symmetrical ganglia of the opposite side. Sometimes the reaction can be observed on both sides *throughout the extent of the spinal cord.* With removal from the place of actual irritation, this reaction only becomes less marked.

---

[1] E. P. Zakaraya. *Arkh. Biol. Nauk*, Vol. 31, No. 2-3, 1931; *Zeitschr. f. d. ges. exp. Med.*, Vol. 80, Nos. 5, 6, 1932.

This led us to the supposition that there must exist a special, hitherto un-known, mechanism of general significance for the central nervous system. A chemical "blow" to one nerve causes the whole system, as it were, "to put itself on guard" and *to develop a number of barriers on paths along which the harm itself has not yet travelled.* This fact alone is evidence that the path through the nerve trunk towards the centre is the path of actual danger.

To prove that we have here actually a specific form of "defensive" reaction, it was necessary to test the question experimentally. The most suit-able process for this purpose is rabies.

The appropriate experiments were carried out by my collaborator G. V. Suslov.[1] The method used was as follows. For each experiment, two dogs were selected. One of them was given a single injection of a small quantity of 5 per cent aqueous solution of formalin into the left sciatic nerve, after which the wound was sewn up. The other dog received no formalin and the animal remained as a control. After 10-16 days both dogs were inoculated with rabies (5 per cent emulsion of *virus fixe*) in the sciatic nerve, but not in the left nerve, where formalin had been previously injected in the experi-mental animal, but into the right (healthy) nerve. After inoculation, the nerve was severed through the middle of the place of injection, and this was followed by a single extraction of cerebro-spinal fluid.

As pointed out above, this method of infection greatly increases the per-centage of dogs developing rabies, as compared with inoculation into the nerve without severing it.

In all, eleven experiments were made on twenty-two dogs. The results were as follows:

Control group. Of eleven control animals, only one did not develop rabies. The initial symptoms of disease in the control animals appeared in two of them on the fourth day, in one on the fifth day, in two on the sixth day, in four on the seventh day, and in one on the tenth day after infection.

Experimental group. Of eleven experimental dogs, six did not develop rabies. The initial symptoms of disease in the five dogs that died appeared in one on the fourteenth day after the infection, in one on the twelfth day, in one on the tenth day, in one on the eighth day, and in one on the fifth day.

It is evident from a comparison of these figures that in the experimental group the *number of dogs that caught the disease and died was considerably less, while the incubation period was perceptibly longer than in the group of control dogs.*

In other experiments, formalin was injected, not into the sciatic nerves of the dogs, but intra-cutaneously or subcutaneously into one or both extremities.

[1] G. V. Suslov. *Arkh. Biol. Nauk*, Vol. 32, No. 2, 1932; *Zeitschr. f. d. ges. exp. Med.*, Vol. 83, Nos. 3, 4, 1932.

We used 2 and 3 per cent solutions of formalin, 2-4 drops of which were injected at various places. Each animal received approximately 4.0-5.0 c.c. of the formalin solution. The consequence of intra-cutaneous injections was a restricted dry mortification of the skin in the form of maculæ. Subcutaneous injections left no traces. After 9-14 days, these dogs, together with an equal number of controls, were inoculated with emulsion of *virus fixe* through one of the sciatic nerves. The conditions of inoculation corresponded exactly to those described above.

In all, fourteen animals were taken for the experiment.

Of seven controls, six dogs developed the disease and died. One remained alive, and this dog could not be considered as fully conforming to the conditions prescribed for the control since it had been used previously in an experiment with injection of another irritating substance into the muscle. In three cases, the incubation period was six days, in one it was seven, in one eight, and in one ten days.

Of the seven experimental animals, three developed the disease and died. Four dogs did not become ill. The incubation period in this group was on the average longer than in the control group, *viz.*, thirteen, eleven and eight days. The disease proceeded more feebly in the experimental dogs and was somewhat protracted.

We also carried out analogous experiments on rabbits. At first they gave no result. Rabbits withstand badly an injury to the sciatic nerves on both sides; besides paralysis of the extremities, the act of defecation and urination is disorganised and many animals die. Then we tried inoculating the experimental and control groups through the sciatic nerve without severing it, but this proved unfavourable. It must be noted that on inoculation with *virus fixe* (Leningrad stock) through the sciatic nerve without previously sectioning it, only dogs give a small percentage of cases of illness, while rabbits easily develop the disease, although not all of them do so. Under these conditions, it is *very difficult to obtain comparable results*. We were constrained to pass to a form of experiment in which both the injection of formalin and the subsequent inoculation of the animals was carried out on one side, but in different nerves, *e.g.*, in the sciatic and femoral nerves (*n.n. ischiadicus et cruralis*). A preliminary test showed that, on injecting formalin into the sciatic nerve of the rabbit, excitability and conductivity along the *n. cruralis* is retained. In addition it was found that on inoculating normal rabbits through the *n. cruralis* and sectioning the latter, about 90 per cent of the animals become ill, in spite of the fact that this nerve is comparatively very thin. In this way, the possibility of comparison was assured.

We took eight rabbits and introduced a small quantity of 5 per cent formalin solution into the left sciatic nerve. After ten days, the rabbits were inoculated in the left *n. cruralis*, followed by section of the latter. Eight control rabbits were inoculated along with the experimental group by the same method.

Of the eight control rabbits, seven became ill and died. Of the equal number of experimental animals, two became ill and six remained healthy.

The data brought forward here show that the reaction which we have observed can be regarded to a certain extent as a "defensive" one. At the same time confirmation was once more obtained of the view that in regard to infection of the nerve system through the nerve trunk, *the action of the irritating agent itself undoubtedly plays a role.*

We possess a number of other facts relating to the same subject, but treating it from a somewhat different aspect. These observations were begun by experiments of my collaborator E. P. Zakaraya.[1] In part, the data obtained by him have already been used above.

The animals experimented on were rabbits. The object of the work was *to study the changes in the nervous system outside the limits of the immediate nerve trauma and during the period immediately following the trauma.* The method consisted in sectioning one of the big spinal nerves, poisoning the centripetal end with croton oil, and subsequent intravenous injection of a 1 per cent solution of trypan blue. The difference in the degree of coloration of the separate parts served as an indicator of the changes that had begun and gave a certain representation of the development of the process itself. The control animals were normal rabbits in which corresponding quantities of trypan blue solution were introduced into the blood at the same time as in the others. After a definite interval (2-3 days), both animals were killed with chloroform. If the experimental rabbit died earlier, the control animal was killed at the same time.

Dissection provided a number of facts for judging the course of the process under investigation, *both in the central nervous system and in the sympathetic chain.*

When croton oil was injected into the nerve on the left side, the *gang. intervertebralia* of the lumbar region were intensely coloured, but considerably more so on the left side than on the right. The dye in the same ganglia of the cervical and thoracic tracts was comparatively weak, but on the left side (*i.e.,* the side of the operation) it was also somewhat more pronounced.

The ganglia of the sympathetic chain exhibited approximately the same changes. The left lumbar ganglia (L_4, L_5, L_6, L_7), corresponding to the

[1] E. P. Zakaraya. *Arkh. Biol. Nauk*, Vol. 31, No. 2-3; *Zeitschr. f. d. ges. exp. Med.*, Vol. 80, Nos. 5, 6, 1931.

nerve traumatised on that side, *exceeded in dimensions the corresponding ganglia on the right side, sometimes by as much as two or three times.* These ganglia were obviously œdematous. On rare occasions we observed here acute hæmorrhage. Their colouring was more intense on the left side than on the right. The extent and degree of colouring of the right and left ganglia in other parts of the sympathetic chain were usually similar.

When the above-described trauma was inflicted on one or two nerves of the *plexus brachialis,* the same changes were transferred to the corresponding nerve tracts. We observed here, for example, that as a result of œdema the *ganglion stellatum* on the side of the operation attained a size of 7 mm. in length and 3.5 mm. in breadth. The corresponding dimensions on the right side were 4 mm. and 2.5 mm. The dimensions and colouring of the inter-vertebral and sympathetic ganglia in the control animals were entirely symmetrical in all cases.

Twice we observed that *the alteration on the side of the injury had affected all the ganglia of the sympathetic chain, from the sacrum to the cranium.* At the same time, *on the opposite, "healthy," side only the sympathetic ganglia connected with the segments of the sciatic nerve were œdematous.* Hence, the process under consideration, starting from a single nerve point at the periphery, had spread over the central and sympathetic nervous system, *both in the frontal and in the sagittal plane,* giving rise to both a symmetrical and non-symmetrical form of affection.

Hence, the above-described method seemed to show that *after trauma of the spinal nerve with croton oil the morphological changes in the central nervous system of the rabbit could be even less intense than those in the ganglia of the sympathetic chain.* These changes were exhibited in the form of œdemata and hæmorrhage. At the same time, the elements of the spinal cord do not exhibit any morphological departures from the normal state. Here the matter is limited to a certain increase in permeability of the "barrier," which can be judged by the occurrence of trypan blue in the medullary membranes and adventitious spaces of the blood vessels of the segments affected. *More pronounced changes in the spinal cord usually set in later on.*

It is worth while dwelling on this fact. It is beyond question that the origin of the phenomena described is not connected with the movement of the irritating agent itself along the nervous system and its direct action on each of the affected elements; indeed, after chemical trauma of the spinal nerve, the sympathetic ganglia suffered destruction not only on the side of the trauma, but also on the opposite, "healthy," side. Moreover, in these ganglia the changes developed in general even more rapidly than in the elements of the spinal cord. But the path for the penetration of the harmful influence to the latter lies open through the nerve spaces; *as regards the ganglia, however, we know neither the paths of transmission nor the forces controlling the movement along them.*

How can one conceive the way in which the sympathetic ganglia are drawn into the process?

First of all, an admixture of sympathetic fibres is present in the composition of the spinal nerves, especially of some of them. The irritating agent can, of course, come into direct contact with these fibres. But this by itself is little enough, for the irritating agent enters also into direct connection with the axis cylinders of the elements of the central nervous system.

Further, it is impossible to assume that the substance used by us was actually selective, *i.e.*, that it was an adequate irritating agent precisely for the sympathetic elements, and indifferent to the central ones. I have already described, in one of the chapters of the first part of this book, the results of our experiments with injections of bile, croton oil, mustard gas solutions, etc., into the cerebral hemispheres. For instance, placing drops of bile on any part of the central nervous system was sufficient to kill the animal (cats, dogs) within a few hours, after a rather long series of convulsive attacks. The same holds good of mustard gas and croton oil. Even a superficial histological analysis of these cases reveals changes of the nerve cells in practically all parts of the central nervous system. Consequently, the fact that the affection of the sympathetic elements outstripped that of the central elements in Zakaraya's experiments *could not be due to a lesser action of the irritating agent upon the central nervous system.*

To understand this phenomenon, it is necessary to recognise the presence of some additional cause. The following series of experiments was undertaken in the attempt to solve this problem.

According to the generally accepted view, tetanus phenomena depend directly on the toxin, which spreads from the place of formation or introduction along the axis cylinders and nerve spaces to the cells of the spinal cord, and affects these. As far as I am aware, the question whether any, and if so, what, role is played here by the sympathetic system has not even been raised.

Suitable experiments were carried out by my collaborator Dr. S. D. Kaminsky.[1] Each experiment involved two dogs. The total number of animals was twenty-eight.

The method was the following. The lumbar and sacral part of the left sympathetic chain was removed extra-peritoneally, under narcosis. Within a few hours, the animals recover completely and do not show any defects in

[1] S. D. Kaminsky. *Arkh. Biol. Nauk*, Vol. 33, No. 1-2, 1933; *Zeitschr. f. d. ges. exp. Med.*, Vol. 88, Nos. 5, 6, 1933.

the motor sphere. After some time (from 30 minutes to 1-2 days) tetanus toxin is injected into the muscles of the left knee of the animal. The dose of toxin varied, but it always exceeded the lethal dose, and the difference in the general features of the process was expressed only in the length of the incubation period. Simultaneously with the experimental animal, a normal control animal, specially selected to match the other in weight and growth, was given the same dose of toxin and in the same place in the left knee.

RECORD OF EXPERIMENT

Experiment	*Control*
Dog No. 161. Weight 16 kg.	*Dog No. 162. Weight 16 kg.*
Dec. 2, 1930. 3 p.m. Extra-peritoneal removal of the lumbar tract of the sympathetic chain.	
Dec. 2. 6 p.m. 3 c.c. of tetanus toxin injected into muscles of the left knee.	3 c.c. of tetanus toxin injected into muscles of the left knee.
Dec. 5. 9 a.m. Local tetanus. Left hind extremity stretched out behind and rigid like a stick. The dog walks on three legs.	Local tetanus. Left hind extremity stretched out behind and rigid like a stick. The dog walks on three legs.
Dec. 7. 11 a.m. Local tetanus. Dog walks freely on three legs.	General tetanus. The dog lies, unable to rise. Marked rigidity of all extremities Head thrown back (opisthotonus). High reflex excitability. The dog responds to touching by reflex convulsions of all muscle groups.
Dec. 8. 9 a.m. Local tetanus. Dog walks freely on three legs. Eats and drinks normally.	Phenomena of general tetanus continue to intensify. Convulsive baring of the fangs. Extremities stretched out like sticks, and tense. Opisthotonus.
Dec. 9. 9 a.m. As before, only local tetanus.	Final symptoms. At 10 p.m. death.

Dec. 11. 9 a.m. First symptoms of general tetanus. Rigidity of hind extremities. The dog moves about the room independently, tottering at times. Slight rigidity of the neck muscles. Eats and drinks normally.

Dec. 12. 9 a.m. The dog moves about the room as before. Eats and drinks. Rigidity of the occipital muscles has increased. Heightened tonus in fore extremities also.

Dec. 13. 12 a.m. The dog is unable to stand up, it raises itself only on the fore paws. Increased tonus of the muscles of all extremities. The dog reacts readily to calling, trying to rise but falling.

Dec. 14. 12 noon. Dog lying down. On calling, it turns its head, it attempts to eat from the hand.

Dec. 15. 9 a.m. Opisthotonus. At night, death.

RECORD OF EXPERIMENT

Experiment	*Control*
Dog No. 185. Weight 11 kg.	*Dog No. 186. Weight 11 kg.*
Jan. 16, 1931. Extra-peritoneal removal of the lumbar tract of the sympathetic chain.	
Jan. 17. 4 p.m. 3 c.c. of tetanus toxin injected into muscles of the left knee.	3 c.c. of tetanus toxin injected into muscles of the left knee.
Jan. 23. 12 noon. Initial symptoms of local tetanus. Heightened tonus of left hind extremity. The latter is not used in walking.	Initial symptoms of local tetanus. Heightened tonus of left hind extremity. The latter is not used in walking.
Jan. 25. 9 a.m. Local tetanus.	General tetanus. The dog staggers in walking. Rigidity of the spine and of neck muscles.
Jan. 26. 9 a.m. Local tetanus.	Symptoms of general tetanus increase.
Jan. 27. 9 a.m. Local tetanus.	Dog lies; unable to rise. Rigidity of the whole body and extremities.
Jan. 28. 9 a.m. Initial phenomena of general tetanus. Staggering in walking. Muscles of the hind extremities tense. Eats, drinks and reacts readily to calling.	Opisthotonus. Convulsive baring of the fangs.
Jan. 29. 10:30 a.m. Dog lying down, only able to raise itself on the fore paws. Eats and drinks normally. Reacts readily to calling. Rigidity of hind extremities further increased.	Dog lying down, with head thrown back. Does not react to calling. All four extremities stretched out like sticks, and tense.
Jan. 30. 9 a.m. Rigidity of all four extremities. Dog lying down. On being placed on its feet, it falls down. Reacts to calling. Rigidity of the occipital muscles has increased, but the dog crawls about the room, moving itself by the fore extremities. Dog killed by chloroform.	Final symptoms. Dog killed by chloroform.

There are eight such records in our possession. In all cases the initial symptoms of tetanus either coincided in the experimental and control animals or the control became ill only a few hours in advance. But in the general picture of the further development of the process a considerable retardation was observed in those dogs which had undergone preliminary removal of the sympathetic chain. Moreover, the tetanus symptoms in them did not attain the same degree of intensity as in the controls. The whole process proceeded feebly, as if the dose of toxin taken in their case had been much less.

Two forms of interpretation of the results obtained suggest themselves: either the absence of the sympathetic ganglia make the elements of the central nervous system less receptive to irritation by tetanus toxin, or the tetanus toxin itself has to draw the sympathetic part of the nervous system into the specific reaction, for the development of the full picture of the disease.

Both these suppositions were tested, but neither was confirmed.

I have already mentioned that in Dr. Kaminsky's first series of experiments we injected the toxin not immediately after the removal of the sympathetic chain but after the lapse of a certain period lasting from thirty minutes to four days. It was noticed in these experiments that the difference between the control and the experiment stood out the more sharply the shorter the interval between the operation mentioned and the injection of toxin. Being interested in the part played by the time factor in the process under investigation, we decided to perform a new series of experiments, separating the time of injection of toxin from that of excision of the sympathetic chain by several days or even weeks.

The results proved to be directly contrary to those observed earlier. The experimental animals developed the disease more rapidly than their carefully selected controls, the process was more sharply marked and death ensued within a much shorter period.

RECORD OF EXPERIMENT

Experiment	*Control*
Dog No. 51. Weight 11.2 kg.	Dog No. 64. Weight 11 kg.
May 12, 1931. 3 p.m. Extra-peritoneal removal of the lumbar tract of the left sympathetic chain.	
May 19. 7 c.c. of tetanus toxin (a weaker preparation than in the experiments of the first series) injected into the muscles of the left knee.	7 c.c. of toxin injected as in the experimental dog.
May 21. 3.25 a.m. Heightened tonus of the left hind extremity. Dog moves about on three legs.	Healthy.

May 22. 10 a.m. Appearance of local tetanus, and almost immediately afterwards (after 3 hours) general tetanus. Rigidity of the hind extremities. Tenseness of the occipital muscles. Reflex convulsions. The dog moves about with difficulty, frequently falling down. Reacts to calling.

First signs of local tetanus. Slight increase of tonus of left hind leg. In walking, the dog sometimes avoids using its left hind extremity.

May 23. 9 a.m. Dog lying down, unable to rise. Head thrown back. Marked opisthotonus. Reflex convulsions of all muscle groups. All extremities tense and stretched out like sticks. Convulsive baring of the fangs. Death.

Local tetanus. Muscles of the left extremity tense. Runs about the room on three legs only. Eats and drinks normally.

May 24. 10 a.m. First signs of general tetanus. Rigidity of hind extremities. Takes food normally. Moves about the room, not using the left hind extremity. At 6 p.m., occipital rigidity.

May 25. 10 a.m. Full picture of general tetanus.

May 26. Death.

RECORD OF EXPERIMENT

Experiment
Dog No. 180. Weight 11 kg.

Control
Dog No. 181. Weight 11 kg.

Nov. 13. 1931. 3 p.m. Extra-peritoneal removal of lumbar tract of the left sympathetic chain.

Dec. 2. 4 p.m. 3 c.c. of tetanus toxin injected into the muscles of the left knee.

3 c.c. of toxin injected as in the experimental dog.

Dec. 4. 10 a.m. Local tetanus of the left hind extremity, which is stretched out like a stick.

Healthy.

Dec. 5. 10 a.m. Initial symptoms of general tetanus. Rigidity of the occipital muscles. Reflex excitability increased. Reflex convulsions of both hind extremities. Dog lying down; put on its feet, it falls down, but it takes food from the hand.

Slight increase of tonus of the muscles of the left hind extremity.

Dec. 6. 10 a.m. Full picture of general tetanus.

Local tetanus of the left hind extremity. The dog walks freely on three legs. Eats normally.

Dec. 7. 9 a.m. Death.

Initial symptoms of general tetanus. Rigidity of hind extremities and occipital muscles. The dog takes food and moves about the room, but often staggers and falls.

Dec. 8. 9 a.m. Reflex convulsions of muscle groups. Dog lying down, head thrown back. Opisthotonus. On touching, the reflex convulsions increase.

Dec. 9. (Morning) Death.

The remaining experiments of this series gave in general the same result.

It may be considered as established, therefore, that the absence of the ganglia of the sympathetic chain does not by itself render the elements of the *central* nervous system less receptive to irritation by tetanus toxin.

Moreover, it was found that the development of the disease does not require direct contact of the toxin with the elements of the sympathetic ganglia. In a new series of experiments, tetanus symptoms developed in our dogs to the full extent in spite of the absence of the corresponding sympathetic chain.

It is also impossible to suppose that during the interval between the operations of removing the left sympathetic chain and injecting the toxin, a replacement of the missing functions takes place by means of the formation of new connections with the ganglia of the right-hand side, which have been preserved in their entirety. Experiments specially performed demonstrated that *removal of the abdominal sympathetic chain on both sides had the same effect on the development of tetanus as removal on one side,* and also that the basic factor, determining the character of the reaction, is time.

A remote possibility that might occur to one is an immediate influence of the removal of the sympathetic ganglia on the tonus of the striated muscles (de Boer, Orbeli, etc.). But, as we have just seen, this would only help in explaining the experiments of the first series. The results of the second series would be in direct contradiction to such an interpretation.

One explanation remains: *viz.,* that on injection of tetanus toxin at the periphery, the elements of the central nervous system experience not only a special form of irritation, but also an ordinary trauma. This is a second process, developing side by side with the first one. The irritation of the spinal elements is handed on from here to the sympathetic parts, drawing them, not into the complex of tetanus phenomena, but into a *pathological process of the nature of nervous dystrophy.* But the sympathetic elements also, becoming altered under the influence of the central elements, *put the latter in their turn into abnormal conditions of life and functioning.* When we remove the cor-

responding sympathetic chain shortly before injecting the toxin, then, in the
first place, the cells of the central nervous system *undergo a certain kind of
shock*, and, in the second place, *they are deprived of the supplementary irritation*, the counter-shock, which under normal conditions they could receive
from the sympathetic elements. On the other hand, if a longer period elapses
between our two acts of interference, the result will be the opposite, since *the
operation of excising the sympathetic chain is itself a nerve trauma, in other
words, is a stimulus for the development of a dystrophic process in other nerve
regions.* We have already seen more than once that this process does not occur
immediately but grows gradually, and inevitably adds something to all the
other processes taking place in those regions. As a result, the tetanus takes a
more serious course.

It is interesting to note that this state of things also is not constant. In
some recent experiments of my other collaborators, I. P. Bobkov and A. L.
Fenelonov, the following observation was made; they injected tetanus toxin
into the neck muscles of two dogs on whom *many months previously* the
operation of removal of the abdominal chain of the sympathetic ganglia had
been carried out on one side. When symptoms of general tetanus developed,
the tetanus was very weakly expressed in the muscles of the hind extremities
on the side of the operation. The process was almost limited to a certain increase of reflex excitability.

It is evident that the intensity of the dystrophic process produced by nerve
trauma can only rarely be altered. For tetanus, conditions are temporarily
created afresh resembling those during the first hours following removal of
the sympathetic chain. The curve of all other processes taking place in the
same nerve regions will vary, depending on the course of the curve of the dystrophic process. *It is precisely this that makes it possible to understand the significance of time as a factor in the change.*

Whatever the properties possessed by the irritating agent and however
isolated the place of its application may appear to be, the consequences express
themselves in a number of nerve structures *which have never been in direct
contact with it.* There is no strict localisation of this process within the limits
of a particular part of the nervous system, since the irritation passes from the
elements of the central nervous system to the sympathetic system and back
again.

In this way, our conception of segmentary affections of the nervous system becomes more precise. It is not a question of *formally delimited segments
of the spinal cord.* We saw that, after trauma of the spinal nerve, alterations
are to be discovered almost from the very start in the ganglia of the sympathetic chain, not only on the side of the injury, but also on the opposite, "healthy,"

side. *Thus, the conception of the segment includes also its sympathetic portion.* The subsequent data demonstrate that nerve parts within the organs also have a definite order in which they are included in the process, and that this order is connected with the point of primary irritation.

It must be stressed that when segmentary nerve changes were found within the limits of, for instance, the sympathetic nervous system, it was often possible to observe also corresponding alterations outside the limits of this segment, the process developing simultaneously in both the frontal and sagittal planes. The same thing holds good also for the central nervous system. If, nevertheless, we do not give up the term "segmentary affections," it is only because this term defines the initial stage of the process, a stage undoubtedly playing a part in its further course. In addition, the extent of functional and morphological changes in the segment that has initially suffered is always small at the beginning.

Summing up these results, we have to recognise that, as regards the development of nervous dystrophy, *the distortion of normal relations among the nerve elements themselves is not of lesser significance than the immediate action on them of the foreign agent.* During the course of our work we frequently observed that the initial changes of a morphological character in the nerve group primarily suffering were inconsiderable. Nevertheless, in definite places at the periphery, the process takes the form of serious destruction of the integrity of the tissues. The immediate irritation by the foreign agent, in spite of its unusual character, *did not kill the nerve cells.* It merely altered their function. The alteration of the normal nerve function, however, resulted in the disease and even *death of tissue elements at the periphery.*

Thus, the nerve trauma by itself does not constitute the direct cause of nervous dystrophy from start to finish. *It merely gives the impulse to the development of a process which subsequently proceeds cumulatively.* Hence, changes arising secondarily in the sympathetic system can later prove to be both more dangerous and more severe.

The facts brought forward have, in addition, a significance from the point of view of method. In investigating nervous functions, the method of irritation and exclusion plays a fundamental role. The disappearance of a particular reaction, on the one hand, or the exhibition of it, on the other, is considered as a positive proof that this reaction is connected with the definite group of nerve elements which were the object of immediate interference. For elementary reactions and short periods of observation, such an attitude is permissible, although with reservations. If, however, we are dealing with a complex process, the external manifestations of which begin only after a certain, often rather prolonged, period, then it is impossible to. judge of its localisation merely by data relating to the place of primary interference. A much greater role may be played here, not by the part which has been subjected to irritation, but by *the act of interference itself, which becomes the originator of a whole group of new processes.* If, in the experiments just analysed, we were to leave the act of interference out of account, we would have to ascribe its consequences (the retardation, intensification and new retardation of the tetanus symptoms) to one and the same object, *viz.*, the sympathetic ganglia themselves. The result would be *the false notion that they are included in the specific part of the reaction, which is actually not the case.*

One cannot help recalling here our experiments on epilepsy, described earlier in the book. Externally similar procedures produced different consequences, while, on the other hand, different forms of interference yielded one and the same result. In the clinic, for example, this is illustrated by cases of traumatic epilepsy, where both repeated closure of the bone defect and repeated removal of the transplanted bones in one and the same patient has a curative effect on each occasion, but the effect is always temporary.

Consequently, on chemical or infectional nerve trauma, a number of different processes of a physiological and pathological character develop in the nervous system. The former are beneficial, the latter find expression in dystrophic symptoms, both within the nervous system and in the peripheral tissues. The dystrophic processes take a cyclic course and may end in the complete restoration of normal conditions. But *in a number of cases they develop progressively.* Commencing in the region of a particular nerve segment, they soon pass outside its limits, embrace other portions of the complex nerve network and culminate in general dystrophy and the death of the animal.

A characteristic property is their incubational or latent period. However, in the process of the work it was established sufficiently clearly that in actual fact there is no latent period. The idea of a latent period is *due to the imperfection of the indicators* used by us. We regard the moment of appearance of local dystrophy in the tissues as the beginning of the process, although it is frequently its final result, and in any case not the first stage.

Independently of whether the irritating agent itself spreads through the nervous system, or whether its action is limited to a single nerve point, there can arise within the nervous system a number of points of unusual irritation, *mutually reinforcing one another and creating new ones.* In the genesis of dystrophic processes, it is this, and not the irritating agent by itself, that plays the fundamental role. This explains why chemical and infectional irritating agents although of diverse nature can produce the same consequences in the final result.

A special nerve "tropism" plays no part here. We have seen that any substance can reach the central nervous system along the nerve trunk. *But one substance may remain indifferent even after having reached there, while another, without even moving from the spot, destroys the nervous system.*

Recently, from Levaditi's laboratory, two works have appeared by Nicolau, Cruveillier and Kopciowska, dealing with the morphological consequences of *virus fixe* vaccination.

Describing a number of changes caused in this way in the central nervous system, the authors estimate them as special reactions (*"réactions speciales"*) to neurotropic virus, as the morphological expression of the *"direct struggle" between the virus and the receptive tissue.*

It is true that this reaction may have a certain defensive significance. But there is nothing special about it. One can easily convince oneself of this by infecting such rabbits intra-cerebrally; they develop disease and die like normal ones. Vaccination for rabies makes the animals resistant only *in respect to infection coming from the periphery*. But it was demonstrated above (Suslov's experiments) that it is possible, without any "struggle" of special elements, to obtain the same results by the aid of a single injection of a few drops of formalin solution into the nerve. In its effect, the reaction here also proved to be "defensive," *but one could hardly regard it as a special and beneficial reaction.*

The same thing holds good in regard to the morphological consequences. If, instead of vaccinating the rabbits with an emulsion of rabised brain, a small quantity of mustard gas is applied to the skin, or a solution of formalin, carbolic acid or other substances is injected into the tissues, *it will be impossible to distinguish the morphological consequences in the nervous system from one another.*

I can venture to assert this, since I have the necessary material in my possession. In our laboratory, B. S. Doinikov and V. G. Ushakov also performed experiments on the vaccination of rabbits with *virus fixe*, and also with the object of studying the morphological changes in the nervous system. The result was in exact accordance with what we observed earlier when we used other irritating agents. Vaccination with emulsion of normal brain produced the same (only slightly weaker) morphological consequences as vaccination with emulsion of rabised brain. This is comprehensible, for the presence of the virus constitutes *an additional irritant*. It is enough to prolong the irritation with normal brain or to increase the dose, and the dimensions of the morphological effect are the same in both cases.

This, above, all, makes it possible to explain the popularity which has been won in many places by Fermi's method of vaccination for rabies. The fact that here a small quantity of carbolic acid is added to the emulsion produces an additional irritation *strengthening the specific immunity by a non-specific addition.* The latter is a reaction to irritation in general, and not specially to the given irritating agent.

CHAPTER XVI

STANDARD FORMS OF NERVOUS DYSTROPHY AND THEIR QUANTITATIVE VARIATIONS

THE propositions laid down in the preceding chapter were further developed in the course of subsequent work.

In setting out this new material, I shall begin with the experiments of my collaborators I. A. Pigalev and Z. G. Kuznetsova.[1] The work was carried out on rabbits and dogs. The irritation was applied to the second and third branches of *n. trigeminus, viz., n. infraorbitalis* and *n. mentalis*. As has already been mentioned, it was the irritation of intra-cranial parts, and in particular of the trigeminus nerve of the rabbit, which provided the early investigators with the first materials for the foundation of the theory of the trophic function of the nervous system (Magendie, Samuel). Since then, many scientists have repeated these experiments in the original form or with variations (Meissner, Longet, Berthold, Kirchner, Schiff, Nasse, etc.). As an indicator of trophic disturbances at the periphery, the majority of these writers employed eye diseases in the form of conjunctivitis or ceratitis, which after a longer or shorter period developed in the rabbits *on the side of the irritation*.

We made it our aim to obtain changes of the eye in one form or another, not merely on the side of the injured nerve, but also *on the opposite, healthy, side*. Moreover, we aimed at obtaining them not from the Gasserian ganglion or the intra-cranial parts of the trigeminus nerve, but from its peripheral branches having no direct relation to the eye.

A number of substances (mustard oil, croton oil, bile, lactic acid, etc.) were tested as irritants. Finally, we adopted croton oil. Following its injection into the substance of the nerve, the latter was severed through the middle of the trunk where it was swollen after the injection. For the experiments, we used the peripheral parts of the second and third branches of *n. trigeminus—n. infraorbitalis* or *n. mentalis*. After making a small cut above the place of exit of the nerve from the bone and exposing the nerve, 2-3 drops of croton oil were injected and the nerve severed. If the wound is sewn up, extensive

[1] I. A. Pigalev and Z. G. Kuznetsova. *Arkh. Biol. Nauk*, Vol. 30, No. 1, 1930; *Zeitschr. f. d. ges. exp. Med.*, Vol. 67, Nos. 1, 2, 1929.

suppuration usually develops. With an open wound, there is only some slight œdematic swelling which quickly disappears. In dogs which underwent extraction of the cerebro-spinal fluid after the injection of croton oil into the nerve, the swelling was always much larger, not only on the side of the operation, *but also in a symmetrically situated spot on the other side.* In all cases, the irritating substance was introduced into the nerve on one occasion only. Individual details of the technique were varied and in this way the experiments were divided into series. Since the results of the separate series differ from one another only in a quantitative respect, I shall permit myself to include them all in a general review.

The injection of croton oil in *n. infraorbitalis* without section of the latter produced in rabbits, even in the first few days, the development of photophobia and conjunctivitis on the operated side. In rare cases conjunctivitis developed on both sides. In these animals, a bluish spot followed by an ulcer appeared within 2-4 days close to the middle of the line where the skin passes into the mucous membrane of the upper lip. The ulcer slowly increased in size and then, in the course of 2-3 weeks, gradually healed.

When we began to sever the nerve after injection of croton oil, the effect was considerably enhanced. In these rabbits, conjunctivitis as a rule developed on both sides, while ceratitis and sometimes ulcer of the cornea frequently developed on the side of the operation. The ulcer on the lip now made its appearance even within one or two days. It rapidly increased in size and did not heal for 5-6 weeks. Very soon an exactly similar ulcer appeared in the symmetrical place of the other, healthy lip, followed by symmetrical ulcers on the tongue. On two occasions we obtained purulent inflammation of the middle ear on both sides, as a result of which the animals died.

In the majority of the rabbits, all these phenomena gradually subsided, which, however, was not a sign of complete recovery from the destruction occasioned in the nerve cells. In a number of cases, at the end of 4-8 weeks, animals which seemed healthy began to exhibit *alteration of the teeth,* at first on the side of the injury and afterwards on the opposite side as well. This was most clearly expressed in the incisors. The change begins with the appearance of discoloured whitish portions which gradually enlarge and fuse, and sometimes occupy the whole tooth. The tooth becomes friable and crumbles. The alteration of the teeth begins earlier on the side of the nerve injury and is usually more pronounced than on the "healthy" side. These changes also are of a temporary nature, since the incisors of the rabbit grow continuously during life. The growing portion proves to be normal, though this is not always so. We observed rabbits in which the incisors remained friable during many months.

Exactly the same thing results if *n. mentalis* is taken for the experiment, except that the eye changes begin somewhat later, the symmetrical ulcers develop on the lower lip and the alteration of the teeth in the lower incisors. On one occasion, besides the alteration of the lower incisors, we observed after some weeks the formation of whitish, and later, carious, portions in an upper incisor, but only on the side of the nerve injury. Ulcers of the tongue were also obtained from this nerve and were also symmetrical. In two cases of this series, we again obtained bilateral purulent inflammation of the middle ear, ending in the death of the animals.

To study in greater detail the nature of the changes observed in the oral cavity and to compare them with corresponding data from the human clinic, the same experiments were once more performed by my collaborator P. A. Glushkov.[1] In 8 rabbits, out of 14 experimented on, it was possible to observe hyperæmia of the gum of the sockets during the days immediately following trauma of the nerve trunk. The hyperæmia was of a stagnant character. It was most pronounced at the neck of the incisors. Very soon the somewhat inflated mucous membrane began to separate slightly from the teeth, forming at the necks of the latter small pockets with the surface of the lip. These pockets subsequently became deeper and crumbs and hairs accumulated in them. On pressure on the gum, pus exuded from these pockets. In two cases, these neck pockets were present as early as the second day after trauma of the nerve; in two other cases on the fifth day, in one on the twelfth day, in one on the thirteenth day and in two on the fiftieth day.

The two last cases are interesting on account of the weak development of the dystrophic process. Only on the fiftieth day was it possible to observe a slight separation of the gum from the necks of the corresponding incisors. In both animals a second nerve trauma was inflicted on the eighty-third day after the first trauma; in the first animal, the sciatic nerve was severed and its centripetal end was subjected to chemical irritation; in the second animal, the left upper cervical ganglion was pricked with a needle moistened with tincture of iodine. *Within a day after this, the separation of the gums from the necks of the incisors markedly increased and pockets were formed with secretion of pus.*

Comparing this general picture with that observed in the human clinic in cases of alveolar pyorrhœa, Glushkov came to the conclusion that there was a *close resemblance between the two processes.* An analysis of the bacterial flora of the pus secreted from the above-described pockets revealed the ordinary micro-flora of the oral cavity (Gram-positive and Gram-negative diplococci and diplobacilli). In alveolar pyorrhœa in human beings the pockets of the

[1] P. A. Glushkov. *Arkh. Biol. Nauk*, Vol. 34, No. 4, 1933.

mucous membrane, formed by the separation of the latter from the necks of the teeth, also contain, as is well known, a quite non-specific micro-flora.

In general features, the same process was also observed in experiments on dogs (Pigalev and Kuznetsova). In these, besides cases of ceratitis and ulcers of the corneal membrane, which were sometimes symmetrical, we observed a series of symmetrical ulcerous developments on the hard palate, tongue, teeth and other parts of the mucous membrane of the oral cavity. The skin affections of the surface of the lips more than once included typical herpes, *i.e.*, the formation of blisters on the reddened and eroded skin *at the corner of the mouth*. Several times purulent inflammation of the middle ear and accessory sinuses of the nasal cavity on both sides was also observed. These symptoms developed both on injury to the *n. infraorbitalis* and on injury to the *n. mentalis*. One must also mention the constant discovery, on dissection, of *hæmorrhages in the lung tissue and in the mucous membrane of various parts of the gastro-intestinal tract*.

In dogs that lived for a comparatively long time after the above-described operation to the branches of *n. trigeminus*, the following phenomena were noticed. In a certain percentage, trophic changes *did not develop at all* or were transient. In other cases, all the disturbances, even if severe, in the region of the corresponding nerve segment passed off and subsequently the dogs *were hardly to be distinguished from normal animals* apart from scars and spots at the place of the former injuries. Finally, some of the dogs after a certain period of apparent health again exhibited trophic changes in the tissues *at the places previously affected*. This was followed by the development of *partial baldness and ulcers in other regions of the body*, which apparently did not have any relation to the segment of the trigeminus nerve. From the time of the single injection of croton oil into one or other branch of this nerve, no other actions were carried out. Extraction of cerebro-spinal fluid also ceased long before the appearance of the signs of generalised dystrophic phenomena. Nevertheless, the dogs grew thin, the hair fell out, the gait was altered, feebleness and general exhaustion developed. All this ended in death.

On dissection, it was possible to discover changes in the brain, in various parenchymatous organs, and also in the bones, which sometimes became very thin and brittle, sometimes, on the contrary, so soft that the ribs, for instance, could be cut with a knife.

The whole picture of the disease including the anatomical changes had much in common with what I. P. Pavlov sometimes observed in dogs that had been kept in a damp place after various operations in the region of the digestive tract.

These and similar observations caused us to endeavour to widen the scope of the work, operating not only on the nerve trunks but also on other parts of the nervous system. Our attention was naturally first given to that part of the brain which is now denoted by the term *hypothalamus*. This region is considered to be the higher centre of vegetative nerve functions. Here are to be found the regulatory centres of water, salt, protein, fat and carbohydrate metabolism, of the circulatory system of the organs of internal secretion, etc. Disease or injury of the hypothalamus may result also in disorganisation in the motor sphere, including even epileptic attacks (Cushing). This region is regarded by some as that of the localisation of the "sleep centre."

Even the earliest investigators, Schiff and Brown-Sequard, in cases of injury to the intermediate and middle brain observed the resulting development of hæmorrhages in the respiratory and digestive organs. The same thing is described by many writers who studied the effect of so-called heat puncture. N. N. Burdenko and B. N. Mogilnitsky observed the development of hæmorrhages and ulcerations in the stomach of dogs in which the part of the hypothalamus behind the infundibulum had been destroyed.

There is no doubt, therefore, that these regions of the brain are connected with many functions of the organism which could be combined in the word "trophic." I shall not give the whole history of the subject. Questions relating to it are in the forefront of attention at the present time, and the basic facts are widely known. Moreover, we are not interested for the moment in isolated facts concerning the physiology and pathology of this particular area of the nervous system, the more so because formal data concerning localisation can hardly be of use to us in obtaining a conception of the course of the dystrophic process within the nervous system. The task was *to elucidate the form of development of the dystrophic process* when the region of the *hypothalamus, in particular the* tuber cinereum *and* substantia perforata posterior *formed the point of primary irritation.*

The chief difficulty of the task consisted in obtaining a really isolated and, moreover, chronic irritation of the *tuber cinereum*. Its deep situation in the middle of the base of the cranium and its close connection with the hypophysis greatly complicated the technique of the operation, in the first place on account of bleeding. It was necessary to change the usual technique in order to avoid any bleeding into the cranial cavity. In consequence of the blood accumulating at its base, the irritation takes on a diffuse character, embracing the whole mid- and hind-brain, and even the upper segments of the spinal cord. This defect is inherent in all the methods. It is primarily on this account that so far we have no exact data allowing us to analyse the complex effect into functions of the hypophysis and functions of the *tuber cinereum*.

Thus the first phase of our work was the question of technique. By altering a number of different technical devices and introducing new ones, we succeeded on the whole in achieving the desired results. We evolved finally a technique combining the following features: 1) all stages of the operation could be carried out in full view; 2) bleeding, both before and after the operation, was absent; 3) injury to the brain was confined exactly within the limits intended and was prolonged chronically; 4) incidental trauma of other cerebral regions was excluded; 5) the dura mater was sewn up without any tension.

Details of this technique have been published in articles by my collaborators M. S. Skoblo[1] and I. A. Pigalev.[2] I shall permit myself to give a description of it here for the benefit of those who might desire to employ it in their work.

It is best to select a small-sized dog for the experiment, since the operation wound is less deep in this case. Young dogs are also to be preferred to old ones; the base of the cranium in them is wider and the middle cranial fossa is flatter.

The operation itself is performed as follows. Under general narcosis a cut is made in the skin and underlying tissues along the medial line of the head from the root of the nose to the second cervical vertebra. On one side of the head (most conveniently the left side) the skin and *platysma* were separated up to the level of the cheek-bone. This is followed by ligature of the blood vessels supplying the *m. temporalis*, the removal of this muscle along the edge of the cheek-bone and careful stopping of bleeding. It is possible to avoid cutting the muscle, by skirting it with a curving cut along the edge of its attachment to the bone, separating it with a spatula from the bottom of the temporal and subtemporal fossæ, and pulling it outwards with a hook. The cranial cavity is opened with a gouge or cutter, the opening is slightly enlarged by the aid of forceps, and the dura mater is separated by a blunt instrument for some distance from the inner surface of the bones.

Following this, *the cerebro-spinal fluid is extracted,* a procedure which plays a very essential role in the further course of the operation. The immediate result is cessation or considerable decrease of bleeding from the bones. In addition the resulting evacuation of the ventricular fluid produces a perceptible *decrease in the volume of the cerebral hemispheres.* In the following extensive opening up of the cranium, the hemispheres not only do not protrude from the edge of the bone opening, but are separated from the bones like the kernel of a nut from its shell. Thanks to this the raising up of the

[1] M. S. Skoblo, *Nauchnoye Slovo,* No. 4, 1930; *Zeitschr. f. d. ges. exp. Med.,* Vol. 73, No. 1-2, 1930.
[2] I. A. Pigalev. *Arkh. Biol. Nauk,* Vol. 32, No. 1, 1932; *Zeitschr. f. d. ges. exp. Med.,* Vol. 82, No. 5-6, 1932.

temporal portion from the bottom of the cranial cavity is greatly facilitated, and a good suture of the dura mater is always assured. Finally, the extraction of the fluid renders unnecessary special removal of it from the region of the middle cranial cavity by gauze tampons, a fact which is also of importance since it is precisely at this moment that there can easily be bleeding from the vessels at the base of the brain, rendering the subsequent results unclear.

After the extraction of the cerebro-spinal fluid, the removal of the dura mater from the bones is continued in all directions, especially below, towards the base. Here it is necessary to beware of injury to the venous sinuses. Following this, the covering cranial bones are removed with forceps below the line joining externally the upper corner of the eye socket to the middle of the *linea nuchæ* (*crista occipitalis* in the dog).

After removing the bones to the level of the cheek-bones, it is necessary *to open widely the mouth of the dog.* By so doing the *processus coronarius* of the lower jaw is moved downwards and draws with it all the muscles, vessels and nerves running from the lateral surface of the cranium to the lower jaw. It suffices now to pass the handle of a scalpel along the bone for the whole lateral surface and part of the base of the cranium to be exposed. The deep-lying part of the covering bones which have been exposed in this way are removed as closely as possible to the medial line. It is necessary to take care that the bone forceps should not grasp the muscles at the bottom of the subtemporal fossa for in the immediate neighbourhood there are the large blood vessels accompanying the second and third branches of the *n. trigeminus.*

When the bones have been removed, a T-shaped cut is made in the dura mater. Its horizontal part runs back from the angle of the eye socket. Its vertical part begins from the middle of the horizontal part and runs below to the edge of the opening in the bone.

Now the operator passes to the opposite (right) side of the operating table. The anæsthetist turns the head of the animal round the longitudinal axis of the vertebral column so that the left side of the operation area passes over to the right. By the force of gravity, the cerebrum separates somewhat from the base of the cranium. At this moment, without further action there will be found to be exposed not only the entire temporal tract but also the *gyrus pyriformis* and even the edge of the *tractus olfactorius.* A slight pressure with a smooth instrument is sufficient to expose the region of the hypophysis in the space between the carotid artery and *n. oculomotorius.*

Immediately after exposing the hypophysis, a previously prepared, small glass sphere, of the size of a pea, is cautiously pushed into the space between the carotid artery and the *n. oculomotorius* and placed immediately behind the back of the *sella turcica.* The head of the dog is replaced in its former position, the hypophysis returns to its place, the brain is let down on the base of the skull and the operation concludes with successive stitching of the wound.

The dura mater is always sewn up. It is not at all necessary to stretch it, since the hemispheres during the operation do not return to their former size. It is, however, necessary to sew it as otherwise the brain substance is bound to protrude through the opening, and thereby damage would be inflicted on parts of the cortex lying close to the base of the brain. It is desirable also that the wound secretion of the external parts of the wound should not penetrate under the dura mater and on to the base of the cranium. By the method described, we had neither bleeding, nor subsequent penetration of the blood from outside parts of the wound. There were no changes in the region of the cerebral hemispheres or at their base, except for restricted tender fusions in the region of the suture of the dura mater.

If, while exposing the hypophysis or at any other moment of the operation, intra-cranial bleeding commenced, we did not finish the operation, but, after waiting for the cessation of bleeding, simply sewed up the wound and excluded the animal from the experiment.

Dissection demonstrated that the glass sphere hardly produces any signs of reaction on the part of the cerebrum or its membranes.

Being situated on the middle line between the anterior ends of the *pedunculi cerebri*, the glass sphere presses on the posterior part of the *tuber cinereum, corpora mamillaria* and *substantia perforata posterior*. Here, a *sore is formed on the brain*, in the form of a circular pit corresponding in dimensions and form to the sphere used. Under the influence of the pressure, the cerebral tissue is atrophied to such an extent that the cavity of the third ventricle is often revealed, remaining covered below merely by the transparent layer of soft and arachnoid membranes. The blood vessels are pushed to one side, as a result of which the bottom of the pit is pale. Instead of a glass sphere, we sometimes used a wax ball or even an ordinary pea, which had been soaked in alcohol for some days before the operation. In these cases, the reaction on the part of the surrounding tissues was considerably greater, and the sphere became enclosed in a capsule of soft scar tissue.

Curiously enough, on using an ordinary pea the dogs in some cases lived for a long while, 1-2 months or longer. Owing to the swelling of the pea, the contact sore on the cerebrum attained considerable dimensions. This, however, did not prevent the animal from walking, eating and even playing, in spite of the presence of various symptoms of a dystrophic nature, such as will be described below. In general such animals soon die. Frequently, even in the hours immediately following the operation, they develop typical epileptic attacks which follow in succession and lead to the animal's death after the lapse of 1-2 days.

Apparently, the associated chemical trauma, *i.e.*, not the pea itself, but the alcohol with which it has been moistened, plays a part here. An argument for this view is that the convulsions sometimes begin within 15-20 minutes after the operation, when the dry pea has not yet begun to increase in size.

In the majority of cases, there were no alterations of the hypophysis which could have developed as a direct result of the pressure of the glass sphere. The sphere is situated behind the hypophysis and cannot be displaced forwards, being kept in place by the posterior edge of the *sella turcica* which is slightly raised above the base of the cerebrum. All the same, in order to avoid the possibility of such injuries, we subsequently altered the technique and began to use, instead of the sphere, a glass ring from which a piece had been removed on one side. The size of the ring corresponds to the dimensions of the pit of the *sella turcica*. Its thickness is 2-3 mm.

At the moment when the cerebrum is lifted up, the *infundibulum* is introduced within the ring, through the break in its circumference, and the rings is turned so that the free ends are directed anteriorly. (Plate 20.) The ring lies at the edge of the pit of the *sella turcica*, leaving the hypophysis in place, without touching it anywhere or putting it under any constraint. When the cerebrum is allowed to fall back again, the ring presses against the posterior and lateral parts of the *tuber cinereum, producing here a semi-circular sore.* The sole drawback to this form of the operation lies in stagnant phenomena in the hypophysis, which sometimes occur as a result of the pressure of the vessels around the *tuber cinereum.*

Using both of these methods, *i.e.*, the sphere and the ring, we have carried out operations on many scores of animals. Here I shall give a general review of the data obtained.

The first two series of experiments were performed by my collaborators M. S. Skoblo[1] and I. A. Pigalev.[2] In the first series the glass sphere was used, in the second the semi-circular ring. The consequences, both as regards the animal's life and the general picture of the dystrophic process, were approximately alike in both series.

In the first place, it must be mentioned that the duration of life of the dogs after the operation varies within very wide limits. Some of the animals die even within the first 10-20 hours, others live some days, while in a third group life persists for weeks and even months (up to a year or more). In

[1] M. S. Skoblo. *Loc. cit.*
[2] I. A. Pigalev. *Loc. cit.*

spite of these variations, the dystrophic phenomena which develop among them are very much alike, differing only in degree.

The first symptom, usually noticed even during the first two hours, is *hæmorrhage of the gum in the region of the parodont.* Swelling, loosening and a dark border of acute hæmorrhages usually make their appearance around the molars of both jaws. The general picture is very similar to that seen in man in the case of scurvy. The process gradually progresses, the border of hæmorrhages around the teeth extends into a continuous strip, the gum separates from the necks of the teeth, revealing the alveolar edge of the bone. In severe cases the ulcerations around the separate teeth fuse and then the whole gum comes away, *laying bare the bone for a considerable distance.* We observed several cases where the mucous membrane of the gum disintegrated ichorously outside the limits of the *processus alveolarius* of the upper and lower jaws. This occurred without signs of reaction on the part of the surrounding tissues, leaving the impression of putrefaction or maceration. Apparently, also, it is not accompanied by any marked painful sensation. The dogs readily permit examination and touching of the altered parts, and they eat and drink without noticeable difficulty. Such severe cases are met with comparatively rarely. Usually, the phenomenon is limited to swelling, loosening, hæmorrhage and ulceration of the jaws around the necks of the teeth. The process can go on for many days and even weeks, gradually subsiding and breaking out afresh.

Other regions of the mucous membrane of the oral cavity are affected at the same time as the gums. Here also *erosions* and *ulcers* make their appearance, especially on the lips, tongue and under the tongue, sometimes on the cheeks, and on the hard and soft palate, more rarely in the pharynx. Here also signs of reaction are often absent. The tissues are flaccid and dirty or, on the contrary, they may have an unnaturally fresh appearance as if the defect had occurred as the result not of ulceration, but of cutting with a knife. In the majority of cases, these changes are superficial; more than once, however, we observed that they began to *progress irresistibly, destroying the mucous, muscular and cutaneous portions of the cheek.* This resulted in an extensive penetrating defect, with the absolutely typical appearance of what pathology and the clinic terms noma or "watery cancer." (Plates 21, 22.)

We were not interested in the question as to what precise microbes were concerned in these processes and what role they played. It was clear that there is only a quantitative difference between the general features of noma and of those ulcers that do not penetrate right through all the tissues. Ulcerations in the oral cavities of our dogs were an invariable consequence of the above-described operations. If any microbes also took part in this process, it can only mean that they were previously present in the organism of the animal as saprophytes, and *the conditions for their activity were the result of a different process. Moreover, their activity or pathogenic character was strictly local.* Thus, it was frequently observed that particular ulcers in the oral cavity, when they had reached a definite size, came to a stop and, as it were, halted, neither advancing nor showing any tendency to disappear. If one speaks of the transition of microbes from a saprophytic to a pathogenic state, then it becomes necessary to *delimit the exact area where this has taken place!* This area, however, has evidently been formed by the action of other forces. The microbes are unable to cross its boundaries. But in that case is their pathogenic character an active property? It is obvious that in the case before us this conception *cannot explain anything and therefore is of no interest to us.*

The next, very characteristic, form of affection is the development of papillomata. These typical growths, in external appearance resembling a cauliflower, can be single or multiple. They are disposed on the mucous membrane of the lips and cheeks, and sometimes on the tongue. Their dimensions vary. Some do not exceed a pin's head in size; others attain the size of a walnut. The time of their appearance reckoned from the moment of the operation is also not uniform, varying from 2-3 weeks up to 5-7 months. After existing for a short time, they become atrophied or fall off, and are replaced by new ones. On disappearing, they leave behind a white spot which is especially visible in those cases where the mucous membrane of the mouth is strongly pigmented. The development of papillomata in our dogs was by no means such a constant reaction as hæmorrhage of the gums and ulceration of the mucous membrane. However, we have already observed it not less than twenty times, and we consider that papillomatosis occurs after the "glass sphere operation" in 15-20 per cent of all cases. In regard to their microscopical features, the papillomata described are in no way different from the usual forms.

Of other changes in the oral cavity, one must mention an *affection of the dentures.* At the beginning, the teeth become covered by a coating of a yellowish-brown or sometimes almost black colour. The appearance of this coating is undoubtedly connected with the hæmorrhage of the gums, but in some cases the coating becomes so strong that it does not disappear even after the cessation of hæmorrhage.

Subsequently, *alterations of the teeth themselves* gradually commence. They become soft, are easily worn away, break off and crumble. The changes mentioned can sometimes be observed even during the second month, sometimes they develop later. After a longer or shorter period, the process may involve all the teeth of an animal, *which up till then had no kind of dental defect.* Usually, however, this process finds expression only in a particular group of teeth, leaving the others more or less untouched. The disease only rarely becomes pronounced, in many cases it is even altogether absent. But sometimes it leads to the complete loss of the dental apparatus. Below is one of the reports of our observations (a case of Dr. M. S. Skoblo).

Dog No. 294. Weight 14 kg.

Oct. 23, 1929. Operation. Sphere of plaster of Paris placed on the *sella turcica* behind the hypophysis.

Oct. 24. Dog in good condition.

Oct. 30. Operation wound has healed. Animal in excellent condition. It is very lively, eats well, and has slightly increased in weight (0.5 kg.). All the teeth are covered by a thick, brown irremovable coating. The guns around the teeth are slightly loosened.

Nov. 3. The coating on the teeth has increased. On cleaning it from the teeth, it is seen that the enamel is rough and has diminished. In various places papillate growths of epithelium, of the size of a pin's head, have appeared on the mucous membrane of the oral cavity.

Nov. 10. Teeth in the same state. The papillomata on the mucous membrane of the lips and cheeks have in part disappeared, in part, on the contrary, enlarged.

Nov. 20. Papillomata in the oral cavity have disappeared. At the places of some of them, only small light-coloured spots (devoid of pigment) remain. Others have disappeared without leaving any traces. Almost all the teeth are decaying. Some of the incisors of the upper jaw have broken off. The right upper canine has crumbled and is loose. The teeth are of a dark brown colour.

Dec. 1. Destruction of the teeth progresses. The upper incisors continue to crumble and to be worn away. They are destroyed to half their size. The right upper canine is also destroyed. The left is attacked by a carious process over the whole surface of the enamel. All the teeth of the upper and lower jaw are covered by a coating of dark chocolate colour. The general condition of the dog is very good. The dog is lively and eats much and readily. Since the operation it has added about 3 kg. in weight.

Dec. 15. The incisors are worn away to the level of the gum. The remaining teeth are affected by dental stone and a carious process. (Plate 23.)

Dec. 27. The dog was killed by mistake.

On publication of these data, they attracted the attention of some stomatologists who then took part in our investigations with the aim of making the facts more precise and elucidating details.

Professor D. A. Entin [1] carried out a series of observations in our laboratory on 43 dogs (ring or sphere operation). The earliest and most typical symptom here was an affection of the marginal parodont. It was observed in a marked form in 34 cases; in the remainder it was expressed less clearly. The process begins with hæmorrhage of the jaws in the region of the molars and premolars, more rarely of the canines. After lasting 10-15 days, the hæmorrhage diminishes and even disappears altogether. In some cases, however, it is followed by *atrophy or retraction of the gum*, around one tooth or several, either after ulcerous stomatitis or without it. The latter proves that the process of atrophy of the bony edge of the alveolæ *does not depend on*

[1] D. A. Entin. *Arkh. Biol. Nauk*, Vol. 34, No. 4, 1933.

cicatrisation of the gum, but takes place simultaneously under the influence of some cause common to both processes.

Simultaneously with the symptoms of parodontitis and in connection with them, the above-mentioned coating is deposited on the teeth. Microscopical examination showed that the coating consists of blood pigments, salts, desquamated epithelium, salivary bodies, leucocytes and various microbes. As the marginal paradontitis subsides, these deposits also diminish, but sometimes they are so considerable that they cannot be removed except by force, thus being converted into *genuine dental stone.* In some cases this is associated with loosening of the teeth and the formation of purulent lacunæ at their roots, *i.e.,* the development of a general picture *very similar to that known in the human clinic as alveolar pyorrhœa.* Hitherto it has not been possible to produce these effects experimentally except by influences exerted immediately on the mucous membrane of the mouth or on the dentures. The data described present, therefore, so much the greater interest, since they were obtained by a nerve trauma in *a remote region of the organism.*

In the same material, affections of the teeth occurred in 13 out of 43 cases. They consisted in the development of spots, erosions and necrosis of the enamel, and in the teeth becoming fragile and easily rubbed away. These changes sometimes developed very early, in other cases much later (after 5-9 months) and then they were usually accompanied by a relapse of pathological phenomena in the soft tissues. It is interesting to note symmetrical *affections of the teeth of a systematic character.* Thus, in dog No. 331, during 25 days, changes were exhibited in three homologous teeth of both jaws.

Returning to the first experiments of my collaborators Pigalev and Skoblo, it is necessary to make the following addition. Besides the above-described changes in the oral cavity, we observed a number of dystrophic processes in other organs as well.

First of all, one must mention *affection of the eyes* in the form of coniunctivitis, ceratitis and sometimes penetrating ulcers of the cornea. Such changes are met with quite frequently, but by no means invariably. They are the same changes that Magendie and Samuel obtained in rabbits by irritating the Gasserian ganglion, and which we observed in experiments with chemical trauma of the peripheral parts of *n. trigeminus* (Pigalev and Kuznetsova). They made their appearance sometimes very soon after the operation with the glass sphere, even within a few days, sometimes much later—after 1½-2 months. Sometimes they take a violent course and end in the loss of the eye. In other cases, the process is restricted to temporary opacity of the cornea with subsequent recovery. (See Plate 24.)

More than once we observed the *symmetrical character of this process, i.e.,* its development on the cornea of *both* eyes. It is impossible for a variety of reasons to consider that the cause of the ceratitis lies in direct trauma of the nervous system of the eye during the operation. In the first place, we always carried out the operation on the left side, because this is technically more convenient; but the development of ceratitis occurred, *not only in the left eye, but also in the right,* and, according to our material, even somewhat more frequently in the right eye than in the left. In addition, even on the left side, the intra-cranial parts of the trigeminus nerve were never subjected to trauma during the operation. It suffices to cast a glance at the base of the cerebrum of the dog and it will be clear that the place where the sphere is put is more than two cm. away from the place where the *n. trigeminus* leaves the pons. Consequently, the above-described ceratitis, which in the clinic has been given the name of nervous-paralytic ceratitis, *is not connected with paralysis in any way.* It is a typical dystrophy, the more certainly so since it cannot be explained as the consequence of vascular changes. The cornea has no vessels, and it is better to leave the process without explanation than to take refuge in the first that comes to hand.

Besides affections of the eyes, we observed on several occasions *purulent rhinitis and purulent inflammation of the middle ear and of the accessory nasal sinuses.*

Attention was also attracted to phenomena sometimes developing *in the region of the operation wound,* which in all cases was hermetically sewn up. Usually, the stitches were removed on the seventh or eighth day and everything afterwards proceeded normally. But sometimes, without any preceding signs of inflammation, on removing the stitches the operation wound *opened to the maximum extent.* At the bottom of it, the tissues had an unusually fresh appearance as if the cut had been made only the day before and not 7-8 days previously. The absence of any signs of reaction persisted on the following days. Such animals died fairly soon, but in certain cases they survived. Then the operation wound also gradually healed by means of the formation of feeble and pale granulations.

Another form of skin dystrophy consisted in *loss of hair,* the bald spots being often symmetrical and occurring on the head, especially around the eyes, where they produced an appearance as if spectacles had been put on.

Even a hasty review of the changes enumerated demonstrates that they are all situated in the region which almost exactly corresponds to the distribution of the branches of the trigeminus nerve (skin of the face and head, eyes, middle ear and accessory nasal sinuses, mucous membrane of the lips, cheeks, tongue, and of the soft and hard palate, teeth, bones of the jaw, etc.). This naturally aroused the desire *to prevent the development of the above-men-*

tioned dystrophy at particular points of the innervation by means of severing a particular branch of the trigeminus nerve.

The experiments performed for this purpose took several forms. In some cases we carried out the "glass sphere operation" simultaneously with severance of the second branch of the *n. trigeminus* where it leaves the cranium, in others the section of the nerve was delayed for several days, in still others, on the contrary, it preceded the first operation. The result of all these forms was alike: severance of *n. trigeminus not only did not abolish the dystrophic symptoms in the corresponding peripheral region but strongly intensified them.* In any case, this was to be anticipated. Trophic ulcers on the lower extremities developed not only *in spite of* severance of the sciatic nerve, but precisely *as a result of* it. The same thing must be said of our experiments with the injection of croton oil into one of the branches of the trigeminus nerve followed by section of it. Here also the first symptoms of dystrophy were exhibited in tissues corresponding to the innervation of the severed nerve branch.

Some would like to regard this as proof that elements of the central nervous system do not participate in the process of development of tissue dystrophy. Quite recently A. Y. Sozon-Yaroshevich carried out a series of researches into the question of the mechanism of development of trophic ulcers on the extremities of dogs as a result of injury to the sciatic nerve or lateral horns of the spinal cord. In cases where the abdominal sympathetic chain was removed simultaneously on the same side, no development of trophic ulcers was observed. From this he draws the conclusion of a direct connection of trophic disturbances with injury or disease of the nerve parts subjected by him to trauma.

The operation of removing various parts of the sympathetic chain, including the abdominal chain, is constantly being carried out in my laboratory for various reasons. Many of my collaborators have worked with this method (Pigalev, Galkin, Kaminsky, Lebedinskaya and Uspensky). It was found that *removal of the sympathetic ganglia not only does not prevent the development of various forms of tissue dystrophy, but often serves as a reason for it.* It is interesting to note that the operation of severing the *rami communicantes* of the sympathetic chain sometimes results in a more severe form of subsequent dystrophy than the removal of the ganglia (experiments of my collaborators S. I. Lebedinskaya and E. A. Uspensky). This must be interpreted to mean that the section of the above-mentioned nerve produces a double trauma *i.e.,* both in the central and in the sympathetic systems. When the sympathetic ganglia are removed, this removes part of the active elements giving an impulse to further generalisation of the irritation.

The act of operation itself, concomitant with trauma of a large nerve tract, forms the starting point for a dystrophic process within the nervous system, as was pointed out in a number of the examples described above. *The chief factor which has to be taken into account here is time.* The result obtained by Sozon-Yaroshevich did not depend on loss of a special function in consequence of loss of special nerve structures, but on the very fact of removal of elements which take part in the functioning of the complex mechanism. Thereby, some of the links in the general chain of phenomena were destroyed.

In concluding the description of the dystrophic consequences of trauma in the region of the *tuber cinereum* by the glass sphere or ring, it is necessary to dwell on one further series of phenomena which are of constant occurrence and decisive importance for the fate of the animals. I refer to affections of the lungs and gastro-intestinal tract.

The changes in the lungs consist of hæmorrhages. These hæmorrhages occur fairly often. Sometimes entire portions of one or both lungs are perfused by blood to such an extent that they give the impression of liver or, at any rate, of that stage of heavy inflammation of the lungs which is termed "*hepatisatio rubra.*" In cases of early death of the animal, we found this reaction occurring even within some hours after the "glass sphere operation." Inflammatory changes were lacking here; consequently, *inflammation could not have been the cause of the reaction.* On several occasions we observed also that the hæmorrhages did not merely involve one particular portion but were *scattered over the entire, normal rose tissue of both lungs,* like spots on a leopard's skin. (Plate 25.)

Changes of the gastro-intestinal tract are so *constant* and *characteristic* that they were subsequently made the subject of a special investigation carried out by my collaborator I. A. Pigalev.[1] They consisted of hæmorrhages and ulcerations scattered over the mucous membrane of the stomach and other parts of the intestinal canal.

Hæmorrhages in the region of the digestive tract after an injury to the mid- and hind-brain were already well known to the older investigators, but the question has not ceased to be of interest even now. A detailed account of the literature can be found in Hauser's book (*Peptische Schädigungen des Magens und Darmes. Handbuch der speziellen pathologischen Anatomie und Histologie*). During a number of years of work, on many occasions we, too, have observed hæmorrhages in various places of the wall of the digestive canal, *but this is not the point at issue here.* In observing a large number of such cases, we could not help noticing certain characteristic features. The most fundamental of these features is the constancy of form and remarkably stereo-

[1] I. A. Pigalev. *Arkh. Biol. Nauk*, Vol. 32, No. 1, 1932; *Zeitschr. f. d. ges. exp. Med.*, Vol. 82, No. 5-6, 1932.

typed disposition of the pathological changes in definite places of the gastro-intestinal canal. They are expressed the more intensely, the quicker the animal dies after the operation; and in cases of the dog's death during the first few days they acquire a catastrophic character.

With the animals of this group, 5-15 hours after the operation, frequent defecations with admixture of blood were observed, in particular instances forming *real intestinal hæmorrhages*, so that the whole floor of the room was stained with blood. In rare cases *vomiting of blood* occurred. On dissection, we found a liquid mass of blood and mucus in the lumen of the stomach, and small and large intestines, and extensive hæmorrhages in their walls. Consider-able portions of the mucous membrane may be destroyed, or desquamated.

In cases which take a sub-acute course, these changes are correspondingly less expressed, the hæmorrhages are more restricted and then the lesions of the mucous membrane *have the character of genuine ulcers*, penetrating not only into the sub-mucous membrane but also into the muscular part of the wall.

Finally, in the group comprising animals that died long after the time of operation, the same changes acquired a more chronic character and bore marked *traces of a relapsing process*. Along with fresh extravasates and ulcers scattered here and there, we found old ones with signs of inflammatory reac-tion and also whitish scars in the places where defects had healed, brown spots and strips—remains of hæmorrhages that had not yet been completely re-absorbed.

What attracts attention, however, is not the form of the process, but its localisation. The latter is absolutely constant in all cases, independent of whether the disease has taken an acute or chronic course.

In the region of the stomach, the erosions, ulcers and diffuse extravasates are situated mainly in the *pars pylorica*. The changes are encountered much more rarely on the remaining extent of the gastric wall. More than once we noticed between the pylorus and the remaining parts of the stomach a sort of boundary at which the process was sharply interrupted. The process attains its highest intensity in the region of the pylorus itself.

The next place that is very strongly affected is the *duodenum*. Most fre-quently it is altered diffusely and has a purple-red colour, being covered with erosions over a considerable area, although ulcers also occur. These changes do not begin immediately from the pylorus but at a little distance from it. Usu-ally the 1-2 cm. of the intestine that are nearest to the stomach hardly bear any signs of affection, forming a pale strip between the two dark purple areas of the pylorus and duodenum.

Further along the small intestine, the intensity of the changes diminishes and its wall often appears normal for a considerable distance. Close to *where the small intestine passes into the large intestine,* the disorganisation is renewed, although by no means to the same extent as in the duodenum. (Plate 26.)

Suddenly at the place of transition itself, *viz.,* in the region of the *valvula Bauhinii,* all the phenomena are sharply intensified. The lips of the *valvula* are so intensely perfused with blood that they have the appearance of a dark cherry-coloured, or sometimes even black, ring. (Plate 27.)

The mucous membrane of the cæcum is also usually strongly affected, but farther on, along the large intestine the intensity of the affection again falls off, *only to be renewed in the region of the rectum.* (Plate 28.)

It is of interest to note that the hæmorrhages, erosions and ulcers in the rectum are sometimes disposed at the top of the folds of the mucous membrane, exactly as occurs in dysentery. Here also, at the boundary of two contiguous affected zones a narrow strip of mucous membrane of unchanged appearance is frequently left. I already mentioned this phenomenon in describing the boundary between the duodenum and the stomach. The same thing can be seen in the transitional region between the small and large intestines in the neighbourhood of the *valvula Bauhinii* and in the final section of the rectum close to the anus.

Consequently, when changes develop in the region of the gastro-intestinal tract after trauma of the *tuber cinereum,* they always possess a well defined localisation and differ in the separate instances only in degree. They are disposed: 1) in the pyloric part of the stomach; 2) in the duodenum; 3) at the place where the small intestine passes into the large intestine (*valvula Bauhinii, appendix*); 4) in the rectum.

When this had been established on the basis of a large amount of material, we compared the result with that which had been obtained previously in dogs subjected to mechanical trauma of the centripetal end of one of the branches of the trigeminus nerve. The corresponding experiments were once more repeated. It was found that the *consequences in both groups of experiments were absolutely alike.* Injury to the region of the *tuber cinereum* and the above-mentioned form of trauma of the *n. trigeminus* are indistinguishable from one another as regards the character of the dystrophic process. It is true that the intensity of the process is usually different and that it is in general greater after the operation with the sphere. But in the latter case also, the factor of individuality enters, and, consequently, the results can only be compared on the basis of large amounts of material.

On this account doubt may arise whether a *direct connection* actually exists between injury to these nerve structures and the above-described peripheral disturbances.

In the first place, we have to recognise here at least two immediate or direct causes; but even so the question is not fully cleared up. If both causes are direct, then their consequences ought to be as inevitable as the contraction of a muscle on stimulation of the appropriate nerve. But, as a matter of fact, in a number of experiments *neither form of irritation used by us was followed by any dystrophic process in the tissues, or the dystrophic process was only hinted at and rapidly passed away.*

It follows that the processes occurring as the direct consequence of the operation served only as an impulse *for some third process,* which was externally manifested by tissue dystrophy. But in that case we are justified in anticipating that many other forms of nerve irritation also, arising perhaps from very remote points of the nervous system, will produce the same picture of peripheral disturbances. It is only necessary that the appropriate mechanisms should be involved in the orbit of the process developing within the nervous system.

This was fully confirmed by our subsequent work. For the sake of convenience, I shall begin by setting out the experiments of my collaborators G. F. Ivanov [1] and S. I. Halperin,[2] although other facts of the same kind had been obtained previously.

The investigations carried out by G. F. Ivanov were stimulated by the results of the dissection of animals that had died within the first two or three days after the operation with the glass sphere. Besides the changes enumerated above, it was noticed that in such dogs the upper cervical sympathetic ganglia on both sides of the body were often hyperæmised and even swollen. To a lesser degree, the same thing was observed also in the lower ganglia. It was found later that very similar changes, *viz.,* increase in volume and hyperæmia, occur also in the suprarenal glands.

G. F. Ivanov carried out a special investigation in order to obtain a more detailed knowledge of the process occurring. A large number of dogs were operated on (using the sphere or ring) and twelve of them provided material for histological analysis. It was mainly those cases which ended in death within 1-4 days after the operation which were selected for examination, since the microscopical features of the changes were here most pronounced. On dissection, the upper cervical sympathetic ganglia and suprarenal glands were cut out. The sympathetic ganglia were fixed in 10 per cent formalin or absolute alcohol and imbedded in paraffin wax. The sections were stained with hæmatoxylin-eosin, according to van Gieson's or Nissl's method. For comparison, corresponding preparations were made from normal animals.

[1] G. F. Ivanov. *Zeitschr. f. d. ges. exp. Med.,* Vol. 74, Nos. 5, 6, 1930.
[2] S. I. Halperin. *Arkh. Biol. Nauk,* Vol. 33, No. 1-2, 1933; *Zeitschr. f. d. ges. exp. Med.,* Vol. 90, No. 1-2, 1933.

The nerve cells of the first cervical ganglion of a normal dog are large circular structures with a nucleus situated eccentrically and with a deeply staining nucleolus. The cells are unipolar or bipolar and the protoplasm contains Nissl bodies. Around such cells and groups of cells one finds elongated cells with an oval nucleus.

In the preparations taken from our experimental animals, the nerve cells were found to be strongly altered in a way *which testified to their rapid destruction*. Among more or less normal examples were cells of an irregularly polygonal or elongated form. They showed no Nissl granulosity and the nucleus was frequently also lacking. In places, all that remained of the cells was merely a granular disintegrated mass, surrounded by layers of circular or drawn-out elements with elongated nuclei. The protoplasm of the cells was basophilic and frequently contained vacuoles. The pericellular spaces were sometimes expanded to such an extent that the deformed nerve cells represented only a small dark clot in one of the corners of an extensive space. The stroma of the ganglia was loosened in all cases. *In the midst of injured and even destroyed nerve elements, normal ones were also found.* In severe cases there were 10-15 altered cells to each healthy one. In lighter cases, 2-3 cells had suffered out of 8-10 healthy ones. (Plate 29.)

As regards the above-mentioned changes in the suprarenal glands, they consisted of marked lipoidosis of the cells of the cortical layer. In the course of a short period, sometimes not exceeding 8-12 hours, these cells were literally flooded with fat, to the same or an even greater extent than occurs in diphtheria intoxication.

For the time being, we will postpone the question of the suprarenals and return to the first cervical ganglion. The essential thing here is that after trauma of the *tuber cinereum* this ganglion becomes involved in the complex process developing in a latent form within the nervous system. Naturally, this instigated us to find out what form the tissue dystrophy would take *if the elements of the first cervical ganglion were made the point of application of the irritation.* The appropriate investigation was carried out by my collaborator S. I. Halperin. The following are two typical records taken from his work.

Dog No. 57. Bitch. Weight 6 kg.

Dec. 1, 1931. A small quantity of bile (in drops) introduced into the substance of both upper cervical ganglia. Wound sewn up.

Dec. 3. At night. Death.

Result of dissection. Completely symmetrical hæmorrhages occupying the entire lower fractions of both lungs. Hæmorrhages *in the wall of the stomach.* Mucous membrane of the *duodenum* clean. *Valvula Bauhinii* heavily hæmorrhagic, with the appearance of an almost black ring. Hæmorrhages in the submucous membrane of the large intestine, *increasing in the direction of the rectum* which is almost wholly black from hæmorrhage.

Dog No. 81. Bitch.

June 13. About one drop of croton oil injected into the left cervical ganglion.

June 14. Left pupil contracted. *Black coating on teeth,* especially on the canines.

June 26. Ceratitis of the left eye. A deep ulcer, larger than a pin's head, on the external half of the cornea. Hyperæmia and protrusion of the third eyelid.

June 27. Ditto.

June 28. Ditto, but to a still greater extent.

July 1. Left eye suppurating, but ulcer healing. Teeth clean.

July 7. Ulcer almost healed. Mucous membrane of the mouth in normal condition.

Even a fleeting glance at these data will show that they are *absolutely similar to those obtained as a result of direct trauma of the tuber cinereum.* Three different lesions, *viz.,* a contact sore on the *tuber cinereum,* chemical trauma of the first cervical ganglion, and similar trauma along the course of one of the branches of the *n. trigeminus* produced the same picture of dystrophic disorganisation in the peripheral tissues. Knowing that this disorganisation only reflects another process proceeding within the nervous system, we are justified in asserting that this latter process *was approximately the same in all the cases.*

The idea of the subsequent series of investigations was as follows. It has already been shown that the constant result of trauma of the nerve structures enumerated consists in affection of the organs of the oral cavity, and in particular of the teeth. It was of interest to determine the form that the dystrophic process would take *if it was initiated by irritation applied directly to the nerve apparatus of a normal tooth.*

For this purpose, my collaborator P. N. Kartashov, together with L. M. Matveyeva,[1] at first in my laboratory and later in the laboratory of the stomatological clinic of Saratov University, carried out a series of special experiments on dogs and rabbits. The basic data were obtained with dogs, since with these animals the general picture of the dystrophic phenomena is richer and develops more consistently and regularly.

In all, over 30 dogs were experimented on. The method consisted in trepanning one or two teeth, most usually a canine and a molar, under narcosis. Into the pulp cavity was inserted a piece of cotton-wool dipped in croton oil or formalin, or some arsenic paste such as is usually employed in dentistry. The opening was sealed externally by quickly solidifying cement. Immediately after the operation, and also on one of the following days, the cerebrospinal fluid was extracted. This procedure was not further repeated since young dogs (puppies) often die as a result of repeated extraction of the fluid.

Adult dogs are much more indifferent to this operation, but in order to

[1] P. N. Kartashov and L. M. Matveyeva. *Arkh. Biol. Nauk,* Vol. 34, No. 4, 1933.

secure comparative results it was desirable to conduct all the experiments under the same conditions. *Not to use young dogs and to carry out the whole work with adult ones was also undesirable, since dystrophic phenomena develop in the former much more rapidly and proceed more intensely.* Control animals were selected as usual; in experiments with puppies they were of the same age as the animals experimented on. Wherever possible, animals from the same litter were used as controls. Trepanning of the corresponding tooth (or two teeth) was also carried out in their case under narcosis, but only cotton-wool dipped in physiological solution was inserted into the pulp and sealed with cement. The cerebro-spinal fluid was extracted from the controls at the same time as from the experimental animals.

The consequences of these operations deserve attention because in them one can clearly trace *the difference between two processes commencing simultaneously.*

One is the reaction of the tissues in the region where the irritating agent is applied. The other is the result of the neuro-dystrophic process which is only historically connected with the irritating agent, or, more accurately, with the point of primary irritation.

The local symptoms are an inflammatory reaction, localised in the immediate neighbourhood of the tooth and consisting of intumescence of the gums, with reddening and local hæmorrhage of the parodont. The tooth gradually becomes loose and sometimes falls out. Subsequently, even the puppies remain externally healthy for one or two months. In adult animals the period may be longer.

One further detail needs to be mentioned regarding the form of the local reaction. With the use of croton oil and formalin, the local changes are usually confined to the limits of the tooth taken for the experiment. If, however, arsenic paste is used instead of croton oil, then, even if inserted into only one tooth, the neighbouring teeth inevitably suffer also, sometimes even all the teeth on the corresponding side and the bony part of the jaw itself.

The conclusion would seem to be inevitable that arsenic is a much stronger irritating agent than either formalin or croton oil; *but the study of the remote consequences of the same methods of interference creates an exactly contrary impression.* In spite of the small local effect of formalin or croton oil, *severe general dystrophy is the rule in their case;* only it does not come about all at once but after a comparatively long period of apparent health. On the other hand, the same experiment using arsenic paste, which produces a greater affection of the denture and jaw in the neighbourhood of the trepanned tooth, *is much more rarely accompanied by subsequent extensive dystrophy.*

We have already encountered and analysed such facts. It is easy to understand them if it is borne in mind that the degree and duration of the irritation is above all bound up with vital processes in the elements concerned. If the irritating agent simply destroys the tissues at the place of its application, then the whole process is limited to this. That is why, in studying the morphological results of chemical trauma of the spinal nerve, it was found that the application of weak solutions of formalin was more effective than strong ones. Approximately the same thing holds good here. In a number of instances, P. N. Kartashov *extracted the tooth, together with the croton oil or formalin contained in it*, after a certain period, but *without waiting for the generalisation of the dystrophic phenomena to begin. This did not save the animal from subsequent extensive dystrophy, and did not even weaken the intensity of the latter*. Hence the process was not connected with continuing irritation of a "croton oil" or "formalin" character, but depended on other causes.

It was pointed out above, that after the liquidation of the local reaction, the animals remained externally healthy for a period of 1-2 months or more. In these cases also, the first sign of the generalisation of the dystrophic process consisted always of those same changes which we have observed so many times: *viz.*, hæmorrhage of the gums, coating on the teeth, ulceration of the mucous membrane of the mouth, and sometimes papillomata, conjunctivitis, ceratitis, etc. The animal loses its appetite and becomes limp and apathetic. Very soon diarrhœa with admixture of blood begins to occur with sharp loss of reactivity, followed by paralysis and death. In other cases, however, all these changes are gradually wiped out, but only to be renewed soon afterwards. In short, *even in the details of its history it is impossible to find a difference between this process and those previously observed by us*. On post-mortem dissection of the dogs, the fundamental affections were found to be localised in the lungs and gastro-intestinal canal. Entire lobes of the lungs were sometimes hæmorrhagic, producing the impression of lobar pneumonia in the stage of *hepatisatio rubra*. In other cases, the pulmonary hæmorrhages were scattered over the whole surface. In the gastro-intestinal tract also the changes were a repetition of those already familiar. They consisted of hyperæmia and hæmorrhages in the pylorus, *duodenum, valvula Bauhinii* with its adjacent parts and, finally, in the rectum. The remaining parts of the intestinal canal either remained normal or were less affected. In those cases where death ensued as the result of a rhythmic development of the disease, traces of old changes were always to be found side by side with new ones. The control animals remained healthy throughout the whole period.

In later experiments, Kartashov was able to observe some further interesting details. He inserted diphtheria and tetanus toxin into the pulp cavity of the tooth in place of croton oil. Controls were organised as usual. The toxin was always given in much less than fatal doses. On injection into other tissues or into the blood such doses would not have produced disease, much less death.

The inclusion of these toxins in the pulp cavity also did not produce disease. *Nevertheless, many animals died after a shorter or longer period, exhibiting typical dystrophy such as has been already repeatedly described.* At the beginning it was sometimes possible to observe signs of a specific reaction. Thus, in two cases with tetanus toxin (dry preparation), P. N. Kartashov observed initial symptoms of local tetanus in the masticatory muscles in the form of trism. The latter persisted for a short time and ended in recovery. After some time, however, both these dogs became ill and died, after exhibiting the whole picture of the extensive dystrophic process with which we are already familiar.

In the preceding chapter, when describing the experiments of my collaborator S. D. Kaminsky, I pointed out that the penetration of tetanus toxin into the tissues gives rise, not merely to a special form of irritation, but also to ordinary nerve trauma, and that the general result is the sum of these two processes. *The example which has just been described is yet another illustration of the same thesis.*

Under the usual conditions of laboratory practice, we study reactions to specific substances but we do not come across processes belonging to the second group. We use large doses so as to obtain the specific effect. In a day or two the animal falls ill; in another day or two, it dies. *The latent period of the processes belonging to the second category is considerably longer*; hence they only become accessible to observation when the specific substance is used in small doses. But, on using a small dose of the substance and not obtaining the special reaction as a result, we become convinced that the process is ended; whatever consequences develop are not connected by us causally with the original operation. Only in those cases where living organisms are selected as the irritating agent, *e.g.*, *Spirochæta pallida,* we admit that the latent period can last for some weeks; to understand the process taking place in those cases, refuge is taken in the rather nebulous conception of struggle between two living factors, the micro-organism and the macro-organism. *But as far as chemical substances are concerned, the latent period of 1-2 months has hitherto been simply unknown.* Consequently, the reaction here described is *a form of relation previously unknown which has up to now never been taken into account.* It is not a response to irritation by a particular substance, and is not connected with any particular properties of the latter.

The general features of this process are now known to us. We must emphasise, in addition, the capacity of the process *for developing at varying rates.* The magnitude of its latent period depends not only on the strength of the irritation, but also *on the sensitivity of the reacting substratum.* With the glass sphere operation or injection of croton oil into the upper cervical ganglion, the latent period of the process is in general considerably shorter than on irritation of the nerve elements of the pulp cavity of the tooth. But even if we take only one of these methods, *e.g.*, the operation with the glass sphere, and compare individual cases, we will see that the material presents a very diverse aspect. In some cases, the latent period lasts 5-10 hours, in others—many weeks. The same thing applies also for each of the other methods enumerated. Yet all this finds no reflection in the form of the process itself, which remains standard, as if predetermined, and varies only in intensity.

More than once, while carrying out diverse kinds of experiments, we observed exactly the same consequences following other forms of operation on the nervous system, *e.g.*, on removing the abdominal sympathetic chain, especially if the operation is carried out by an inexperienced worker and consequently accompanied by excessive trauma. The same thing was also observed sometimes after experiments associated with trauma of the spinal cord or cerebrum, or even of the sciatic nerve.

A typical picture of generalised dystrophy after trauma of the sciatic nerves was noted several times in experiments performed by my collaborator I. A. Pigalev. As soon as the process took on an extensive character, changes appeared *in the oral and nasal cavities, in the lungs and at the usual places in the gastro-intestinal tract.* These consequences, however, were by no means so constant as after trauma of the *tuber cinereum,* the upper cervical ganglion or branches of the *n. trigeminus.* But they are interesting in another respect. They once more confirm the thesis that *any portion of the nervous system can become the starting point for processes of a neuro-trophic character.* Moreover, it must be mentioned that with certain changes in technique it is fairly easy to obtain a marked increase in the percentage of cases where the dystrophic process, starting from the sciatic nerve, passes into the standard form of extensive dystrophy. Thus, another of my collaborators, V. S. Galkin, obtained this result *by replacing croton oil by an emulsion of normal brain, which was introduced into the centripetal end of the severed nerve of a dog.* His observations include crateriform ulcers of the stomach with calloused edges—typical "round ulcers," piercing almost all the layers of the gastric wall. In other cases he noted hæmorrhage of the gums, and along the course of the gastro-intestinal tract ulceration in the oral cavity, etc. It is interesting that even when the emulsion is prepared from the brain of an animal of the same species, the dystrophic consequences of its introduction, both in the region of the corresponding segment and outside the limits of the latter, is frequently expressed even more intensely than on using croton oil.

Facts of this nature must be well borne in mind. It is impossible to decide the question of the harmfulness or non-harmfulness of a particular substance merely on the basis of data on the direct effects or immediate consequences. The strength of the irritating agent is the degree of irritation; and *the degree of irritation is the sum of many processes developing one after another, and they must all be taken into account to the end, i.e.,* to the moment of actual extinction of all the phenomena. Then it may prove that *the harmfulness of an irritating agent, the original action of which is weak, is in the long run not less and may possibly even be greater than that of a strong one.*

Having constantly before our eyes the previously described changes in the gastro-intestinal tract, we cannot help becoming interested also in other pathological processes in which gastro-intestinal hæmorrhages are observed, but which have not been considered dependent on influences of a neuro-trophic character. I am not referring here to operations on the nervous system of the visceral organs themselves, such as, for example, section or cauterisation of the *n. vagus* close to the stomach (Zironis), injury to the suprarenals with their complex innervation (Finzi), trauma of the organs themselves, of the *n. splanchnicus* (Pazenkov), or of separate sympathetic ganglia and plexuses. Such operations are often accompanied by hæmorrhages and ulceration in the gastric wall, but these facts have been well known for a long time, although hitherto they also have had no real explanation. Much greater attention is merited by other processes, *whose cause lies in so-called general intoxication e.g.,* by the salts of the heavy metals—sublimate, lead, antimony—and also by infectional processes such as rabies.

The origin of gastro-intestinal hæmorrhage and ulceration in intoxication is usually connected with the paths of excretion from the organism of the salts of the heavy metals, which takes place through the intestinal walls. As the result of the particular substance accumulating here, it is supposed that it produces a direct effect on the tissues.

An attempt has been made to explain affections of the gastro-intestinal tract in the street form of rabies by aid of the same mechanism. With this aim in view, Puntoni made a search for the virus in the gastro-intestinal canal of animals that had died from rabies, and actually discovered it there.

We made it our task to study the *form and distribution of these changes in different parts of the digestive canal.* My collaborator, I. A. Pigalev, made a large number of investigations of this sort. He poisoned dogs through the blood by various doses of salts of heavy metals (mercury, lead, antimony) and dissected the animals after death. It was found that hæmorrhages in the substance of the mucous membrane, erosions and ulcers were disposed *in exactly the same places as after the operation with the glass sphere, chemical trauma of the first cervical ganglion, etc.* In more severe cases, the mucous membrane was affected throughout the extent of the digestive canal, but even then the degree of alteration was greater in the usual places. In cases of average severity, we always found corresponding changes in the oral cavity, pyloric part of the stomach, *duodenum, valvula Bauhinii,* appendix and rectum. If the alterations did not occur in all the places enumerated at once, they were invariably found on some of them, *e.g.*, in the mouth, stomach and rectum, or in the *valvula Bauhinii* and rectum, and so on. *It was impossible to distinguish the process either macroscopically or microscopically, from that previously observed by us.* One can, of course, describe each of these separately as gastritis, colitis, or bauhiniitis, but this can hardly be said to facilitate in any way an understanding of the essential nature of the processes taking place. (Plate 30.)

Exactly similar data were obtained on dissection of bodies of dogs that had died from the street form of rabies. Subsequently, I. A. Pigalev tried introducing into the circulatory system of dogs other viruses, non-pathogenic for these animals, but in doses which caused death (*b. typhi* or *b. coli*). Both live and dead cultures were used. In such cases, the disease also found expression in general weakness of the animal, hyperæmia and hæmorrhage of the gums, and liquid stools with admixture of blood. On dissection, changes were discovered in the oral cavity, lungs and gastro-intestinal canal. *In form and disposition, the changes could not be distinguished from those described above.* (Plates 31, 32.) Weighing up all the material mentioned, it is difficult to suppose special peculiarities in the mechanism of origin of each case. *This mechanism is a nervous mechanism, and the changes in the organs are indirect.*

In elucidating the genesis of changes in organs topographically remote from the point of primary irritation, the question naturally arises of the possibility of the biological or chemical irritating agent being transported from the region of the primary focus by the blood and lymph. In this case, the affection of the tissue elements in the remote parts would also be direct. In deciding the question however, it is essential to take the whole complex of conditions into account and not merely the fact that a foreign agent is found within the focus; otherwise it is easy to fall into error. The irritating agent by no means always appears in the region of the secondary focus as a result of its passive transport; it can be retained at the point of entry owing to mechanical causes (embolism, valvular and filtering systems of the organism). We are now well acquainted with the fact that a particular irritating agent often "selects" secondary foci in the organism. To explain the selective character of these affections and the fact that not all tissues were altered to the same degree, the theory of "tropism" was put forward—the theory of a special sensitivity or affinity of definite organs and whole systems for definite irritants.

The capacity of many tissue elements to take up and retain foreign particles that have penetrated into the organism is not constant. The process is strongly intensified in regions of inflammatory and generally altered foci. When such a focus is formed anywhere, then not only chemically active but also absolutely indifferent substances, *e.g.*, India ink, will be taken up and deposited precisely at the spot. Hence, *we have the right to speak of selectivity or affinity only when we are convinced that at the moment of entry of the irritating agent into the tissues, the latter are absolutely normal.* In many cases, the presence of a foreign substance is no evidence of its active role, for its appearance here may be a secondary effect. It is possible that in this case the development of the local process is aggravated; but this is quite another question, relating *to the course of the phenomenon and not to its origin.*

What are the conclusions that must be drawn?

In the first place, it is necessary to recognise at least the role of the nervous system as the organiser of peripheral pathological foci, since the order in which organs and tissues are affected is often merely the reflection of the dystrophic process proceeding within the nervous system.

As already mentioned more than once, the study of the matter from this point of view showed us that the incubational or latent period is one in which the process develops in a hidden form within the nervous system. *In judging the genesis of local pathological foci, this is the first thing that must be taken into account.* If a more or less considerable period elapses between the moment when the foreign agent penetrates into the tissues, and the occurrence of the reaction, this alone is sufficient to cast doubt on the immediate nature of the tissue reaction and on its direct connection with the irritating agent.

The generalisation of the dystrophic process begins with a segmentary affection of the nervous system (of its central and autonomous parts). At this stage, the dystrophic reactions in the tissue can still be distinguished from one another by the place where the process began.

At the next stage, we find that the process has already passed beyond the limits of the injured segment. This action also is not of an arbitrary character, but it is much less closely connected with the point of the initial affection, and it has its constant or "standard" form.

At the next stage, we find that the process has already passed beyond the first moment of their origin, do not occur arbitrarily, but in certain systematic and constant forms. A particular final result depends to a considerable extent on the magnitude of the original irritation.

It must not be forgotten, however, that an easy transition to generalised dystrophy is obtained only in the experimental conditions employed by us. These conditions are, of course, exaggerated and therefore unsuitable for studying the physiological stage of this process; we adhered to them only because we had no alternative.

Moreover, our immediate interest was centred precisely in an analysis of nervous dystrophy, in estimating its role in the genesis of various pathological processes. But even under these conditions, it was by no means always possible to obtain a uniform level of development in the picture of the dystrophic symptoms. *The quantitative aspect varied within wide limits.* Even though we used the same technique and made a careful selection of animals, etc., some animals died within a few hours, others remained outwardly healthy for months and even years.

On summarising the results of a large number of observations, it was found that the whole material could be divided into the following six groups:

1. In animals of the first group, dystrophic disturbances at once take a progressive course and acquire catastrophic rapidity with a fatal outcome in the hours immediately following the experiment.

2. The second group contains animals in which the same phenomena last longer and end in death after 7-10 days.

3. In the third group, the initial symptoms agree with those observed in the two preceding groups. Subsequently, they gradually subside and are not renewed; after many weeks and months the animals are still to all appearance healthy.

4. The fourth group of animals is allied to the third in that here also the initial symptoms, after lasting a certain time, disappear. Later on, however, without any kind of new external influence, the symptoms reappear in the old places. This process can take place rhythmically, being repeated several times in one form or another. Sooner or later, the animals die.

5. In the fifth group, our introductory operations were not followed by any dystrophic process in the tissues. At first sight, the animals seemed to have remained healthy. However, in the majority of cases they proved unsuitable for any further chronic experiments, since they easily perished as a result. In the development of the new disease, derangements were always exhibited by them and in precisely the same form and at the same places where these derangements ought to have occurred as the result of the first experiment.

6. Finally, one further group could be diagnosed. These animals have the highest power of resistance to generalisation of the dystrophic process. Like the animals of the fifth group, they do not respond to the "first blow" to the nervous system; but in addition they withstand subsequent operations in approximately the same way as normal animals.

However diverse the results as shown by the groups of the list given, it is easy to prove that the difference *is an indicator merely of degree and not of form.* The cause of quantitative variations of the process lies in the individual properties of the animal experimented on, properties made up of many ingredients which at the present time are still not susceptible of objective analysis.

We can count on obtaining a constant effect only when studying more elementary reactions, such, for instance, as contraction of a muscle separated from the organism, secretion of an isolated gland, etc.; whereas in studying the same reactions within the organism we are dealing with one of the fundamental properties of the nerve cell—the property of summation. *The higher we go up the ladder of complication of reflexes, the greater the difference will be.*

This becomes especially clear in the case of higher nervous activity. The complexity of conditioned reflexes and the variability of the neural combinations composing them have the result that the effect of one and the same irritation can be different, both in quantity and in quality. The results of experiments, after the most accurate equalisation of all external conditions, are here often so variable, that in order to systematise them it has been necessary to create a *whole theory of types of nervous constitution in dogs* (I. P. Pavlov). Only then could the material be arranged in proper order.

The analysis of neuro-trophic phenomena has also led us to recognise the need for introducing appropriate subdivision, in view of the exceptional complexity and mobility of nerve combinations.

The normal nervous function naturally ceases with the cessation of the cause that has evoked it. A pathological process of the same category *can itself become its own cause,* and in its progressive development draws strength from itself. It is capable of subsiding, but after a certain period, when it is apparently entirely extinct it may reappear without any new instigation on our part. The general picture is usually a repetition of what occurred the first time, since the changes reappear at the old places and in the old form. After a certain time has elapsed, they disappear again. In some cases, the relapse in the places previously affected is followed by general dystrophy and death. It is clear that the disappearance of pathological symptoms after the first trauma was no proof of the complete restoration of the nerve elements that had suffered. It is evident that *a new pathological focus had been created in the nervous system.* The fact that we are not always able to connect the relapse with a new external influence does not mean that there was no such influence. I have already brought forward data relating to the cause of trophic ulcers in the human clinic. Pulmonary grippe during the post-operation period was here one occasion for relapse. There is no doubt that some little-noticed influence operated in the case of our animals.

This led us to suspect that those animals which do not respond to nerve trauma by the obvious development of dystrophy cannot be considered normal. A number of observations confirmed this. A series of special experiments were then organised *with the object of elucidating the nature of the phenomenon known in the clinic as "predisposition"* (experiments of my collaborators A. A. Vishnevsky and K. P. Golysheva [1]).

The material for the experiments consisted of dogs that had already undergone nerve trauma without any special consequences, or had fully recovered their health after a short period of illness. We kept such animals under observation for a long time, and then took them for a new experiment. For the second nerve trauma (the second "blow") a nerve region was selected which was topographically remote and not directly connected with the place of the first trauma (the first "blow"). In some cases, the first blow was inflicted in a region of the central nervous system (operation with the glass sphere or ring, introduction of chemical substances into the upper cervical ganglion), in others the experiment began with chemical and mechanical trauma of one of the spinal nerves. The second blow was also inflicted on various parts of the central and peripheral nervous system.

In the majority of cases, *typical dystrophic symptoms developed even within a short period after the second blow and precisely in those places where they had appeared before or where they ought to have appeared as a result of the first blow.* Thus, if the first blow had been the glass sphere operation, then the introduction of a drop of croton oil under the nail of one of the toes of the forepaw was sufficient to produce the development of stomatitis, papillomata in the oral cavity, ulcerous ceratitis, typical hæmorrhages in the gastrointestinal tract, etc. On the other hand, if the first blow was trauma of the sciatic nerve, then the operation with the glass sphere produced a renewal of ulceration in the old scars on the hind extremities. In this case, of course, changes typical of the glass sphere operation appeared as well, but the affection of the extremities sometimes even preceded them. During several years' work we made a large number of such observations. All my collaborators repeatedly met with such cases.

This fact must therefore be considered as firmly established. Its interpretation cannot cause any special difficulty. The physiology of the nervous system is acquainted with examples of a similar kind, although in other spheres of investigation. I. P. Pavlov's works on the cerebral cortex in dogs, and later those of A. A. Ukhtomsky on other nerve structures, have shown that a cell, when in a state of excitation, "attracts" excitations arising in any other part of the nervous system. At the present time a large number of facts of this sort

[1] A. A. Vishnevsky and K. P. Golysheva. *Arkh. Biol. Nauk*, Vol. 33, No. 1-2, 1933; *Zeitschr. f. d. ges. exp. Med.*, Vol. 89, No. 1-2, 1933.

have become known. They caused Professor A. A. Ukhtomsky to develop the theory of so-called "dominants." Magnus, studying postural reflexes, came to the same conclusion from a somewhat different aspect. He observed cases when a definite postural reflex evoked by a definite stimulus is for some reason inhibited. If now the animal comes under a new stimulus normally producing an entirely different motor reaction, the effect will be, not the reaction typical of this new stimulus, but the first reaction which for some reason had been inhibited. The first stimulus produced no visible effects, but the nervous system retained traces of it, or, according to Magnus's terminology, it acquired a "readiness" for the reaction. In our experiments, we have a *fourth variety of nervous activity; this activity is peculiar in function and purpose, but takes place under the same conditions as the first three, viz.,* the "conditioned reflex," the "dominant," the "readiness" of Magnus. This demonstrates once again that *not only the basic principles of construction of the nervous system, but even the details of the functioning of its various parts, have much in common and are linked by a common plan.*

The dystrophic process arising within the nervous system is capable sometimes of subsiding completely without leaving lasting traces behind it. Sometimes, however, it is preserved in a latent form, and then the application of any new stimulus may call it into life. In the peripheral tissues, there will be a reproduction of the reaction, corresponding in dimensions and form to the process which had already taken place there. We may encounter in this way vascular phenomena (œdema), or inflammatory phenomena (ceratitis), destructions (noma, gangrene, ulcer), new formations (papillomata), that is to say, in the final analysis, *all the forms of local pathological processes known to us.* Acquaintance with this category of phenomena turns upside down all the old conceptions of the genesis of local pathological processes, shatters a number of the notions created by cellular pathology, and casts doubt on the actual value of classifying diseases according to the organs and systems of the body. As a matter of fact who would have believed, even recently, *that it is possible to blind a dog by acting upon the sciatic nerve or to kill an animal through the pulp cavity of the tooth,* producing intestinal hæmorrhage by means of one drop of formalin, two or three months *after not only the formalin, but the tooth itself had been removed.* Undoubtedly, this also strikes a blow at the standing conception of the so-called ætiology of diseases. Scores of extremely diverse irritations, applied at various points of the organism, may in the final result bring about the same consequences. On the other hand, externally identical influences may turn out to produce differing results. We observed this in all our experiments with a second nerve blow. Trauma of the sciatic nerve sometimes produces trophic ulcers of the hind extremities and sometimes papillomatosis of the mucous membrane of the mouth. The operation with the glass sphere acts approximately in the same way. If we had not known in advance the history of each of our animals, the effects produced might have seemed chaotic and fortuitous.

We are now coming to the question of qualitative variations of nervous dystrophy. The study of these variations is possible either when the primary irritation is comparatively weak, or when the nervous system of the animal employed in the experiment is more than usually stable. If the process has gone beyond the limits of definite nerve groups and definite nerve combinations, then its generalisation proceeds in standard forms. With weaker degrees of the process, the individual peculiarities of the given nervous system have an opportunity to manifest themselves. These individual peculiarities can be compared with a multitude of nodes scattered throughout a complex network, where all the parts are joined so as to form a unity. *Each new node that is added to this plexus alters the tonus of separate parts and of the whole network.* The formation of the nodes is bound up with an endless number of causes and the presence of every node in the network may be temporary or permanent. They may not become manifest during a long period, and afterwards find expression in a sudden deviation from the usual reaction. To foresee these deviations even in part, it is necessary to know *the history of each individual nervous system.* This is the reason why in our experiments we are of late feeling more and more the *difficulty of choosing suitable animals as controls.* Here we have a concrete application of the motto of the great physicians of the past: *"There are no illnesses, there are only ill people."*

QUALITATIVE VARIATIONS OF NERVOUS DYSTROPHY

CHAPTER XVII

ACUTE IRRITATION (INFLAMMATION)

OUR subsequent work in studying neuro-dystrophic processes was determined by the three following propositions:

1. For the development of dystrophic symptoms in the nervous system, it is not essential that the point of primary irritation should be a nerve trunk or nerve ganglion. The changes produced in the nervous system by the irritation of nerve-endings within the peripheral tissues (skin, cellular tissue, muscles, etc.) can be quite as severe as those due to the direct injury of complex nerve structures.

2. The form of development of dystrophc processes wthin the nervous system is not fundamentally dependent on whether a purely chemical irritating agent or a biological (infectional) one is employed.

3. At any point of the nervous system, a process can commence which finally results in the phenomena of general dystrophy in their standard forms.

The last sentence must not be taken to mean that the point of primary irritation has no influence on the form of development of the dystrophic process. We have repeatedly seen that the process often begins segmentarily, *i.e.*, *during the first stages, at least, its form is definitely connected with its starting point.* The inclusion of other nerve tracts also takes place by stages. The greater the irritation, the more difficult it is to trace any order in the course of its development; but this by no means signifies that there is no such order.

It is clear from this that, if we endeavour to study *the whole course of the process and not only its starting point and final result,* we must adhere to a technique involving only weak forms of irritation. This instigated us to experiment with biological agents, in particular with some varieties of pathogenic microbes. At the same time, another aim was also kept in view here, *viz.,* the solution of the old controversy *concerning the role of the nervous system in the process of inflammation.*

This question arose simultaneously with the general question of the trophic function of the nervous system and was decided along with other problems in the general course of our work. Hence its history repeats all the stages of our work on our main subject. Moreover, from the time of the creation of cellular pathology, investigators have chiefly devoted their attention to the study of tissue elements and the forms and dimensions of their inherent reactions. The part played in these phenomena by the nervous system was ignored or even categorically denied. But the reality of experimental evidence does not tolerate the asseverations of arm-chair science, and the clinic is raising anew the question of the role of the nervous system in the process of inflammation.

In 1906, Spiess drew attention to the fact that the use of anæsthetics in some cases of acute inflammation not only alleviates the course of the process, but sometimes interrupts or prevents it. He regarded the reflex nerve impulse preceding inflammation as the basic factor. According to his observations, removal of this primary factor altered the whole character of the subsequent inflammation. Spiess's observations have been confirmed by other investigators.

Subsequently, in 1921, the work of Laqueur and Magnus appeared, dealing with the consequences of phosgene poisoning in cats. In the action of phosgene, the most serious changes are observed in the lungs. Preliminary severance of the vagus nerves in the neck either entirely averts these changes or very considerably diminishes them.

At the same time, A. G. Molotkov published a number of clinical observations on the history of certain inflammatory processes after severance of the corresponding nerves. On the basis of his material, he arrived at the conclusion of the prime significance of the nervous system in the genesis of these processes.

Shortly afterwards (1924), however, Shimura carried out a large number of experiments which provided evidence that the inflammatory process develops in the same way in denervated as in normal tissues. From this he drew the conclusion that all the features constituting inflammation are the independent response of the tissues themselves to immediate contact with the irritating agent. The same opinion is held by Lubarsch, from whose laboratory Shimura's work was issued.

An energetic protest against this was uttered by Ricker who pointed out that in the intact organism the inflammatory process ought not to develop exactly in the same way as in denervated tissues. Along with a critical summary of previous data, Ricker brings forward experimental material, mainly his observations from practice as a pathological anatomist. Ricker's work has been subjected to criticism. This was an easy task for his opponents, in view of the abstract way in which his views were expounded; but it was *absolutely unjustifiable from the point of view of unbiassed valuation of his data*. The attacks against Ricker are the more incomprehensible as his ideas were very modest and did not go beyond the recognition of the "play of vaso-motors" as an action preceding the development of local pathological processes.

It is a curious fact that even such ideas still encounter resistance!

At the present time, I repeat, things have become more tranquil on this front, but it is not because the question of the role of the nervous system in the process of inflammation has actually been settled. Even now, the local inflammatory focus is looked upon as something independent, governed by its own separate laws; even now, the process of inflammation is explained as a result of the capacity of local tissue elements to react directly to the irritating agent. Altogether, the question of the role of the nervous system in inflammation is so unpopular that, for example, *the chapter on inflammation in textbooks simply passes it over in silence.*

As far as purely scientific articles are concerned, they also treat the question timidly. The nervous component of the inflammatory reaction is admitted *as an auxiliary factor* capable of exerting an influence indirectly, and only on the course of the inflammation, but not by any means on its genesis.

Until recently, moreover, formalism has also prevailed in regard to methods of work. The basic task has been the study of inflammation in denervated tissues. A great deal of labour has been expanded on this, and in general without result, since neither interruption of spinal or sympathetic paths, nor extirpation of nerve ganglia is able entirely to remove nerve elements and nerve influences in the tissues. These influences can be partly exerted along the neuro-humoral path and also through local axon-reflexes (Langley), as has already been established for inflammatory processes in a number of works of Brücke, Alpern and others.

In our experiments, we approached the subject from another aspect. While pursuing the aim of studying the role played by the nervous system in the development and history of inflammation, we at the same time began to investigate *the role played by inflammation in the functioning and state of the nervous system.*

In a complex organism, influences are reciprocal. Moreover, inflammation as such is not a constant phenomenon. We have here a manifold mobile substratum, and the factor of time, in the course of which the process continuously changes. During this time, a series of different events connected in some way with one another, take place both in proximity to and far away from the local focus. By analysing both aspects of the phenomenon, we could expect to observe what had been previously concealed.

At one period, we attempted to carry on this work just as all the others had done, in particular Shimura. The method consisted in attempts to exclude from a definite region the possibility of nerve action on the inflammatory process. The results of the experiments, in their external aspects, were closely analogous to the results obtained by Shimura; for us, however, they did not represent a categorical solution of the problem.

We have seen that the inflammatory process in the tissues evokes dystrophic symptoms within the nervous system *and by means of them returns to the periphery in the form of various sorts of local changes.* These reflected processes are often symmetrical, but they may be situated also outside the limits of the segment primarily affected. *The basic cause for their formation is the destruction of normal nerve conditions in a definite tissue region, connected by a chain of nerve links with the originator of the whole process, i.e., with the primary focus.* It is evident from this that even in the primary inflammatory focus only the first steps can be looked upon as the immediate result of the encounter of the tissues with the foreign agent. After a short time, the direct action of the irritating agent itself *is supplemented by an additional factor of irritation on the part of the corresponding nerve structures.*

From this moment, the general picture and history of the primary process itself ceases to be confined within the bounds of local conditions and partial laws, and it is absolutely unknown which of the two basic components of the irritation will gain the upper hand at any particular moment.

By bringing in this way the inflammatory process and nervous dystrophy into close relation with one another by means of the nervous component, we obtained a new field for experiment and had a justification for employing pathogenic micro-organisms to excite, not only inflammatory symptoms, but also neuro-dystrophic processes. In the new form of work, the microbes as irritating agents have the further advantage over chemical and physical agents that they are not so easily washed out of the tissues.

Selecting the microbe irritants according to the degree of their virulence, we hoped also to prolong the neuro-dystrophic process and thereby to obtain a more detailed idea of its development.

In making it our aim to elucidate some details concerning the influence of the place of primary irritation on the form of development of the neuro-dystrophic process, we naturally turned back to our previous observations.

In the first instance, we must refer to the *changes occurring at definite points of the gastro-intestinal tract.* In the experiments described above, these points were the result of a secondary action—the result of a process that had begun in an entirely different region. *Now, however, we decided to make them the point of primary irritation.*

The appropriate experiments were performed by my collaborators, first by P. V. Manenkov and subsequently by I. A. Pigalev. The animals used were rabbits. As irritating agents, we used various stocks of staphylococcus in doses which did not produce death when introduced into the blood.

Dr. Manenkov's experiments [1] were as follows. Two normal rabbits were subjected to laparotomy. In one of them, staphylococcus was injected under the serosa of the stomach, in the other (control) animal, the same dose of the microbe was introduced under the serosa of the large intestine approximately at the middle of its length, *i.e. remote from the cæcum and rectum.* After this the operation wound was sewn up.

The result showed that all the rabbits inoculated in the gastric wall perished within a period of 8-16 hours. Of the rabbits inoculated at the same time in the wall of the large intestine, many remained alive, while others survived the first group by a period of several days. Yet another interesting circumstance was noted in the experiment: on dissecting the rabbits inoculated in the gastric wall, the inflammatory changes were found not only in the region where the virus was injected, but *throughout the stomach.* Besides this, symptoms of general peritonitis were always present, in the form of blood-serous and even purulent exudation and hyperæmia of the vessels of other visceral organs. Purulent inflammation had previously been rarely noted, for the animals died before it could develop.

On dissecting the control rabbits which had died after inoculation in the wall of the large intestine, symptoms of general peritonitis were found *very rarely,* so that the official cause of death here must be regarded not as peritonitis, but sepsis. More than this, the local reaction at the points on the large intestine where the virus was introduced was always *sharply defined.* If the rabbit died within the first two days, then swelling and redness could be seen round the place of injection. If, however, death occurred after some days, then very frequently nothing could be found here beyond small fusions and a limited amount of pus of the size of a pin's head. The neighbouring parts had an obviously normal appearance.

In the following series of experiments,[2] staphylococcus of low virulence was introduced under the serosa of the stomach, small or large intestine, uterus, parametrium, bladder, and also into the substance of the parietal and visceral folia of the peritoneum.

Sometimes, the virus was injected into the organs of the same rabbit. In the majority of cases, however, we used several rabbits and injected virus in one organ of each. If one rabbit died, then all the others were killed with chloroform, after which a study was made of the *character and intensity of*

[1] P. V. Manenkov. *Kazan. Med. Zhurn.,* No. 1, 1929; *Zeitschr. f. d. ges. exp. Med.,* Vol. 64, Nos. 1, 2, 1929.

[2] P. V. Manenkov. *Zeitschr. f. d. ges. exp. Med.,* Vol. 66, Nos. 3, 4, 1929.

the local reaction. It was found that under similar conditions the most serious and extensive changes, in the form of swelling, infiltration, hyperæmia and hæmorrhage, were observed in the gastric wall. In the small intestine, the reaction was much weaker, being limited usually to the vicinity of the injection. Sometimes it was not even possible here to find the place where the virus had been injected. As regards the degree of reaction, the bladder is affected to approximately the same extent as the stomach.

On injecting the virus into the *corpus uteri* or into the *tubæ* near the *corpus,* the local reaction is usually weak. During the first period a limited reddening is observed, after which one finds only a purulent spot at the place of the puncture. It is interesting to note that if the virus is injected into the parametrium at the bottom of the pelvis, inflammatory changes of the *corpus uteri* are much greater than on immediate inoculation of this organ.

This fact is very noteworthy. The virus, when introduced into the organ itself, proves to be almost indifferent to it. *The same virus has only to be caused to act externally for the immune organ to lose its resistance* and to develop signs of severe inflammation. The microbe alone is not a satisfactory explanation for such a phenomenon!

Four years later, some of these experiments were repeated by Scholer, in part using a different technique. He produced inflammation in rabbits by the method of local anaphylaxis and noticed that it developed easily in the gastric wall but that it was not possible to obtain it in the wall of the intestine.

Our study of the standard forms of nervous dystrophy had shown us that the selective affection of certain points of the gastro-intestinal canal is due to nervous influences; when we tested the same points for the degree of their reactivity in the process of inflammation, *here also they stood out quite distinctly.* Hence, the connection between the two processes is at once apparent.

The supposition arose that not only the intensity of the local inflammatory reaction (for instance, of the stomach) but also the extension of the process outside these limits, with the development of extensive peritonitis, is dependent on nervous influences. If the peculiar reaction of a given point depends on the peculiarity of its nervous connections, *it ought to be sufficient to alter these connections by some means or other for the reaction to be altered.* The external construction of the innervation in the gastric region permitted simpler technical methods of work; hence, for our experiments, which were of theoretical importance, we selected the stomach.

These experiments were carried out by my collaborators I. A. Pigalev and M. P. Bushmakina.[1] The observations were made on rabbits which had

[1] M. P. Bushmakina and I. A. Pigalev. *Arkh. Biol. Nauk,* Vol. 28, No. 3, 1928; *Zeitschr. f. d. ges. exp. Med.,* Vol. 63, No. 1-2, 1928.

undergone preliminary bilateral vagotomy on the œsophagus immediately below the diaphragm. If certain experimental conditions are observed (as little incidental trauma as possible) and a special diet is given (without oats or hay), the rabbits tolerate the operation very well. However, they gradually become thin, less mobile and less "clean." Some of them die from pneumonia or perforation of the stomach, especially if given dry, coarse food. After 10-15 days, when the operation wound had healed and the injuries in the œsophagal region were becoming cicatrised, the rabbits were inoculated not in a particular organ but *in the free abdominal cavity,* using for this purpose a culture of "septic" staphylococcus specially virulent for rabbits. For two years previously we had already carried on work with this culture, which we obtained from I. M. Gakh in Kiev. Throughout this time its virulence had in no way diminished. On intravenous injection, 1/100 of a 24-hour culture of this staphylococcus killed a rabbit in 10-20 hours. The same effect was obtained with 1/20-1/30 of a 24-hour culture on inoculation in the abdominal cavity. In the doses mentioned, there were no cases in which the inoculated rabbits remained alive. Nevertheless, we adopted a dose amounting to 1/15 of a 24-hour culture, as a more than fatal dose, giving a result before the expiry of 24 hours. As controls, we took normal healthy rabbits of the same weight which were inoculated intra-peritoneally at the same time as the experimental animals and with the same dose of virus. The results can be seen from the following tables.

TABLE 1

Rabbit No.	Weight (Gm.)	Date of inoculation	Dose	Outcome	Duration of life
325	1,650	12.4.28	1/15-1/20	Death	18 hours
464	—	—	„	„	About 24 hours
660	—	—	„	„	Less than 24 hours
675	1,770	—	„	„	„ „ 15 „
667	1,950	—	„	„	About 15 hours
201	1,550	4.5.28	„	„	„ 10 „
665	2,050	—	„	„	„ 12 „
671	2,100	—	„	„	„ 10 „
668	1,750	9.5.28	„	„	Above 8 days
469	2,750	—	„	„	„ 14 hours
672	1,700	—	„	„	„ 3 days
224	1,100	15.6.28	„	„	„ 11 hours
664	1,250	—	„	„	„ 13 hours
370	2,270	—	„	„	„ 13 hours
282	2,230	—	„	„	„ 5 day

TABLE 2

Rabbit No.	Weight (Gm.)	Date of vagotomy	Date of inoculation	Dose	Outcome	Duration of life
514 · · · · · ·	1,850	23.3.28	12.4.28	1/15-1/20	Recovery	(Observed 23 days)
988 · · · · · ·	1,500	3.3.28	12.4.28	,,	Death	15 hours
347 · · · · · ·	1,700	11.4.28	4.5.28	,,	,,	7 days
673 · · · · · ·	1,950	18.4.28	4.5.28	,,	,,	4 days
501 · · · · · ·	1,720	—	—	,,	Recovery	(Observed 14 days)
669 · · · · ·	1,700	19.4.28	—	,,	Death	2 days
658 · · · · · ·	2,770	20.4.28	9.5.28	,,	Recovery	(Observed 12 days)
513 · · · · ·	2,350	—	—	,,	Death	20 hours
374 · · · · · ·	1,700	24.5.28	15.6.28	,,	,,	36 hours
404 · · · · ·	1,340	1.6.28	—	,,	Recovery	(Observed 9 days)
293 · · · · · ·	2,500	2.6.28	—	,,	Death	4 days
451 · · · · · ·	1,500	1.6.28	—	,,	Recovery	(Observed 9 days)

Comparison of these two tables shows that vagotomy below the diaphragm in these rabbits increases the resistance of the visceral organs to infection; in other words, *it creates conditions hindering the generalisation of inflammatory phenomena.* Out of 12 rabbits, 5 even recovered, although, I repeat, with the dose indicated we never observed a single occasion throughout the period of our work where a normal rabbit was able to withstand the infection. If, moreover, it is taken into account that rabbits deprived of the vagus nerves cannot be considered healthy, generally speaking, and in fact easily perish from a variety of causes, the difference pointed out acquires still greater significance.

In the experiments described, a circumstance was repeated to which I drew attention previously, in the chapter on standard forms of nervous dystrophy. It was found that if the rabbits were inoculated immediately after vagatomy or within the following 2-3 days, they died just as soon or even sooner than the controls. We observed something of the same sort when the "glass sphere operation" was combined with section of one of the branches of the *n. trigeminus*, with the aim of preserving the tissues from development of dystrophic symptoms. Instead of being prevented, they were sharply intensified. In other experiments of my collaborator A. S. Vishnevsky,[1] the reverse result was obtained. When, within a shorter or longer period after irritation of the sciatic nerve in dogs, he had secured the development of trophic ulcers on the extremities, severance of this nerve above the place of injury frequently cured the disease. The same thing was obtained in the human clinic by Molotkov, Shamov, Brüning and others. But the clinic is now well aware that exactly the same operation of neurotomy *in some cases easily cures ulcers of many years' standing, and in others acts as a cause provoking them.*

[1] A. S. Vishnevsky. *Vestn. Khirurg. i Pogr. Obl.*, Vol. 39, 1928.

This is impossible to understand if the result is connected only with the particular form of operational interference—if, for example, it is reduced to mere section of the paths of the pathological reflex.

It must be remembered that the object acted on is the nervous system. Influences exerted on it can remain local (*i.e.*, disappear without going beyond the simple reflex arc) only in cases of so-called physiological stimuli, and even then only if the intensity of the stimulus does not exceed a certain degree. *Unusual forms of stimulation bring into action a number of nerve mechanisms.* Inhibiting some functions, we excite others, we distort their normal course of development, *we transfer the process into new nerve regions.* One must add here also those individual peculiarities which, left behind in the form of traces of past stimuli, can alter both the direction and strength of stimuli newly encountered. To be able to foresee the result with certainty, one must have a good acquaintance with the substratum, but the latter is different in different animals and moreover, is continually changing. *This is the reason why the factor of time stands out so conspicuously in our experiments.*

Hence, in estimating the results of the experiments with intra-peritoneal inoculation after vagotomy of rabbits, we must connect them not only with section precisely of the *n. vagi* but also with the fact of the destruction of the normal state of the nervous system as a whole, particularly in the given region. *After severance of the nerves, the organ is changed.* The staphylococcus culture now produced in it a new form of reaction. The generalisation of the process within the nervous system encountered greater obstacles, and general peritonitis did not develop.

In the course of subsequent experiments, we became convinced that the organ (the stomach) actually became different as a result of vagotomy.

It was pointed out above, that on injecting staphylococcus culture into various organs of the abdominal cavity of rabbits, the part most seriously affected is the stomach. It was of interest to determine if this phenomenon is altered after cutting the vagus nerves and, if so, in exactly what way.

With this aim in view, P. V. Manenkov [1] selected pairs of rabbits and severed the vagus nerves in one rabbit of each pair. The control rabbit, in order to equalise the conditions of the experiment, also underwent a "test" laparotomy, a pull being given to the stomach. After two to three weeks, both rabbits simultaneously underwent a second laparotomy and were inoculated with identical doses of our staphylococcus, *not in the free abdominal cavity but in appropriate places under the serosa of the stomach.* The dose of staphylococcus was 1/200-1/500 of a 24-hour culture. We obtained the same result from the experiments of this series as from the preceding one, *viz.*, the normal rabbits

[1] P. V. Manenkov. *Zeitschr. f. d. ges. exp. Med.*, Vol. 66, Nos. 3, 4, 1929.

perished. The vagotomised rabbits either survived or considerably outlived their controls. But even in those cases where the vagotomised rabbits perished, *it was not only impossible to note general peritonitis but even local symptoms remained localised to the vicinity of the injection.* No inflammatory changes were produced in any part of the gastric wall. It is interesting that the rabbits inoculated through the stomach after vagotomy nevertheless perished sooner than the rabbits which P. V. Manenkov inoculated in the wall of the large intestine during the preceding series of experiments. In neither case did general peritonitis develop; consequently, some special factor must have played a role here.

The staphylococcus that we used is distinguished by its special pathogenic character for rabbits, whatever the method of introduction and especially if introduced intravenously. It might be thought that, on its injection into the gastric wall even of a vagotomised rabbit, the infection substances get into the blood sooner than in the case of injections into the wall of the large intestine.

To test this, the following series of experiments were carried out on normal rabbits.

The animals, as usual, were selected in pairs. Both rabbits underwent laparotomy simultaneously. One of them was given an injection of 1/200-1/500 of a 24-hour culture of staphylococcus in the gastric wall. In the other, to equalise the experimental conditions, the stomach was only pulled out through the wound and then replaced and the wound sewn up. This second rabbit received an injection of the same dose of staphylococcus directly in the blood (through the auricular vein). As a result it was found that *all the rabbits inoculated in the gastric wall died very much sooner than rabbits in which the virus was injected into the blood.* Consequently, if sepsis took place here, it took a more severe course when it began from the gastric wall and did not penetrate directly into the blood.

Returning to the facts described above of the development of the inflammatory process in the abdominal cavity, we shall have to draw the conclusion that general or extensive peritonitis in our animals developed not only (or, more correctly, not so much) owing to the microbe spreading through separate tissues and organs, as owing to generalisation of the process of irritation through the nervous system. The microbe came along afterwards and infected the organ already destined for infection beforehand. It is evident that what has been said applies also to sepsis.

It also becomes clear from the experiments that it is not merely the rate of absorption into the blood that alone determines the danger of peritonitis in general and of " upper peritonitis" in particular. Everything that we have observed makes us connect the difference pointed out with differences of nervous constitution of the organs themselves.

Morphology and physiology furnish many proofs that not only connections with other nerve tracts but also the structure of nerve parts within the organs are different here. Interesting in this respect is the work of Professor B. I. Lavrentyev and his collaborators on the question of the morphology of the nerve elements of intramural ganglia of the mammalian digestive tract.

The origin of these researches was as follows. It was shown by A. S. Dogel that two sharply differentiated types of nerve cells could be observed in the intramural ganglia of the digestive tract. From his study of the character and course of the processes of nerve cells of these two types, Dogel put forward the supposition that the cells of the first type receive stimuli from central neurones (neurones of the first order), while their axons are connected with smooth muscles. Cells of the second type can bring about purely local autonomous reflexes for the given organ, being connected with the mucous membrane on the one hand, and with cells of the first type on the other.

The researches of B. I. Lavrentyev confirmed, in the first place, the existence of two sharply differentiated types of nerve cells in the intramural ganglia of the mammalian digestive tract. At the same time, on the basis of a great deal of histological material (cats, dogs, cows, rats, camels) he succeeded in establishing that the cells of these two types were not distributed uniformly along the digestive tract. Using the mathematical signs $>$ and $<$, the relations can be expressed in the following two formulæ:

Cells of the First Type

Œsophagus $>$ stomach $>$ small intestine $<$ rectum

Cells of the Second Type

Œsophagus $<$ stomach $<$ small intestine $>$ rectum

Experiments showed that bilateral vagotomy in the neck leads to degeneration of the pericellular apparatus of cells of the first type. Their presence in large quantity in the rectum led to the supposition that here also they are connected with the parasympathetic path. Bilateral section of *n. errigentis* fully confirmed this supposition. After this operation, there is degeneration of the pericellular apparatus of the cells of the first type in the rectum. Further investigations of B. I. Lavrentyev provide reason for thinking that some concentration of cells of the first type occurs also in the transition region between the small and large intestines.

Consequently, the distribution of cells of the first type along the digestive tract coincides fairly exactly with the points of the gastro-intestinal canal noted by us during our study of nervous dystrophy and inflammation.

We saw that on generalisation of the *"pure neuro-dystrophic process,"* the intensity of tissue changes is maximal at definite points of the gastro-intestinal canal. If, however, the primary irritation is applied to these points, then the *"pure inflammation process"* arising here will also be distinguished, both in its intensity and its tendency to generalisation, from the corresponding process in neighbouring portions. Experiments with section of the vagus nerves provide grounds for thinking that this difference is connected with neuro-dystrophic processes which are produced more easily at the point indicated, and, *combining with the inflammation, aggravate the latter to a marked degree.*

To make the nervous component of the inflammation evident in the given case, it was necessary to produce at the same points another process of an undoubtedly *nervous character, but which would be neither a pure inflammation nor a pure dystrophy.* For this purpose we fixed on anaphylaxis.

The syndrome of anaphylaxis is the syndrome of epilepsy, *i.e.,* it is certainly of a nervous character. In addition, in order to obtain it, it is desirable to make the first injection of the irritating agent not into the blood, but *directly into the tissues.* Whatever may have been said of the significance of immediate contact of the irritating agent with various tissue elements, we must not forget that these elements include also nerve endings, *i.e.,* that the nervous form of irritation *arises here at the very start.* Finally, the onset of anaphylaxis, no matter whether passive or active, *is preceded by incubation.* In the case of passive anaphylaxis, it is merely shorter. The large number of observations described above has caused us to approach with a certain caution the valuation of any phenomena that are preceded by incubation. We have already come to regard the latter as a signal that we are dealing with a phenomenon of a nervous nature.

The probability of a close relation between the nerve mechanisms of two such apparently dissimilar phenomena as the neuro-dystrophic process and anaphylactic shock can also be presumed on the basis of the following observations. In guinea-pigs that had died from anaphylactic shock, especially in protracted cases, we repeatedly observed *hæmorrhages in the mucous membrane of the stomach and rectum, i.e.,* exactly in the places typical for the standard form of the generalised neuro-dystrophic process.

With the object of elucidating this question, my collaborator I. A. Pigalev performed a series of experiments on guinea-pigs. Sensibilisation was carried out by means of horse serum. In some animals the injections were made in the gastric wall, in others in the wall of the small intestine, at about the middle of its length. A minimal dose of serum was given: one drop. In guinea-pigs, the wall of the small intestine is so thin that to insert the needle into it without piercing through it is by no means simple. All the same, the needle must be inserted in the substance of the intestinal wall to the greatest distance possible, otherwise the serum will run back through the channel of the puncture into the abdominal cavity. It is essential to be very much on guard against this, since sensibilisation through the abdominal cavity is the most certain path for producing anaphylaxis. If it were to take place, we should not have any difference as regards the point of primary irritation between our two groups of animals. To guarantee against such a mistake, we used an extremely fine needle, inserted it as deeply as possible between the layers of the intestinal wall and rigorously controlled that the penetration of the serum was actually into the tissue. This control is not difficult since the intestinal wall is almost transparent. If there was the slightest doubt, the guinea-pig was excluded from the experiment.

In all the animals, the decisive dose of serum was injected into the blood three weeks after the beginning of sensibilisation.

Forty-six guinea-pigs were sensibilised in the gastric wall, with the following results:

	Number	Per cent
Fatal shock	34	74
Non-fatal shock	11	24
No shock	1	2

Thirty-eight guinea-pigs were sensibilised in the wall of the small intestine, with the following results:

	Number	Per cent
Fatal shock	8	23
Non-fatal shock	13	33
No shock	17	44

These figures speak for themselves. If we add that it was never possible to push the needle as far into the layers of the small intestine as into the gastric wall, that is to say, that the danger of the serum getting into the abdominal cavity was much greater in the former case, then the difference becomes even more significant.

I have no intention of basing an analysis of the whole mechanism of such a complicated and little-understood phenomenon as anaphylaxis merely on the results given above. We probably do not take into consideration very many circumstances without which it cannot be explained. There is no doubt, however, that *in the nervous part of the mechanism of anaphylaxis there is something closely allied to the mechanism of nervous dystrophy, since it also arises from a focus of primary irritation, also proceeds along a complex path within the nervous system (incubation) and is also completed by a definite constellation of reactive properties of the organism.*

As a result the convulsive syndrome is, as it were, prepared in advance and only awaits the signal. Such a signal is considered to be the reciprocal action of the antigen and the sensibilisin, which in the opinion of A. M. Besredka, Lumière and others, takes place at the surface of the cells of the central nervous system and destroys their equilibrium.

The correctness of this idea is doubtful. In the first place, *it is not at all essential for irritation of the corresponding nerve structures that they should be brought into immediate contact with any particular irritating substance.* In the part of this book dealing with the genesis of convulsive processes, many examples were described of fatal convulsive states developing in dogs that possessed a constant point of irritation within the nervous system as a result of maximal extraction of the cerebro-spinal fluid.

In the second place, we have in our hands material which provides evidence that in the sensibilisation of animals (rabbits and dogs), sensibilisins *do not make their appearance* in the region of the central nervous system, in particular in the cerebro-spinal fluid. Consequently, they cannot encounter the antigen at the surface of the central nerve cells. These data were obtained by my collaborators A. V. Ponomarev and A. A. Kanarevskaya[1] in experiments on passive anaphylaxis. For obtaining anaphylactic anti-bodies, rabbits and dogs were used, while guinea-pigs were used for demonstrating them (heterological passive anaphylaxis).

The experimental method consisted in repeated injection of the antigen in large doses into the abdominal cavity or veins of the animals. Egg albumen or horse serum was used as the antigen. At the end of eight days after this procedure, cerebro-spinal fluid and blood were taken from the animals. Serum was prepared from the latter. Some of the guinea-pigs were given an injection of the serum in the abdominal cavity, others received an equal quantity of cerebro-spinal fluid.

Since the quantity of fluid in rabbits is very small, and maximum withdrawal of it is impossible, it was necessary to use the fluid of several rabbits for one guinea-pig, so as to avoid admixture of blood. With dogs, of course, this was not necessary. After 24 hours from the foregoing preparatory injection, the guinea-pigs received a definite amount of the appropriate antigen (egg albumen or horse serum), injected directly into a vein. As a result, all the guinea-pigs treated with serum of rabbits or dogs experienced pronounced

---

[1] A. V. Ponomarev and A. A. Kanarevskaya. *Arkh. Biol. Nauk.*, Vol. 36, No. 3, Series B.

anaphylactic shock which ended in death in the majority of cases. There was not a single case of anaphylactic symptoms in any guinea-pig treated with cerebro-spinal fluid.

Hence, sensibilisins accumulating in the blood in response to the introduction of the antigen, do not pass into the region of the central nervous system and consequently their subsequent *contact with the antigen cannot take place at the surface of the central nerve cells.* The process takes place at the nerve periphery, which becomes changed in a special way and involves central parts of the nervous system in the reaction, *not through the spreading of the irritating agent till it reaches these parts, but through the irritation.* This is precisely the reason why the phenomenon of anaphylaxis can be observed in the organs of sensibilised animals even after they have been isolated and drained of blood!

We repeat that we do not pretend thereby to have cleared up the nature of anaphylaxis. Our attention was centred only on the participation of the nervous system in the complex mechanism of anaphylaxis. *We succeeded in studying this participation under the same technical conditions as neuro-dystrophic processes,* and this could not help giving rise to the conception of some kind of kinship between them.

The local inflammatory process, and with it the fate of the organism, is therefore, undoubtedly dependent on the form in which the nervous system is drawn into this process and the extent to which this takes place. *It is impossible to consider the influence of the nervous system here as merely negative.* We know very well that in the vast majority of cases acute inflammation ends in recovery. If the inclusion of the nervous component were always an aggravating factor, every local inflammatory focus would inevitably lead to the animal's death. A trauma inflicted on the nervous system in a portion of the tissues altered by inflammation, would be repeated in the form of a neuro-dystrophic process. The state of the affected portion would become still worse, and this in its turn would be bound to increase the nerve trauma. The result would be a vicious circle from which there would be no exit.

Since no animal is guaranteed against petty lesions and the inflammation accompanying them, the evolution of the animal world would be rendered quite impossible. However, we find a different state of things. Consequently, the nervous component of inflammation can be a positive, *i.e.,* a trophic, factor. We find it to be dystrophic in our experiments because the conditions under which we study the process are heavily exaggerated.

Moreover, even in our experiments, this factor was not always negative, *e.g.,* in the experiments with vagotomy. Under certain conditions, alteration of the nervous state of an organ resulted in the inflammatory process taking a favourable turn. *But in that case, one must also presume the presence of influences on the nervous system in all other means of treatment and pro-phylaxis of inflammation.* Hence, an experimental solution of this problem was of great interest.

The appropriate experiments were carried out by my collaborator A. V. Ponomarev.[1]

The subject of our analysis was active local immunisation by means of anti-virus, according to Besredka's method. The animals used in the experiments were rabbits.

As is well known, A. M. Besredka produced local immunity in a portion of the skin of the animal by the application of a bandage dipped in anti-virus If a large area of the skin is moistened in this way, the exhibition of local immunity can be noted not only in the area taken, but over the whole surface of the skin. It must be remarked, however, that in portions not immediately subjected to the action of anti-virus, local immunity is shown to a much weaker extent.

It is difficult to understand the fact of the generalisation of the process over the whole skin if, as has been done, the circulation of the lymph is made the basis for its explanation. There are no data in favour of the existence of a special system of lymph-circulation connecting all the lymphatic spaces of the skin. On the contrary, the facts indicate, that the lymphatic system of the skin is regional. We saw in the case of scarlatina that a generalised affection of the whole skin is easily liquidated by influences proceeding from the region of the central nervous system. It is permissible to believe that in the experiments with anti-virus we are confronted by an analogous process.

How are the experiments with "anti-virus" usually performed?

First of all, the animal's hair is shaved off. But shaving does not mean only removing the hair. It implies scraping the skin and exposing those parts of the epithelial layer which are usually furnished with nerve endings. After shaving, the anti-virus has the possibility of coming into contact with the nervous system of the skin and thus irritating it.

For our experiments, we took two rabbits. In both of them we shaved the skin of both ears and severed all the receptor and motor nerves of the left ear. The receptor nerves were severed at the neck—the facial nerve, immediately where it emerges from the bone, since it is here that its branches run towards the ear. In one of the rabbits, bandages with anti-virus were applied and fastened to both ears. The bandages were moistened at regular intervals during 24 hours. After this period both rabbits were inoculated simultan-

[1] A. V. Ponomarev. *Arkh. Biol. Nauk*, Vol. 28, No. 4, 1928; *Zeitschr. f. d. ges. exp. Med.*, Vol. 63, Nos. 1, 2, 1928.

eously with an equal quantity of staphylococcus culture introduced into the skin, and partly under the skin, of both ears.

The control rabbit, to which the bandage with anti-virus had not been applied, developed inflammatory changes which were almost *absolutely alike in the normal and in the denervated ear.* Within 24 hours, both ears were equally swollen, red and hot to the touch. After 48 hours, necrotic portions were exhibited by both ears.

In the experimental rabbit, however, the reaction was quite different in each ear. *No inflammatory symptoms were noted in the right ear,* the nerves of which were entire, apart from insignificant thickening of the tissues at the place of injection. The ear was pale, not swollen and cold to the touch. At the same time, the inflammatory reaction in the left ear, where the nerves had been severed, was very great and in no way different from the inflammatory reaction in the two ears of the control rabbit (swelling, redness, heightened temperature, necrosis). The experiment was performed several times under the same conditions, and always gave the same result.

Thus, the anti-virus proved capable of evoking local immunity *only in tissues in which the nerve state was normal.* The destruction of the nerves radically altered the whole reaction.

In this series of experiments we encountered a curious contradiction. Severance of the auricular nerves, it is seen, proved to have almost no influence on the development of inflammation in the ear. When Shimura made his experiments, it was precisely this which impelled him to deny any participation of the nervous system in the inflammatory process. Further observations, however, have made it clear that the matter is by no means so simple.

Immunisation of local elements was not obtained by the use of anti-virus unless the normal nerve connections of the organ were preserved. Severing them created conditions preventing the development of immunity; consequently, it must be admitted that the nervous system has the power to destroy inflammation. It would be strange if it could fulfil this function without playing any part in the process itself!

There is only one conclusion to be drawn: we are far from knowing everything about the intricate morphological and functional complex of inflammation. Basing our estimate of a phenomenon on some external characteristics, we lose sight of the others, and as a result our knowledge is incomplete. Each year brings new facts in the sphere of nervous physiology and morphology. Many of them can only with difficulty be inserted into the framework of old conceptions; some of them indeed, for instance the experiments of Paul Weiss, are altogether incompatible with the rest.

In dealing with the severance of nerves, it must not be forgotten that the severed fibre bundles are not all equivalent. Thus denervation of the ear in the rabbit produces a quite different result from cutting the vagus branch to the stomach. Our information about the vagus nerve in general is very elementary. Recently, the researches of B. A. Dolgo-Saburov in the laboratories of Bushmakin and Tonkov have enriched our knowledge with a number of new and interesting facts. It was found, for instance, that on section of the vagus nerve at any *level* (cervical, thoracic or abdominal regions), regeneration was observed not only in the central but also in the peripheral stump. It was proved also that it is impossible to include the regenerated fibres of the severed peripheral portion in the category of "specially resistant," as previously described by Ramon J. Cajal, De Castro and others. Resistant fibres are observed only during the first 5-7 days after the severance; later they disappear. Here, however, they were noted after 13-19, and even after 30, days. Regeneration of the peripheral nerve stump was especially clearly marked in Dolgo-Saburov's experiments in regard to the abdominal region of the vagus. This work is only in its early stages, but it promises to alter radically our conceptions of the morphology and physiology of this nerve, which itself is a complex part of the nervous system.

Hence, it is not surprising that it is more difficult to establish the dependence of inflammation on nerve influences by experimenting on the ear of the rabbit than on parts of its gastro-intestinal tract. If Shimura had only transferred his experiments to another region of the nervous system, his negative conclusion as to the role of the latter in the inflammatory process would have become less categorical.

The experiments with anti-virus aroused the desire to obtain the same effect in another way, by transferring the contact of the anti-virus with the nervous system to another region of the nervous system, for example the subarachnoid space (experiments of my collaborator A. V. Ponomarev).

For this purpose, we prepared in the usual way a "polyvalent" staphylococcus anti-virus, diluted with 3-5 times its volume of physiological solution, and injected it into the rabbit subarachnoidally. Undiluted anti-virus must not be used since it produces severe convulsive phenomena and the animals die.

Immediately following this, or even beforehand, various quantities of staphylococcus culture are injected into the skin and partly under the skin of the stomach. We used a double control. One control was a normal rabbit infected at the same time as the experimental rabbit, in the same manner and with the same dose of culture introduced into and under the skin of the stomach. A third rabbit, prepared beforehand by the application during 24-48 hours of bandages with anti-virus to the shaven skin of the stomach, was infected at the same time as the others and in the same way.

The results showed that local symptoms after infection in the rabbit which had received injection of anti-virus into the subarachnoid space were not only less than in the simple control but were sometimes less than in the rabbit that had been treated by direct application of anti-virus to the skin; and this although we infected the experimental rabbit almost simultaneously with the introduction of anti-virus into the subarachnoid space.

When we tried introducing the anti-virus into the blood, in order to avoid the poisonous effect, and followed this by "pumping," the result obtained was in general even more pronounced.

The experiment was so arranged that each of two rabbits received 5.0 c.c. of anti-virus in the blood, after which one of them underwent "pumping." Both these rabbits, as well as a third one, which had been prepared by a 24 hours' application of a bandage with anti-virus, were infected simultaneously and identically. In these cases, it was sometimes observed that in the rabbit which had undergone "pumping," there were still almost no local inflammatory changes after 24 hours from the time of infection, while in the other two they were always clearly marked, although to a different extent.

We did not determine how long "local" immunity of the skin lasts after the action of anti-virus applied, in one form or another, to the central nervous system.

A. M. Besredka considers that, after the immediate application of anti-virus to the skin, local immunity lasts as long as the anti-virus remains in the cellular elements of the skin. It is possible that the action here on the nervous system lasts longer than on being directly introduced into the medullary region from which all foreign substances are very rapidly removed. But rabbits, treated for 24 hours with anti-virus by Besredka's method, also gave a diminished local reaction only in the first days after infection. Many of them subsequently died. We observed the same thing in our animals. In order to obtain from the anti-virus more prolonged exhibition of local immunity under the usual conditions, the bandages must be applied to the skin for 2-4 days.

Moreover, the question of the duration of immunity in this case did not interest us, since, of course, we did not propose to draw any practical conclusions, much less proposals, on the basis of our experiments. Nor did the question of the specific nature of the phenomena of "local immunity" that were obtained have any importance for us. *Whether the penetration of the anti-virus into the region of the central nervous system produced a special form of irritation of the latter or not, the fact remains that, as a result of the nerve transformation connected with this, the development of inflammation at the periphery took a different course.* From this we are justified in drawing the conclusion that *the nervous component of the inflammatory process is a positive (physiological)* factor. Its passage into a dystrophic (pathological) form depends on an excessive degree of irritation.

As early as 1927, Professor V. V. Chirkovsky became interested in our experiments on active local immunisation and, together with his collaborator L. A. Dymshits, he repeated them in a somewhat special form.

The object used for the experiment was the eye of the rabbit. Introduction of anti-virus under the conjunctiva or into the anterior chamber of the eye did not produce immunisation towards staphylococcus. When, however, this was combined with the procedure of "pumping," a positive effect was obtained in 10 cases out of 14.

Weighing up all these data, we are bound to come to the conclusion that *the mechanism of local immunisation is not confined to the action exerted directly on the underlying tissue by the immunising agent.* Chemotaxis, as a cell reaction underlying immunity, undoubtedly occurs; however, we observe that the extent of this reaction depends on certain influences from the centre, *i.e.,* that the nervous system controls to a certain extent the functions of the mobile elements which play a role in immunity.

S. I. Metalnikov, by immunising caterpillars to the cholera vibrio, has established that the development of immunity in them is bound up with the integrity of one of the nerve ganglia, and he also declares in favour of recognising the influence of the nervous system on the phagocytic elements.

In the course of the above-described experiments a large number of problems relating to general pathology have been touched on; but essentially our attention remained concentrated on one of them. It may be formulated in the following way.

The locus of primary irritation determines, at least for a certain period, the form of development of the dystrophic process within the network of the nervous system.

If the degree of irritation exceeds a certain strength, then each nerve cell that is involved in the process becomes itself a source of irritation and creates new foci for the latter. The process develops violently and rapidly attains the stage of general dystrophy. This is also the basic obstacle in the way of an investigation that attempts to analyse the process and study its stages.

It does not follow from this, of course, that the only conditions determining the whole process from beginning to end are the locus and strength of the primary irritation. We have repeatedly had occasion to observe, that in spite of identity of locus, and possible equality of strength, in some cases a pure neuro-dystrophic form of tissue-change developed, in others—inflammation, in a third—anaphylactic shock, and in a fourth—Schwarzmann's phenomenon, and so on.

Definite special features are to be noticed in the general picture of the irritation in each case; but in regard to the nervous mechanism all these, externally so diverse, phenomena *have something in common which unites them all.*

The extent of functional changes in the elements of the nervous system results in the primary inflammatory focus acquiring all the features of a secondary one that develops as the result of the generalisation of the neuro-dystrophic phenomena. Microbes will occur in both the one and the other. In both cases they can be regarded as pathogenic, *i.e.*, as contributing something to the process; this process, however, may progress even in their absence and may terminate favourably even in their presence.

CHAPTER XVIII

CHRONIC IRRITATION (INFLAMMATION)

DURING recent years, the study of chronic forms of irritation (inflammation) has not offered us any difficulty, since the material previously obtained had already provided us with all the fundamental prerequisites for this study.

I have more than once had occasion to mention periodic or rhythmic development as one of the forms of the dystrophic process observed in our animals Pathological tissue changes that had temporarily disappeared were renewed, and usually at the places previously affected. We also learned how *to provoke* these relapses easily. Consequently, there must have been established in the organism some kind of permanent points *which continued to retain traces of the past injury.* Temporary recovery was no evidence of the final liquidation of the process. Since the cause, *not only of the original changes, but also of the relapse of the process and of the provocation of this relapse, lay in agencies of a nervous nature, while the changes themselves merely reflected at the periphery another process that developed within the nervous system, the conclusion followed of itself.* By this means, the real value and concrete content of the concept of sensibilisation and also of the strange notion of "dormant infection" could be estimated.

For the tissues at the periphery to be in a state of continuous irritation, in a state of "readiness" to pass into an obviously pathological condition, it is by no means necessary that the irritating agent should be demonstrably external, or that it should be possible to find it among the injured elements, and to isolate it and extract it from them. In regard to this foreign agent, one must not demand obvious "ocular" proofs. *In a formal respect, it may easily remain invisible, which does not prevent it from being actually external in regard to the tissues.*

The microbes that were discovered in chronic non-healing ulcers in our animals were secondary and accidental colonists. Their presence did not intensify the process, nor did their removal abolish it. Nevertheless, these ulcers *are nothing less than foci of chronic inflammation.* One can easily convince oneself of this by carrying out the appropriate morphological analysis.

Hence, *local distortion of the nervous influences is sufficient both for giving rise to and for maintaining foci of chronic inflammation.*

However, a large number of examples are known in pathology where such foci have certain features which confer on them a special or, as is usually said, specific character. In such foci are always or almost always to be found definite, and not accidental, micro-organisms, to which, therefore, it is difficult to deny the role of responsible agents. One must mention here in the first place tuberculosis virus and *Spirochæta pallida* of syphilis.

In making experiments on animals with these, one obtains as is well known, local changes typical for the irritating agent used. In regard to tuberculosis, one further important circumstance has to be taken into account. At the present time, methods exist for infecting tissue cultures *in vitro* with tuberculosis (Timofeyevsky, Maksimov and others). The disease develops in the cultures with the formation of tubercles. All this takes place of course, in the absence of any nervous influences. An impression is created that not only the tuberculosis disease itself but also the form of reaction to it are independent processes having no sort of connection with the functions of the nervous system.

But when we turn our attention to spontaneous tuberculosis, we, strangely enough, observe something quite different.

From a very early period, the clinic has attached a high importance to the nervous system in this process. Since the time of Spiess, laryngologists have frequently and successfully employed various forms of local anæsthesia and also neurotomy of *n. laryngeus superior* in treatment of tuberculous ulcers of the larynx (Verkhovsky).

A. G. Molotkov has already accumulated a large amount of material on the treatment of tuberculous ulcers of the tongue by neurotomy of *n. glossopharyngeus.* In my opinion, among his observations a case stands out especially clearly where an extensive and dirty ulcer of the tongue rapidly healed and became covered with epithelium, while isolated tubercles remained visible in the depths of the tissue through the fine transparent layer of new epithelium. *For some reason, these tubercles ceased producing additional reactions in the surrounding tissues.* Biopsy of such portions showed the presence in them of typical tissue elements and microbes which subsequently only gradually disappear. Hence, *first the inflammation came to an end, and only after this came the liquidation of the "causes" which had produced it.* This should provide material for reflection for those persons who are convinced that the inflammatory reaction of the tissues is independent of nervous influences!

Yet another circumstance remains not entirely comprehensible. We know from laboratory experiments that it is possible to infect almost any organ with tuberculosis by direct injection of the virus. In the spontaneous form of this process, however, or on infection through the blood, the organs of an animal are affected selectively and in some definite sequence. One cannot help thinking that, on injecting virus into an organ, besides the introduction of a special irritating agent, *there is also the infliction of an ordinary trauma.* In cases where the virus penetrates into the same tissues through the blood, this additional factor does not exist or is considerably less.

Hence, simple encounter with the virus is not enough. It is necessary also that the so-called "resistance" of the given organ to the virus should be diminished. Consequently, the place for the focus is prepared either in advance or simultaneously, but, in any case, *by the action of some other agent.* It was natural to seek here for the participation of precisely those processes which have been studied by us under the name of nervous dystrophy.

I shall pass on now to set out the data obtained in this connection (experiments of my collaborator A. V. Ponomarev[1]).

The animals experimented on were rabbits. They were infected in the lower lobe of the right lung by means of Vallée culture, the virulence of which was somewhat diminished. Following this, one of the *n. vagi* was severed in each animal—in some cases the right nerve, in other cases the left. Normal rabbits, infected under the same conditions, served as controls. After 4-5 weeks, the rabbits were killed and dissected.

The results showed that the development of tuberculosis was to be noted in all cases in the right lung (the one in which the infection had been introduced) and also in its pleura, but in the left lung it was found very rarely— *much more rarely and more feebly developed than in the controls.* Consequently, severance of one of the *n. vagi* in the neck of the rabbit hindered the development of tuberculosis in the left lung, in spite of the fact that the right lung and pleura contained a large tuberculosis focus. An alteration in the state of innervation of one organ of the pair found expression also in the other. Both lungs became more resistant to hæmatogenic tuberculosis no matter whether the left or the right vagus nerve had been severed.

Subsequently, experiments were performed using the technique described in the preceding chapter (experiments of my collaborators, I. A Pigalev and G. S. Epstein [2]). The object of these experiments was to trace the development of tuberculosis after infection of various points of the gastro-intestinal tract.

For infection, we used one of the weakest cultures, *viz.,* BCG. The rabbits received injections of virus in the same quantity and in the same number of places in the wall of the stomach and in that of the large intestine, re-

---

[1] A. V. Ponomarev. *Arkh. Biol. Nauk,* Vol. 29, No. 4, 1929; *Zeitschr. f. d. ges. exp. Med.,* Vol. 70, Nos. 3, 4, 1930.

[2] I. A. Pigalev and G. S. Epstein. *Arkh. Biol. Nauk,* Vol. 29, No. 4, 1929; *Zeitschr. f. d. ges. exp. Med.,* Vol. 70, Nos. 3, 4, 1930.

mote from the rectum. The rabbits were killed at the end of a month and dissected.

In every case without exception, *changes in the gastric wall were much more pronounced than in the wall of the large intestine.* In the stomach, infiltration and œdema always occurred for some distance around each of the points of inoculation. The infiltrate attained the size of a pea, or even of a hazel nut. Sometimes we observed ulceration of the mucous membrane of the stomach above the infiltrate. In the case of the large intestine, however, it was always rather difficult even to find the places inoculated, *sometimes indeed it was simply impossible.* These places were defined by hyperæmia or a "purulent point" at the puncture. In the gastric wall, we sometimes observed the formation of inflammatory infiltrates outside the place of injection as well, which *never occurred in the wall of the large intestine.*

It must be mentioned that microscopic investigation of pieces cut out of the inflammatory infiltrates from the wall of the stomach and large intestine demonstrated the absence of typical tuberculosis tubercles. With this virus, therefore, a specific tuberculous reaction did not develop in the tissue, the result being restricted to simple phenomena of chronic inflammation.

In another series of experiments, infection of the rabbits by BCG culture was carried out in a somewhat different way, *viz.,* the virus was injected into the wall of the stomach and small and large intestine, not of the same, but of different animals. The amount of virus used and the number of places of injection was always the same. Under these conditions, it was found that the inflammatory changes in the wall of the large intestine, and especially those in the wall of the small intestine, were still less than in the experiments of the first series; *out of 5-6 punctures it was hardly possible on dissection to find even 2-3,* usually in the form of a small scar trace on the surface of the serosa.

The following fact was noted in these experiments. On dissecting rabbits that had been killed 4-5 weeks after infection in the gastric wall, we frequently found in the lungs inflammatory phenomena of an acute (but not tuberculous) character. We did not observe any such affections of the lungs in rabbits infected in the wall of the large intestine. Hence, *irritation of the gastric wall produces a heightened receptivity towards non-specific inflammation in another organ of the same nerve segment, i.e., it sensibilises the lung.*

In another series of similar experiments, we used virulent Vallée culture and obtained the same result. It was somewhat less pronounced, since thin culture produces affections extending outside the limits of the place of injection, not only in the stomach but also in the large intestines.

In further experiments with Vallée culture we made the following observations.

Three rabbits of like weight were included in each experiment. In one of them, both *n. vagi* were sectioned. After two weeks, all three underwent laparotomy, and equal quantities of virulent Vallée culture were injected into the gastric wall. The places of injection were alike in number and disposition in all three animals. About 2-3 weeks after this, one of the two rabbits infected in the normal gastric wall was also subjected to vagotomy. At the time of the operation, the visceral organs were closely examined and a record made; already it was always possible to note fairly severe and extensive changes of the wall of the stomach, epiploon and duodenum. After a further 2-4 weeks, all three rabbits were killed and dissected.

The result showed that the most serious alterations of the stomach, epiploon, liver, parietal peritoneum, etc., were always to be found in the normal rabbit. In its case, the epiploon was strewn with separate tubercles and their conglomerates, and was sclerosed and frequently shrivelled into a lump. The stomach was affected to almost the same extent. It was impossible to determine the point of injection of the virus here, since both neighbouring and even remote parts of the gastric wall were approximately equally affected. A large number of tubercles were also observed on the parietal peritoneum, especially in its diaphragmal part. The visceral peritoneum of the small and large intestines, and their mesenteries also, were much less affected. (Plate 34.)

In the rabbits in which both *n. vagi* had been severed below the diaphragm, *the whole process took a different course.*

Only isolated tubercles could be seen in the epiploon, which was not sclerosed and not fused with the neighbouring parts. The places where virus had been injected in the gastric wall could always be easily determined, since outside them the stomach was affected only to an insignificant extent. In this organ, tubercles could be found only in isolated places. The parietal peritoneum usually suffered to the same extent as in the rabbits of the first group, but the visceral peritoneum, including the mesenteries of the intestines, was almost entirely clean. (Plate 35.)

It is interesting to note that the rabbits which underwent vagotomy 2-3 weeks after infection gave almost the same result *as the rabbits subjected to vagotomy before infection.* Even those changes which had been noted at the time of the operation to the vagus nerve not only did not become intensified but often became considerably weaker. In some cases, the result of vagotomy following infection was even better than where it preceded it. (Plate 36.)

Interesting data were also provided by another series of experiments, also performed with Vallée culture. In every case where the rabbits were infected in the free abdominal cavity, and especially in the gastric wall, they developed severe affection of both lungs. It can be said that in the syndrome of the disease this affection quickly becomes the most important feature. The tubercles penetrate both lungs to such an extent that the pulmonary tissue is hardly visible between them. If, simultaneously with infection or shortly afterwards, vagotomy is performed, not under the diaphragm, but in the neck, and only on one side, *the process in both lungs is hindered*. In the lung tissue of such animals, at the end of the same period it is possible to find only isolated scattered tubercles at a distance from one another. We sometimes even found both lungs free from tubercles, while the lungs of the control rabbit were affected all over.

Consequently, tuberculosis of the gastric wall sensibilises the lungs in the rabbit, *provided the normal relations in the nervous system are maintained*. Alteration of the latter produces, even if only temporarily, increased resistance of the lungs to tuberculosis.

Severance of one of the *n. vagi* in the neck has the same effect on both lungs. Consequently, *such severance not only acted by itself but also served as a stimulus leading to the creation of new conditions within the nervous system*. This caused a change in the bio-chemical properties both of those tissues with which the severed nerve was immediately connected and of those connected with the other half of the given segment of the nervous system. Hence, here also there was a repetition of the rule (already noted previously on many occasions) that, in estimating the effect of a particular procedure applied to the nervous system, it is necessary to take into account not only the form of this procedure but also *the act of interference itself* which originates a whole group of processes.

In order to bring out clearly how the order of development of tuberculous infection in the organs depends on processes developing in the nervous system, it is necessary to arrange an experiment in a region where it is possible to analyse the complex mutual relations in the nerve apparatus, utilising at least data from the history of development. We can find such a region in the genito-urinary system.

The testicle, epididymis and kidney are topographically and functionally closely connected, but arise from different sources. In the human clinic, these three organs are often affected by tuberculosis separately and simultaneously, but the connection between these separate processes has not yet been established. In spite of much research by experimental and clinical workers, the problem has remained insoluble, or the solutions given are extremely contradictory. One can easily convince oneself of this by a glance at the literature on the subject (Baumgarten, Kramer, Sawamura, S. P. Fedorov, Kholtsov, Küttner, Wildbolz, Israel, etc.).

The question has been decided almost exclusively *on the basis of data from the study of the morphology of the paths for various liquids—blood, lymph, urine and semen—and the mechanism of the movement of these liquids.* Arbitrary assumptions were made of the direct and reverse flow of these liquids, on which the distribution of the virus was supposed to depend. An explanation of symmetrical affection of the second epididymis was sought in anti-peristaltic movements of the *vas deferens.* The result is that, as before, the movement of the microbe from the region of the primary focus along the tubular pathways *is regarded as the sole cause of the spreading of the process.* It is well known, however, that the latter only very rarely passes from the epididymis to the testicle, in spite of their very close association, while, on the contrary, it very often affects the contralateral epididymis, the path to which is a long and winding system of tubes.

In planning our experiments, we took the following observations for our starting point.

By whatever route tuberculosis virus is introduced into the rabbit, whether in the subcutaneous tissue, blood or peritoneum, generalisation of the process by extension to other organs is assured. It has long been known that the organism is by no means uniformly affected in this way. In rabbits, irrespective of the place of primary infection, it is always very quickly found that *the organ suffering most is the lung,* followed in decreasing order by the epiploon, spleen and ligaments of the liver. General tuberculosis of the visceral organs begins much later, even if the infection itself took place along this route.

The kidneys are affected at a still later stage. The disease can only be observed in them in protracted cases, where the rabbit lives 3-5 months after infection, or where a highly virulent culture is employed causing the generalisation of the process to proceed with great rapidity. If, however, the rabbit dies or is killed 30-50 days after infection, it is hardly ever possible to find tuberculosis of the kidney, although by this time other organs may already be affected to a very considerable extent. This circumstance is the more peculiar in that the distribution of tuberculosis virus from the place of injection takes place through the blood, and it is precisely through the kidney that the latter becomes cleansed of microbic impurities.

Starting out from the conception that the formation of new local foci does not occur accidentally but is predetermined by certain tissue derangements taking place in advance, *we made it our aim, in regard to the kidney, to bring about such derangements artificially in the organism, but without directly touching either the organ itself or its autonomous nerve apparatus.*

Our experiments were guided by the following considerations. The kidney in mammals is embryologically the metanephros. It develops from a special portion of the connecting lamina between the ventral and dorsal sections of the mesoderm. The neighbouring portion of the same lamina gives rise to the parenchyma of the testicle (and ovary). As is well known, there is a close connection between the circulatory systems of these organs. It is probable that their nervous systems are also in close relation to one another. If this is so, we may expect that *by acting on the nervous elements in the testicle, we shall involve the nervous system of the kidney as well.*

The experiments were performed by my collaborators I. A. Pigalev and G. S. Epstein,[1] the virus being injected into the parenchyma of the testicle in the rabbit in the same quantities as used previously for injection into other places. Subsequently, after 4-5 weeks, *i.e.*, a period within which the kidneys were not affected after using other methods of infection, the rabbit was killed.

As a result, we obtained tuberculous affection of both kidneys *in 100 per cent of our experiments.* Here, of course, the lymphatic transference of the virus was out of the question; for, in that case, we should have to assume, not merely a reverse flow of lymph from the lympathic collectors which it has in common with the testicle, but also a reverse flow of lymph within the parenchyma of the kidney. In addition, it must be pointed out that on unilateral infection of the testicles *we always obtained bilateral affection of the kidneys.*

However, in order to make this experiment absolutely irreproachable from the technical point of view, another variation of it was performed.

Here we argued as follows. The testicle, in origin and in composition, is a complex organ. Its two chief constituent parts—the glandular elements and the ducts—are entirely distinct in ontogeny and phylogeny. They develop from different sources and from different regions of the body. They become united secondarily. The circulatory system of each is independent. *The same view must be adopted of their nervous systems.* In that case infection through the epididymis should not produce tuberculous affection in the kidney.

This was actually confirmed by experiment. Tuberculosis of the kidneys after introducing the virus into the epididymis was only observed when, at the moment of infection or after it, the tuberculosis virus penetrated into the parenchyma of the testicle. In such cases we always had, not an isolated focus in the epididymis, but a joint affection of epididymis and testicle. If the infection was carried out cleanly, and the primary focus was localised in the epididymis, the kidneys remained healthy.

The same experiments were performed by another of my collaborators, Dr. Feigel, on female rabbits, but using weakly virulent staphylococcus culture instead of tuberculosis virus. *The operation was performed on the ovary.*

Here, almost without exception, *unilateral infection of the ovary resulted in the development of multiple purulent foci in the parenchyma of both kidneys*

[1] I. A. Pigalev and G. S. Epstein. *Arkh. Biol. Nauk*, Vol. 32, No. 2, 1932.

(carbuncle of the kidney). The difference from the preceding experiments consisted in the process developing much more rapidly (within 3-5 days).

A final solution of the question as to the nature of the phenomena described was obtained through the experiments of my collaborators A. T. Dolinsky and D. S. Chetvertak.

After confirming the results obtained by Feigel with female rabbits, they proceeded to a new modification of the experiment.

They injected 1-2 drops of a 2 per cent solution of formalin into the tissue of one of the ovaries of a rabbit. Three weeks later, 0.1 c.c. of a suspension of staphylococcus of low pathogenic value for the rabbit (a 24-hour culture washed into 2.0 c.c. of physiological solution) was introduced intravenously. After one month, the rabbits were killed and dissected.

In the ovary, at the place of injection of formalin, there was found only fine bands of connective tissue and sometimes a small cyst containing a transparent fluid. No changes were found in the other organs and cavities of the body, *with the exception of the kidneys, where the formation of multiple purulent foci always took place, penetrating the parenchyma of the organ mainly in the cortical portion.*

This experiment, combined with those described above, leaves no doubt that in associated affection of separate parts of the genito-urinary system, the connection of these parts through any kind of tubular pathways *cannot play any decisive role*. The selectivity exhibited in the affection of particular organs is founded on processes of a nervous nature. If the so-called sensibilisation were the result merely of influences directly affecting the tissue elements, and not through the medium of the nervous system, the ovary would be the first or even the sole organ involved in the pathological process. But the changes we observed were sharply distinct from the changes in the kidneys.

If the irritation of the ovary produced a change in the nervous system of the kidney, the nervous system of the ovary could not remain intact! Nevertheless, the kidney was not affected by staphylococcus. It follows from this that the process produced by the immediate *irritation of a particular point of the nervous system becomes the originator of dissimilar tissue changes of a biochemical character in various other points of the organism.*

One further experiment, the result of a chance observation can be added to the experiments demonstrating the connection between the point of primary irritation and the order of development of the dystrophic process in the nerve network. In carrying out a large number of intra-peritoneal infections of rabbits it is natural that technical failures should sometimes occur. It happened to us on a few occasions that on making the injection, the point of a blunt needle pushed the abdomen in front of it and, without penetrating into the abdominal cavity, *remained in the substance of the sub-peritoneal tissue.*

An isolated tuberculous focus gradually developed at the place of injection. When, at the end of a certain period, the rabbits were killed and dissected, we found, besides slight tuberculosis of the lung, *an isolated affection of the serosa and mesenteries of both testicles.* The process was sharply demarcated at the edge of the mesentery of the testicle, as if there was an invisible boundary between the mesentery and the parietal peritoneum which it could not cross. Other organs of the abdominal cavity, not excluding the epiploon, remained unaffected. Three such observations were made. This made us wish to reproduce the phenomenon intentionally, and I charged my collaborator L. N. Fedorov, with the performance of the experiments.

A number of rabbits were infected with tuberculosis virus in the substance of the abdominal wall along the medial line, halfway between the pubis and the *processus xyphoideus.* Vallée culture of diminished virulence was used for inoculation. This is indispensable for all experiments the object of which is to study the sequence in the development of the process, since the use of strong cultures causes violent development of the disease, in which case it is much more difficult to trace the sequence looked for.

The injection of the virus is carried out in such a way as to cause infiltration of part of the wall as far as the subperitoneal tissue.

Very soon, an infiltrate begins to be formed at the place of injection. After 1-1½ months, the rabbits were killed and dissected. Even while the animals were alive, it was possible, by simple palpation of the testicles, to diagnose tuberculous affection. This was confirmed on dissection. In all cases where the infiltrate occupied the whole thickness of the abdominal wall, and not merely the subcutaneous connective tissue, *the serosa of the testicles and their mesenteries were affected all over.* For a fairly long time the process is of an isolated character and is very sharply interrupted at the edge of the mesentery of the testicle. In addition, tubercles are scattered in enormous quantity *on the parietal peritoneum of the internal surface of the scrotum,* i.e., on the *tunica propria.* Here also, the affection is *suddenly and sharply interrupted at the edge of the internal inguinal ring,* and the remaining part of the parietal peritoneum, even in the immediate neighbourhood of this ring, remains completely healthy. In the epiploon there are either no tubercles or very few. In any case, it is very much less affected than the scrotum, the testicles and their ligaments. We obtained cases in which the affection of the serosa and mesenteries of both testicles had already progressed very far, *at a time when it was not possible to determine the presence of tubercles even in the lung.*

The following point deserves special notice. In the previously described experiments, tuberculosis of the testicle, caused by the direct injection of virus into it, was always accompanied by bilateral affection of the kidneys. In the present case, however, when the testicles were affected by tuberculosis secondarily, the kidneys remained without alteration. Consequently, the processes were fundamentally different in the two cases, although both were manifested by one and the same indicator—*viz.*, tuberculosis tubercle.

All these experiments once more confirm that the form of development of the dystrophic process, *at any rate in its first stages, is connected to a considerable extent with the place where the process began.*

To the material given above we must add experiments demonstrating the comparative intensity of affection by the virus of tuberculosis in the separate tissues and organs that develop the disease simultaneously. Here we must include two series of experiments performed by my collaborators, one series belonging to I. A. Pigalev[1] and the other to V. S. Galkin.[2] The first of these authors studied the degree of change in organs of the abdominal cavity, on intra-peritoneal infection by tuberculosis; while the second made it his aim to draw up a picture of the distribution of India ink, also introduced intraperitoneally.

The experimental animals used were cats and rabbits; for the ink experiments, dogs also were included. The animals were killed after a definite period from the beginning of the experiment. It was found that the records of dissection in these essentially diverse types of experiment were so much alike that *one could be substituted for the other, merely putting the word ink in place of tubercles, and vice versa.*

The greatest degree of tuberculosis affection was noted in the region of the large and small epiploon, the serosa of the stomach, and the rectum and its mesentery. In addition, the ligamentous apparatus of the testicle and ovary was always affected. The mesentery of the testicle and the broad ligaments of the uterus also were in all cases thickly strewn with tubercles. There was a sharp line of demarcation of the process at the boundary of these structures. The small intestines and their mesentery remained almost free from tubercles. The amount of tubercles on the serosa of the large intestine markedly increased as it approached the rectum.

Enumerating the organs in which ink accumulates on being introduced into the abdominal cavity, one must mention—*the large and small epiploon, mesenteries of the duodenum and rectum and also the ligaments of the ovaries and testicles. The mesenteries of the small, and of the greater part of the large,*

[1] I. A. Pigalev. *Arkh. Biol. Nauk*, Vol. 31, No. 6, 1931; *Zeitschr. f. d. ges. exp. Med.*, Vol. 80, Nos. 3, 4, 1932.
[2] V. S. Galkin. *Zeitschr. f. d. ges. exp. Med.*, Vol. 94, No. 1-2, 1934.

intestine remain absolutely free from ink.

It is evident from this that the distribution of these so very diverse substances in the organs of the abdominal cavity can hardly be dependent on *the existence of special properties in the substances themselves.* Moreover, it is quite obvious that we are dealing here with those *same places which have been mentioned more than once in describing dystrophic changes along the course of the gastro-intestinal canal.*

It is a question, therefore, of properties belonging to the organs themselves. These properties are variable. But their variability is connected with influences of a nervous nature. The virus, in spreading from the primary focus, does not accidentally lay hold of one organ or another.

It is now a well-established fact that the presence of bacilli in the blood of affected organisms is a phenomenon of constant occurrence, both in conditions of artificial infection of animals and in spontaneous tuberculosis in man. The presence of streptococcus, staphylococcus and of intestinal and tuberculosis bacilli in the blood of healthy persons is also not rare. This, however, does not necessarily result in the formation of foci of inflammation. In the vast majority of cases, *the organism easily frees itself from bacterial impurities.*

When we infect an animal artificially, we not only establish a depot of live microbes, *but also inflict a trauma.* Along with the tissue elements of the particular organ—surface of the serosa, cellular tissue, inner surfaces of vascular channels, etc., the nerve elements innervating these tissues also undergo irritation, *i.e., an impulse is given to the development of nervous dystrophy.* In this way, not only the microbe employed for irritation, but others as well, *e.g.,* those that have hitherto circulated harmlessly in the blood stream as accidental germs, may acquire a local or general "pathogenic" character. Thus, in the above-described experiments of A. G. Dolinsky and D. S. Chetvertak, the staphylococcus proved to be pathogenic *only for the kidneys,* although under other conditions the kidneys would have been *the last* to suffer.

In observing the development of symmetrical trophic ulcers in dogs after unilateral chemical trauma of the sciatic nerve, we made the following observation: *the process only rarely begins directly from the skin.* At the beginning, an œdematous swelling usually appears; the centre of this swelling rapidly softens. If, without waiting for spontaneous opening of the focus, a section is made through its thinned surface, the tissues will be found in a state of disintegration.

Although the focus does not contain pus, it is usually never sterile. However, *opening and emptying it does not cause healing. Neither will there be progressive growth of the focus.* On reaching a certain size, it becomes stationary, although there will now be more microbes in it than before.

To what an extent the occurrence of microbes in such chronic inflammatory foci can actually be accidental is evident from the experiments of Dr. Kashkin from A. G. Molotkov's clinic. Studying the micro-flora of chronic ulcerous foci before and after neurotomy, he established that section of the corresponding nerve by itself *brings about a radical change in the micro-flora.* Forms that were present before the operation disappear and are replaced by new ones, which for a time become just as constant as the old ones. Thus, from being an active participant, or even the producing agent, the microbes are degraded to a subordinate position.

All this, however, must not be taken to imply that the microbes do not play any role as initiators of inflammation, or are not capable of maintaining it.

For the microbe to be actually both the producing and supporting agent of inflammation, a number of conditions must be simultaneously fulfilled. Above all, *it must be an irritating agent,* and for chronic inflammation it must also be a weak irritating agent, as far as the nerve cells are concerned. If the irritation produced by it is a large one, a violent reaction will result which will either rapidly put an end to the microbe or, equally rapidly, end in the death of the organism.

With weak degrees of irritation, the process may begin imperceptibly. We have seen above that an externally weak irritating agent of this kind is capable *in the final result* of proving far more dangerous. The functions of the irritating agent are imperceptibly transferred to the nerve cell which becomes the source of new irritation that progressively develops within the network of the nervous system. At this stage, not only the maintenance of the inflammation, but also its transition to a chronic form and the creation of new local foci, *is brought about by other mechanisms.*

For the microbe subsequently to retain even the mere role of an *indicator,* conferring particular, special features on the inflammation, it must find the conditions necessary for its existence in the altered tissues. The new local foci that have appeared at the periphery as a result of nervous dystrophy will in that case be colonised by the microbe which was the initiator of the whole process only if the physico-chemical conditions of the environment are suitable *precisely for this microbe* and for no other. If this is not the case, the disease, which *began under the action of one irritating agent, will continue under the ægis of another*—perhaps even an innocent one; in the meantime, the physician, reasoning from the obvious, will ascribe to this other agent both the initiation and the whole responsibility for the subsequent course of the process.

One has only to change the state of innervation of an organ which was hitherto an easy "prey" to the virus, for instance to sever the *n. vagi* of a rabbit's stomach, for the character of the tuberculous process to change accordingly. The temporary character of this change makes the matter only more evident; we know, indeed, that *precisely the nervous system cannot be changed in a definite fashion, and once for all.* Our operation stimulates a whole series of processes, which develop progressively and do not rapidly die out. *In the secondary foci,* therefore, the fate of the virus, and with it the characteristic features of the whole process, is connected with the state of the tissues which preceded the appearance of the microbe and gave the latter the possibility of exhibiting its actual or apparent activity. But the state of a tissue, both in the sense of what constitutes its environment and in the sense of the energy of its living elements, depends on mobile influences of a nervous nature; consequently *the nervous factor in the process is decisive from beginning to end.*

When tuberculosis is studied in conditions of *laboratory experiments,* both the impulse to the development of the process and the infection of the secondary foci proceed from a single source. *In the clinic,* the impulse may be malaria, grippe, processes of a rheumatic type like *erythema nodosum,* physical factors, etc. The formation of secondary foci is not connected here with the infection from which the disease obtains its name.

This makes it possible to understand the divergence in the course and outcome of laboratory and spontaneous tuberculosis. *However many rabbits we take, using the same form of infection, the resulting picture of the disease in them will be alike.* Departures from the general norm are rare and mainly quantitative. *Yet the human and animal clinic is not acquainted with any other disease which can compare with tuberculosis for variety in form, course and outcome.*

I desire to emphasise that the analysis which has been made aims at regarding the question from the point of view of general pathology. Tuberculosis was taken not on its own account but solely because it includes the most typical features of chronic inflammation in general. We find another example in syphilis.

Here also, according to the generally accepted view, the spirochæte is the cause of the process from beginning to end. With such a simple way of deciding the question, it would seem that no doubtful points ought to arise. And yet the very necessity of reckoning with the spirochæte at every moment makes the current views on the pathogenesis of syphilis a purely verbal exercise in attempts to escape from a mass of contradictions.

I shall not set out any details about the pathogenesis of syphilis and immunity in this disease. They are well known to everyone, or—more correctly —are not known to anyone. Matters here are far worse than in regard to tuberculosis. There is hardly any other process in which verbal superstructures to the experimental data are so inevitable. One cannot help coming to the conclusion that there is some mistake at the very foundations of the theory, not of *syphilis, but of inflammation in general,* making it impossible to arrange the factors in a definite logical order.

The successes obtained in the prophylaxis and clinical treatment of rabies, tetanus, anthrax and especially diphtheria, gave rise to a natural endeavour to increase the number of processes dealt with. These efforts did not bear the anticipated fruits, but previous successes still prevent the basic theses from being shaken. Changes in organs during the infectional processes are still regarded as the result of contact of the organs with a specific irritating agent, and also as evidence of mutual struggle between the two factors. We have already repeatedly seen that such a conception can by no means always be justified in fact. *The strength of one of the factors—the microbe— is considerably weaker than is usually thought; on the other hand, the other factor— the injured organism—is capable of inflicting damage on its own tissues and organs to a much greater extent than is done by the microbe.*

The strangest fact in the pathogenesis of syphilis must be considered the absence of "actual" immunity, although we possess a number of data showing that the spirochæte is a real antigen and that "theoretical" immunity in the form of a whole series of specific reactions *in vitro* and *in vivo* does occur.

After the lapse of a certain time from infection, further inoculations in rabbits are not accompanied by development of sclerosis. This signifies that the spirochæte has now ceased to be the specific irritant that it was before, and that to a certain extent it has been rendered harmless ("infectional immunity"). *Is it not surprising that the rabbit, after developing immunity and rendering the spirochæte harmless, may nevertheless perish as a result of severe "syphilitic" destruction of its tissues with development of a mass of new local foci, which just before it was supposed to be incapable of forming?* Can one rest satisfied with an explanation of this based on such definitions as immunity to chancre (*Schankerimmunität*) or special immunity for the skin alone, an explanation which *attempts to legitimise the fact by a purely verbal formulation?*

The fact is also noteworthy that, with the continuing development of syphilis in a human organism, the local symptoms become increasingly more severe (roseoles, papulæ, pustules, gummata), while the amount of the immediate irritating agent continually decreases in these affected areas, so that, for instance, in the gummata the spirochæte can only be discovered with difficulty.

Experimental syphilis in rabbits is in its general picture very closely analogous to that in human beings. After inoculation there is *a prolonged incu-*

bational period, followed by sclerosis and subsequent remittent development of the disease.

Kolle's experiments showed that repeated inoculations in rabbits during the first 90 days after infection also cause formation of chancre. If they are produced by a different stock, the period is prolonged to 120 days. After that the "skin" rather suddenly loses its "sensitivity" to the virus, although during the whole preceding period its sensitivity was for some reason growing all the time, judging by the fact that the incubational period of each subsequent infection progressively decreased. *For both these phenomena we have nothing but the verbal conceptions of anergy and allergy,* in which we have to take refuge at each period of alteration of the syphilitic phenomena.

Another fact must be mentioned in regard to experimental syphilis in rabbits. A certain percentage of animals on inoculation develop neither sclerosis nor any other syphilitic symptoms. This does not mean, however, that the rabbit is not infected. It is only the *picture* of the disease which is lacking; at the same time the spirochæte can be found in its tissues, and its lymphatic glands provide excellent material for infecting other animals. Such rabbits are called *"nullers."* Kolle gave a method for producing them at will. For this purpose, he introduces insoluble compounds of bismuth (creating a bismuth depot) into the rabbit's tissues. Infection of such rabbits is not accompanied by sclerosis or subsequent symptoms of syphilis, but in these cases also the spirochæte is easily discoverable in the tissues. Kolle terms this state symptomless infection (*symptomlose Infektion*). A similar phenomenon was noticed by Nicolle and Lebailly in guinea-pigs infected with virus of *typhus exanthematicus* and termed by them *"infection inapparente."*

What has been said by no means exhausts all the perplexities encountered in studying the pathogenesis of syphilis, but I do not think it is necessary to give a full enumeration of them. *It is not part of our task to study this process as a specific pathological form.* After observing in the case of tuberculosis the fundamental features of the general questions relating to the nervous factor in chronic inflammation, the direction taken by our work on syphilis followed automatically.

Even on a first acquaintance with the experimental work on syphilis, the question of "nullers" could not but attract our attention. The data obtained by Kolle in this respect acquired a special meaning for us. We could only regard them in the following light: to obtain the full picture of the disease in rabbits, *not only infection, but also a focus of primary irritation in the nervous system is necessary.* Consequently, the experimental problem consisted in establishing *whether in syphilis the nervous system participates in the formation of the primary and secondary foci, and if so, to what extent.* The solution of this question provided us with the clue to a number of other problems.

The appropriate experiments were performed by my collaborator I. A. Pigalev. The work was carried out on rabbits, and we used for infection Truffi's stock, obtained from Professor V. M. Aristovsky. Observations on the course of syphilis in rabbits have been carried on by us for more than four years, and the basic features have been fully elucidated.

The first thing that must be mentioned here is that after inoculation into the skin of the scrotum of normal rabbits, in 95 per cent of cases we obtained typical sclerosis *even before the lapse of 35 days.* In 3-4 per cent, the incubational period was longer than this, and in 1-2 per cent we had "nullers." Sclerosis progressively increased until it attained certain definite dimensions, whereupon, after persisting for a certain period, it gradually disappeared. A pause then occurred, after which a period began marked by secondary symptoms appearing in typical places (eyelids, lips, nose, anal region).

Having thus obtained an idea of the course of the process in normal animals, we passed on to experiments with various kinds of nerve injuries, consisting at the beginning in severance of the nerves relating to the scrotum.

Our aim was not the denervation of the tissue, but the infliction of a nerve trauma causing a corresponding mobile change of the state of innervation in the given region. Most frequently we sectioned the *n. pudendus* in the gluteal region and the *n. genitofemoralis* on the dorsal wall of the trunk (extra-peritoneal method). Sometimes we included also the *n. cutaneus femoris lateralis.* In some cases the nerves were severed only on one side of the body, in other cases on both sides; it was found, however, that this did not play any essential role as regards the general consequences observed—unilateral and bilateral nerve injuries gave the same results. This further strengthened us in the conviction that *the important question is not so much the severance of the particular nerves selected, as the infliction in general of a nerve trauma in the given region.*

The operation itself is carried out by means of incisions in the lumbar and upper gluteal region, *i.e.,* in regions remote from that of the future infection —the skin of the scrotum. Each experiment was accompanied by a control. Infection of the experimental animals was carried out 5-15 days after the operation, under exactly the same conditions as for the controls and *always in the same places of the skin of the left scrotum.*

As was to be expected, under these new conditions we only rarely obtained the usual form of response.

In the first place, there was a marked change in the incubational period. It was pointed out above that in 95 per cent of cases sclerosis developed in normal rabbits after 35 days from the time of infection; *the latent period never exceeded 40 days.* Under the new experimental conditions, the incubational period was noticeably longer: *it reached 50-70 days, and in some cases even 90 days (rabbit No. 61).* Subsequently, the development of sclerosis frequently assumed an abortive form. Instead of the usual, sharply delimited compact infiltrate, about the size of a large nut, there developed a flat callosity of the skin, having the form and dimensions of a lentil, or somewhat larger. Such a sclerosis could not be used for inoculation. After a short time, the infiltrate began to regress and within 3-4 weeks vanished without leaving a trace.

But the most interesting phenomenon was the appearance, in almost half the total number of cases, after a certain period from the appearance of sclerosis on the left side, of *symmetrically situated typical sclerosis on the right scrotum (which had not been infected).* This phenomenon sometimes occurred after infection of normal rabbits, but it was a rarity. In fact, in working with normal rabbits *we only obtained it two or three times during a number of years.*

The symmetrical sclerosis of the contralateral scrotum was usually of considerably larger dimensions than the primary one. It appeared after various periods, on the 45th, 70th, 80th and *even the 150th day,* sometimes at a time when the primary sclerosis at the place of infection had already faded. It is interesting to note that such a late formation of secondary sclerosis was noted in some rabbits in which the primary sclerosis had appeared only on the 90th day.

Another interesting case was the following. Rabbit No. 15 was infected in the skin of the left scrotum 5 days after bilateral severance of the *n. pudendus* and *n. genitofemoralis.* On the 30th day, a small thickening developed at the point of infection, about the size of a lentil, which persisted unchanged until the 110th day, when a flat, slightly ulcerated, infiltrate appeared also at the symmetrically situated place on the right scrotum. Following this, the original left sclerosis began to increase in size rapidly, and in a short time it grew to the size of a large bean.

Among incidental observations, it is worth noting that after infecting rabbits that have undergone severance of the corresponding nerve, swelling at the place of inoculation is practically lacking even during the first days; while in the control animals it lasts for a long time, frequently until the moment when sclerosis begins.

It follows that when a nerve trauma is added to the usual form of infection of rabbits by syphilis, the form of development of the process undergoes a pronounced change. This finds expression in a number of special features. The most important of these is the development of symmetrically situated affections having all the characters of the primary reaction, *i.e.*, sclerosis, but developing in places where the virus was not injected. These affections are not accidental, for they practically never occur among the controls.

The time of appearance of secondary sclerosis—70-90-150 days after inoculation—is also evidence that we are faced here with some special combination of conditions not usually occurring.

The question arises: *Did not exactly the same phenomenon occur in all our experiments with the usual forms of nervous dystrophy?* We obtained in these experiments, after chemical or ordinary infectional trauma of the nervous system, a segmentary affection of the nervous system with the formation of symmetrical pathological foci in the tisues. The secondary foci *on the healthy side exactly reproduced the picture of the changes primarily exhibited on the side of the trauma.*

A second series of experiments were performed by Dr. I. A. Pigalev under somewhat different experimental conditions.

An account has already been given above of the general features of development of tuberculosis in rabbits in cases where the primary focus was artificially created within the tissues of the anterior abdominal wall close to the medial line. In the development of the disease, *one of the first places to be affected is the scrotum* (*viz.*, the *tunica propria*). The process is sharply interrupted at the level of the inguinal ring and does not cross this boundary.

In other experiments, while studying the action of certain skin irritants, we also had an opportunity of convincing ourselves of the specific character of the reactions exhibited by the rabbit's scrotum in response to irritation (experiments of my collaborators N. A. Astapov and I. P. Bobkov,[1] I. A. Pigalev and A. K. Pukhidsky [2]). The data obtained can be briefly summarised as follows:

As is known, the scrotum of the rabbit consists of two separate halves, which are fused only at the roots. If a platinum loop with lewisite is applied to the distal area of the left or right scrotum then, after a certain time, the skin of this scrotum becomes mortified throughout its extent. The mortification can spread also to the skin of the other scrotum, *but it does not pass to the skin of the stomach* if the latter is protected from immediate contact with the place affected. Exactly the same thing is observed if lewisite is applied to the root of the scrotum close to the inguinal ring. In this case, the mortification spreads downwards and involves the whole scrotum, but *does not cross the boundary of the inguinal canal to the stomach*, in spite of the latter being topo-

[1] N. A. Astapov and I. P. Bobkov. *Med. Sanit. Vopr. Protivokhim. Zaschit.* [*Medico-Hygienic Questions of Anti-Chemical Defence*], Symposium, No. 1, 1932.
[2] I. A. Pigalev and A. K. Pukhidsky. *Ibid.*

graphically so close. Finally, if the same quantity of lewisite is applied to the skin of the lower portion of the stomach in close proximity to the inguinal ring, the mortification advances upwards and involves an extensive area of the skin of the stomach, *while the scrotum remains intact.* (Plates 40-42.)

It is very easy to change all this; all that is required is to perform laparotomy 1½-2 weeks before the experiment, drawing the testicle into the abdominal cavity and separating it from the scrotum. After this, inflammation and mortification passes easily both from the scrotum to the abdominal wall and in the reverse direction.

In the rabbit, the connection of the testicle with the scrotum is very weak. It is represented by some fine bundles of connective tissue running from the *caput epididymis* to the bottom of the scrotum (relics of the *gubernaculum Hunteri*). Separation of the bundles is performed by the means of a blunt instrument and does not cause any bleeding. Nevertheless, *this alone is sufficient to change the properties of the scrotum.*

The experiments on tuberculosis provided grounds for considering that the characteristic-features of the development of the inflammatory process in the scrotum of the rabbit are connected with nervous processes. In that case, the loss of these charactistic features also could only be the consequences of *nervous changes.* Hence, we must regard the operation of separating the *caput epididymis* from the scrotum as a special kind of nerve trauma. This gave us the possibility of drawing a comparison with the data of our other experiments where the course of a particular process showed divergences after what was certainly a nerve trauma. *Our experiments on syphilis were of this kind.*

We decided now to repeat them, substituting for the operation of severing the nerves the separation of the connection between the *caput epididymis* and the scrotum. For the rest, the experiments were performed under the same conditions as before. Controls were selected as usual, infection of the experimental animals was carried out 5-15 days after the operation in a fixed and invariable place of the skin of the left scrotum; in one-half of the experiments, disjunction of the testicles from the scrotum was carried out on one side, while in the other half it was carried out on both sides. The results of the experiments were not noticeably different in the two cases and therefore I include them both in this review.

The operation was made by means of laparotomy. The operation was performed in the middle of the belly, *i.e.,* in a region sufficiently remote from the point of infection. The testicle of the rabbit, deprived of its connection with the scrotum, is not let down again and remains in the abdominal cavity, although the scrotum does not shrivel and the way to it remains open as before.

These experiments *repeated in full the data of the first series.* Here again, we encountered an incubational period two or three times in excess of the normal. The latent period, instead of 25-30 days, was prolonged to 50-70-90 days and above; *this was the rule* since it occurred in more than half the experiments. In accordance with this, we observed an abortive form of sclerosis, regressing very shortly after its appearance. Finally, we not only frequently observed here the development of sclerosis at a symmetrical place on the other healthy scrotum, but we obtained cases where sclerosis *appeared directly at the symmetrically situated place on the right side, while on the left side at the point of actual infection there were no signs of specific reaction.*

Specially interesting in this respect is the case of one rabbit in which the testicles were disconnected on both sides. The primary (in reality, of course, secondary) sclerosis here developed not on the left side at the point of inoculation, but at the symmetrically situated place. Its appearance was first noticed on the 90th day. Gradually increasing in size, it reached the dimensions of a pea but afterwards regressed and disappeared on the 180th day. Beginning from the 210th day, sclerosis began to develop spontaneously in the same rabbit in an absolutely typical form, *and again at the root of the right scrotum.*

It must be mentioned that we obtained several cases in the experiments of this series *where the process was accelerated instead of slowing down.* Thus, in rabbit No. 37 sclerosis was noticed on the left side at the place of infection as early as the 17th day—and on the 40th day symmetrical sclerosis appeared on the right side.

Whatever criterion is applied to these experiments, it is clear that the general picture of syphilitic sclerosis in the rabbit can be obtained *not only at the place where the virus is introduced, but also at the symmetrically situated place on the other side.* This sclerosis, like the first one, contains a large amount of spirochætes. It would be difficult to explain the mechanism by which they get here and their subsequent fate, as well as their participation in the development and maintenance of tissue changes, by applying the concepts of direct inoculation, of the struggle of the two agents, *viz.,* the micro-and the macro-organism, of temporary victory of the former and new temporary victory of the latter, or by having recourse to any other of the views that are generally put forward for the more or less ingenious analysis of the pathogenesis of syphilis.

We obtained absolutely typical sclerosis in intact tissues which were connected with the point of primary irritation through the corresponding segment of the nervous system. This sclerosis was undoubtedly secondary; but since it arose within a short period of time and moreover in the same nerve segment, *it repeated in all details the general picture which was found, or ought to have been found, at the primary focus.*

By what means the spirochæte appeared there, maintained itself and multiplied, is another question. There is no doubt that special conditions for its life were produced in the changed tissues. It need not even be the sole inhabitant. We confirmed by experiment that in the sclerosis of the rabbit it is always possible to discover not only the spirochæte but also an ordinary flora, even in very large quantity. It is interesting that these ordinary microbes are *also confined within the limits of the sclerotically altered tissues,* without producing any additional inflammatory symptoms in the neighbourhood, although they easily produce extensive suppuration on inoculation at any other point of the body of the same animal.

In making it his aim to determine, not only the cause, but also the course of a particular pathological phenomenon, the physician, for some reason, adopts different methods of work in studying these two aspects. *The cause is regarded as something invariable, given once for all, while the course or development of the disease, on the contrary, is looked upon as a sequence of reactions.* Time is concretely taken into account only in the second division of the work, and not in the first. This is a mistake. *The cause, like the consequence, changes with time.*

The development of the reaction is a chain of separate links connected in a definite order. Each of the links in the chain cannot have the same cause as the preceding one. It is clear that *as the process develops, its driving force also continually changes.*

In order to recognise that a muscle cell is a mesodermal cell, it is necessary to pass in review mentally the whole cycle of transformations undergone by the latter. The first and last stages of this development, taken separately, are not comparable, *since apart from their history they have nothing in common.* We encounter exactly the same state of affairs if we try to compare the causes of the initial and final reactions in any other complex biological process. *The connection between them can even be entirely lost.* Not knowing the paths and stages of transformation of the cause, up to the present time we are still unable to understand why, for instance, the common cold in one case produces grippe, in another—pneumonia, in a third—nephritis, in a fourth—inflammation of the cerebral membranes or tuberculosis of the knee, and in a fifth —nothing at all.

The materials analysed by us demonstrate very clearly, not only the development of the pathological process, *but also the evolution of its causes.*

Chemical and infectional trauma of nerve structures results in nervous dystrophy; this, in its turn, gives the impulse for the development in the tissues of other kinds of pathological change, *including those of an inflammatory character*. Their disposition at the periphery can be *predicted by us in advance*, and their boundaries *remain unchanged*, often throughout long periods.

It is considered that the basic cause of inflammation is some external "injurious influence." It is clear from our cases that the injurious influence was only such for particular points of the organism and became impotent even in neighbouring portions. Such a state of things would be inconceivable if the "injurious influence" was actually brought in from outside. Consequently, other causes are concerned, lying concealed in the primary change of the tissues themselves at particular points.

A local change of the state of the nervous system is, above all, a local change of the environment, a destruction of the normal physico-chemical state of the given region. However this destruction comes about—whether by a foreign agent or processes of an internal nature—the character of the reactions exhibited will be one and the same, for now *the damaged elements of the organism themselves become a foreign agent for it.* Consequently, the nervous system is itself capable of being the organiser of inflammation, of creating the "injurious influence" which produces the inflammation.

It seems to me that the above-described observations categorically decide the question of the participation of the nervous system, *not only in the course but in the genesis of the inflammatory process, and that as far as principle is concerned, the matter can be regarded as settled.*

An infectional or toxic focus, exactly like an irritating agent of a physical nature, produces changes in the organism both locally and at a distance. These changes may pass away without leaving traces, but this is not always so. Where the nervous system is drawn into the process, the fate of the primary focus and the generalisation of the process cease to be dependent on local causes alone. A new additional cause makes its appearance, as a result of which the original cause easily becomes obscured, and finally loses its importance.

This is especially pronounced in processes of infectional origin, where the immediate irritating agent may be both annihilated and neutralised by a series of specific and non-specific reactions. We have seen that if microbes are present chronically (often for a number of years) in the pathologically altered tissues, this is far from being proof that the organism is incapable of coping with them. On the contrary; the microbe is neutralised, it does not itself irritate the tissues any longer, *and precisely for that reason its physical destruction becomes impossible.* At the same time, such destruction is useless, since, *after the microbe has ceased to be the cause of the disease,* the destruction of the microbe does not abolish the disease.

If, in our analysis of the general complex of conditions of acute inflammation, lasting hours or days, we were compelled to put the nervous system in the forefront, its role in chronic inflammation must be still more marked. Indeed, in chronic inflammation *both the maintenance of the primary focus and the formation of secondary foci become nothing less than a new pathological function of the nervous system.*

It is no wonder that up to now we have not had any theory of chronic inflammation. We have been brought up to believe that the nervous system does not play any essential role in this phenomenon. *How could we guess that in the final analysis it is just the nervous system that is its fundamental cause?*

CHAPTER XIX
SPECIFIC REACTIONS

We have still to analyse one question which we have hitherto deliberately omitted from consideration. This question concerns the quality of the irritating agent, in other words, the property of the foreign agent to evoke in the organism a reaction which is distinguished by special features typical of this particular agent. This is a very complicated question. At the same time it is a fundamental one, *since it is precisely the problem of quality which forms the object of study of special pathology, as distinct from general pathology.*

The difficulties that arise in its solution depend not so much even on the complexity of the subject, *as on the absence of correct basic propositions.* We have already had to point out more than once that, in judging the consequences of irritation, the whole chain of subsequent reactions is often considered as the result of the direct action of the irritating agent on each of the reacting elements and that this conception is erroneous. We reached the conviction that the agent commencing the reaction very soon transfers its property of irritating agent to parts of the organism itself.

In this way, a whole mass of reactions arise from a single point. Not all of them are specific. For the investigator to be able to filter out just those processes which are actually connected with a definite and special action, it is necessary to begin by *excluding everything accidental and subsidiary*; in other words the field of work has to be cleared. This naturally restrained us from proceeding directly to the study of specific reactions, and for a number of years caused our attention to be concentrated *on the study of their nonspecific features.*

We saw that rabies, a sore on the *tuber cinereum* produced by a glass sphere, irritation of any branch of the *n. trigeminus* by croton oil, injection of formalin into the pulp cavity of a tooth or of bile into the upper cervical ganglion, introduction of foreign protein or various vaccines into the blood, poisoning by salts of the heavy metals, *e.g.,* corrosive sublimate, etc.—all these are capable of producing in a number of organs changes that are *absolutely constant and so much alike that it is impossible to distinguish them from one another.* It is clear that we cannot connect the production of these changes with special qualities of the irritant used, otherwise we should have to compare a glass sphere with corrosive sublimate and the latter with rabies virus. It is clear that the presence of the irritant, *e.g.*, corrosive sublimate, in the foci of acute local affections cannot alter our point of view on this subject, since we obtain exactly the same foci, in the same form, and at the same places, without using any poisonous substances.

Nor is importance to be attached to the fact that in cases of chronic poisoning (mercury, lead), particles of the heavy metals are deposited in chronic inflammatory foci. It is interesting to note that these places are very constant. The chief proof of the theory of "tropism" is derived from this fact. But, as we have already shown, *this topographical constancy casts suspicion on the whole interpretation.* We saw in our experiments that a glass sphere placed on the *sella turcica* "selects" for local peripheral foci exactly the same places as lead or corrosive sublimate. Are we not then justified in thinking that these places have been prepared by another process and that their *origin is only historically connected with the immediate irritating agent?*

This is the reason why it is necessary at the outset to become acquainted with the constant features which do not depend on the properties of the irritating agent and are exhibited equally in all cases of irritation.

In analysing this aspect of the matter we found that the time factor is prominent above all, for without taking it into account all other data lose their value. Additional irritations on the part of the nervous system soon convert the reaction into a complex of direct and reflected actions. It then becomes impossible to speak of special properties of the irritating agent, since even its complete removal is often powerless to arrest the process.

Nevertheless, this process in some strange fashion is capable of preserving its qualitative peculiarities throughout many months and years! The explanation of this contradiction is simultaneously also the key to the problem of quality in pathology.

Concrete work in this direction can be reduced to the analysis of two propositions.

The first is connected with estimation of the time factor. If qualitative characteristics are inherent in a pathological process, then (as was shown by examples taken from the sphere of chronic inflammation) they must be communicated to it *in the first stages of the action of the irritating agent.*

The second proposition is of much greater theoretical importance. We have seen that the irritating agent can be withdrawn from the organism or neutralised, and yet the process preserves its specific features. Consequently, for a certain time, changes produced in the organism by the irritating agent can remain in it, *not simply in the form of ordinary irritation, but in a special —qualitatively distinct—form of this irritation.*

It is generally believed that this peculiar form of irritation is preserved by the elements that have already come into immediate contact with the irritating agent.

Weighty considerations in support of this view are derived from the study of experimental malignant neoplasms. At the present time, methods exist for converting normal tissue cultures into cultures producing malignant tumours under the influence of chemical irritation (Fischer, Carrel, Laser). As a result of a number of consecutive transfers, a culture of normal cells becomes "cancerous," with all the inherent characteristics thereby involved, and retains its new properties even when the irritant is no longer applied. All this takes place *in vitro*; no nerve influences are required. The experiments mentioned give a negative answer to the question of the role of the nervous system in this process, and any attempt to prove that it does play a part here is condemned to failure in advance.

However, this is the situation only on a hasty view. In experiments on tuberculosis in tissue cultures *in vitro*, we encountered an essentially similar phenomenon. This did not put a stop to our study of the role of the nervous system in tuberculosis and, as was shown, *led to an affirmative answer to this question.*

The basic premise consists in the inadmissibility of analogies between processes taking place in a complex organism and in tissue cultures. Even if an epithelial cell is converted into a cancer cell in consequence of immediate contact with the irritant, it is still necessary to discover *whether there is anything in the organism which is capable of facilitating or preventing such a transformation.*

The first experimental data on the question of the connection of neoplasms with a definite functional state of the nervous system were provided by Spiess. In the case of cancer in mice or cancer of the throat in man, he succeeded in showing that repeated local anæsthesia results in inhibiting the growth of neoplasms and sometimes even causes them to disappear altogether.

That the nervous system must possess at least some influence on the development of neoplasms can be considered experimentally established by the experiments on so-called tar cancer. First Ischikawa and Kotzareff, and afterwards Tsunoda and others, by severing various nerves of the ear in rabbits, sometimes obtained a considerable increase in growth of tar papillomata, and at other times, on the contrary, inhibition of their development. Even before this, A. G. Molotkov had obtained in some cases rapid cures of cancer of the cheek and upper lip in man by severing the second branch of the *n. trigeminus*. Ricker also put forward a number of data from his observations providing evidence of the connection of neoplasms with changes in the nervous system. The histological researches of Argaut, Ischikawa and others revealed the presence of nerves in cancer tumours. Martynov proved their considerable development in stages preceding the formation of tar cancer in rabbits. The clinic has long known that cancer is frequently accompanied by pathological symptoms of a nervous character.

Consequently, there is no doubt that some connection exists between neoplasms and the nervous system. However, a formal indication of the participation of the nervous system in this process is not sufficient. The nervous system, being connected with almost every cell of the organism, must as a matter of course be involved in all pathological processes. *The problem is to determine the form and extent of this participation.*

A series of experiments, described in preceding chapters of this book, have shown that the nervous system is not only involved in, but *organises and determines* many pathological forms which hitherto have been regarded as independent of nervous influences. We bore these conceptions in mind when approaching the study of tar cancer.

We carried out operations on various parts of the gastro-intestinal tract of rabbits. The irritant used was coal tar, obtained from the Moscow Gas Works (experiments of my collaborator I. A. Pigalev [1]).

In the first place, we tested the action of coal tar *on those regions of the gastro-intestinal tract which had previously attracted our attention during the study of other processes.*

It was not a matter for surprise that in this new form of experiment approximately the same result was obtained. In the course of 3-4 weeks, a drop of tar, introduced once under the mucous membrane of the stomach, caused cauliflower-like tumours, sometimes of considerable size, to develop in the immediate vicinity. Microscopical examination demonstrated the presence of adenoma with atypical growth of epithelium, which invaded the *muscularis mucosae* and had lost its normal morphological structure (absence of the chief and covering cells, the epithelium passing into a high cylindrical form). The growth of the adenoma sometimes proceeded very rapidly. We obtained cases where, even within 20-25 days from the moment of injection of tar, the adenoma reached a size of 5-8 sq. cm. with a height up to 1 cm.

In other, rarer cases, the process was limited to a feeble ulcer of the mucous membrane at the point of injection.

In many scores of experiments, on the introduction of tar under the mucous membrane of the small or large intestine, we never observed any but ordinary inflammatory changes. Only on repeated application of tar tam-

[1] I. A. Pigalev. *Arkh. Biol. Nauk,* Vol. 28, No. 4, 1928; *Zeitschr. f. d. ges. exp. Med.,* Vol. 63, Nos. 5, 6, 1928.

pons *in the rectum* of rabbits did we obtain in two or three cases the formation of small adenomata in the substance of the mucous membrane and papillomata on the skin around the anus.

To clear up the question, it was desirable to put it experimentally in a sharper form. This involved obtaining an answer to the question whether the epithelium actually reacts to the tar only as a result of direct contact with it.

The mucous membrane of the stomach is very sensitive to this irritant: within 3-4 weeks we often obtained an adenoma of considerable size. Consequently, the reaction must have begun here from the very beginning. *If it were to be shown that even in the first stage the reaction was governed by changes in the state of the local innervation, then the question would be automatically settled.*

The experiment was arranged by us in the old form that had previously proved its worth (experiments of I. A. Pigalev). A series of observations were made on rabbits in which we severed both trunks of the *n. vagi* at the œsophagus before injecting tar into the stomach. The animals were killed at various periods—from 3 weeks to 1½ months. *Atypical growth of epithelium was now not obtained in a single case.* Sometimes a feeble, slowly cicatrising ulcer made its appearance. In the later periods, we succeeded in noting the formation of shagreened portions of the mucous membrane but the development did not go so far as adenoma.

We should like to emphasise once again the resemblance between these results and those repeatedly obtained by us in other experiments.

This resemblance goes even further. It was once more confirmed here that it is not on account of the denervation of the tissues that vagotomy has an influence on the process of development of tar adenomata. *It is a question of nerve trauma, i.e.,* of temporary change in the state of the nervous system.

It was found that after vagotomy the development of the adenoma is only retarded, but not abolished. When we tried killing the rabbits after a long period (2½-3½ months), we discovered in many cases atypical growth of epithelium in the locus of the old ulcer with its calloused base. The edges of the ulcer were raised, giving a cauliflower-like appearance. Microscopical analysis revealed adenoma with atypical growth of epithelium. It should be remembered that in our experiments during the study of acute and chronic inflammation, something very similar was noted. We were compelled to connect the result with a change in the character of nervous interrelations. *Consequently, both categories of processes have one thing in common, viz., their nervous component.* If there is anything that must be demonstrated, it is not the participation of the nervous system in these processes, but, on the contrary, our right to regard local elements (epithelium, muscles, connective tissue, etc.) as independent originators of special forms of response to irritation.

Experiments on the development of "malignant" properties by cells in tissue cultures *in vitro*, under the influence of chemical actions, cannot in any way contradict this thesis. The effect which is produced in tissue cultures *in vitro*, by a chemical agent introduced from outside, is performed *in vivo* by a different agent, also foreign and also chemical in nature, but arising in this case as a result of an abnormal state of the nervous system.

Everyone is acquainted with cases where, after the ear of the rabbit has been smeared with tar several times, this operation was for some reason or other discontinued. Inflammatory changes of the skin, in the form of desquamation rapidly disappear. The rabbit remains healthy for many months. But sometimes, without any visible cause, tar papillomata and genuine chancroids suddenly appear on the ear. *Thus, the trace of the former irritation proves to have been preserved here in exactly the same form as originally.*

The fact that the character of the reaction is determined during the first stages of irritation and that the nervous system plays a decisive role in this process, permits us to answer the question put at the beginning of this chapter: what are the elements in which the traces of the special form of irritation are preserved?

Let us assume that under laboratory conditions, when a really foreign agent artificially introduced from outside begins the reaction, the nervous system only creates accessory conditions which are, nevertheless, essential for the course of the process. This signifies that if the local nerve conditions at any point of the organism are changed by some other cause, *but in the same way* as by the action of the foreign agent, *the consequences will inevitably be identical.*

From this we can draw two conclusions:

1) The quality of an irritating agent is expressed in its capacity to evoke a special form of nerve irritation;

2) The nervous system can retain for some time traces of such irritation without changing the characteristic features of the latter.

It is necessary to test these propositions by the investigation of some process where the specific properties of the irritating agent are unquestioned.

The most suitable process for this purpose is tetanus. If it had not been for tetanus toxin, the idea of the quality of the irritating agent would never have attained its present form. In this regard, tetanus toxin is even more interesting than diphtheria toxin. In animals, the use of the latter produces a non-typical picture of "general" disease, ending in death. Tetanus toxin also produces death, but before this it gives rise to a series of symptoms which are very characteristic and *comprise a definite cycle of pathological symptoms.*

At the present time, the whole pathogenesis of tetanus is looked upon as the result of the direct contact of each reacting element to the irritant. According to the generally accepted point of view, the toxin advances along the nerve from its place of formation or introduction to the corresponding cell structures of the spinal cord. Acting directly on them, it sharply increases their reflex excitability. At the beginning, this is observable within the limits of one or two nerve segments. As new portions of the toxin arrive, the toxin spreads upwards and downwards along the spinal cord, involving the corresponding elements of neighbouring regions. The process terminates in generalisation of the tetanus symptoms throughout the central nervous system.

Hence, the whole thing is reduced to a simple and almost mechanical factor; all nerve elements drawn into the process are connected directly with the toxin; if the toxin did not move along the nerve and spinal cord, we should not know what tetanus is. In full accordance with this view, *it is believed that the only way to put an end to the symptoms of tetanus is by removing or neutralising the toxin.*

As already noted, this view enjoys general recognition. It is based on absolutely direct experiments, the chief of which can be divided into two series. The first series comprises experiments demonstrating the progressive accumulation of the toxin at various levels of the nerve trunks connected with the place of injection. The second establishes that preliminary section of the corresponding spinal nerves safeguards the animal against the disease, even when active and fatal doses of toxin are injected into the tissues. Other researches have aimed only at supplementing these data with further details.

The matter seemed settled without leaving any doubts or reasons for new experiments. Such was the state of affairs before we had arrived at the necessity of dividing the mechanism of movement of various substances along the nerve trunk into two forms, passive and active.

If the active form of movement is the result of chemical interaction between the toxin and the nerve tissue, then *irritation begins from the first stage of the process and not merely from the moment when the toxin reaches the nerve cell and enters into combination with it.* This circumstance has somehow been left out of account. We directed attention to it for the first time in the experiments described above, performed on dogs, in which we injected the toxin into the muscles of the knee after unilateral or bilateral removal of the abdominal sympathetic chain. The influence on the course of the tetanus process of the new conditions thus created was then obvious. It became clear that, other conditions being equal, *changes even in remote nerve regions are capable of sharply altering the form of response of elements in which the process appears to develop selectively.* All this caused us to doubt the correctness of the orthodox conception of the pathogenesis of tetanus.

Direct grounds for such doubt were furnished by a chance observation described in the work of my collaborator Dr. S. I. Lebedinskaya,[1] belonging to the period when we were studying the consequences of nerve trauma inflicted repeatedly after various intervals of time. As has been shown, the reaction obtained by no means always corresponded to the character of the repeated irritation. Frequently it gave rise to a process which had developed or ought to have developed as a result of the primary irritation.

On one occasion we used a dog which had recovered after injection of a small dose of tetanus toxin into the muscles of the left knee. During the illness it had suffered only from tetanus of the left hind extremity. This developed seven days after injection of the toxin and gradually increased, but did not pass to the region of other muscles and persisted about twenty days. After that, the animal regained the power of using the affected organ.

Five days after the final extinction of the disease symptoms, the dog was accidentally included in another experiment which at the time did not have any relation to the study of tetanus. The animal underwent trepanning, and a glass sphere was placed in the region behind the *sella turcica* (*tuber cinereum*). The consequences of this operation, as described many times above consists of various forms of dystrophy, generalised throughout certain tissues and organs. In this particular case, *the consequence of the operation was the re-establishment of the tetanus symptoms which had disappeared not long before*. Within 24 hours, the dog underwent tonic cramps mainly in the hind extremities, which after 48 hours resulted in the typical syndrome of segmentary tetanus. This was followed by heightened reflex excitability, rigidity of the vertebral column, opisthotonus and death.

There can be no doubt that the tetanus was renewed here *without any participation of the specific toxin*. The "glass sphere operation" was carried out more than a month after the injection of toxin, *i.e.*, after a period fully sufficient for the development of immunity. Moreover, the animal had been ill and had recovered, and it is usually considered that recovery is only possible if the toxin has been removed or neutralised.

But the most important feature is that we obtained here *something more than a simple relapse*. The original character of the disease consisted only in local tetanus of one of the hind extremities. The relapse not only gave a repetition of the same symptom, but also segmentary, and subsequently general, tetanus.

The inevitable conclusion to be drawn is *that local tetanus can pass into general tetanus without the spreading of the toxin from the region of the primary focus throughout the central nervous system.*

[1] S. I. Lebedinskaya. *Arkh. Biol. Nauk*, Vol. 34, No. 4, 1933.

In our case, the local symptom was merely the first stage of a complex nervous process having *its own definite cycle of development*. With an original irritation of small magnitude, the process was capable of coming to a stop halfway. When, however, the strength of the irritation exceeds a certain limit, the process develops to the end. Underlying it, therefore, is the ready-prepared nervous mechanism, *where each new part that is set to work determines thereby the functioning of the succeeding part.*

If this particular case can be explained in this way, it is surely possible to extend the explanation to all other forms of spontaneous and laboratory tetanus. The question thus raised acquires exceptional importance not only for the pathogenesis of tetanus but *for pathology as a whole*. It was natural that we made this the subject of special investigation.

First of all, it was necessary to test whether a nerve trauma of accidental origin (a "second blow"), applied shortly after the liquidation of tetanus symptoms, was actually capable of re-establishing the process in one or another of its forms.

The corresponding research was conducted by my collaborators I. P. Bobkov and A. L. Fenelonov.[1] Cats were used as the experimental animals, since with dogs it is in general difficult to select a dose of toxin which gives only local tetanus without its subsequent generalisation. In cats, the process develops more slowly, easily stops at the stage of local tetanus and quite often ends in recovery.

It was established by preliminary experiments, that on introducing tetanus toxin *into the anterior chamber of the eye, and especially into the corpus vitreum*, cats are easily able to cope with the disease, even if the toxin is injected in more than fatal doses. In addition, the disease is deprived of its characteristic features. The symptoms of local tetanus are lacking or, in some strange fashion, *they are transferred to the opposite end of the central nervous system*. Thus, we frequently observe the first local symptom in the caudal region and muscles of the hind extremities. On stroking the animal, rigidity was increased to the degree of tonic cramps. Subsequently, rigidity of the vertebral column developed, but it rarely reached a high degree.

All these symptoms usually persist for a comparatively short time, 3-7 days and disappear without leaving traces. Of nine cats, *only one died*. When the same toxin, but in a dose only one-sixth to one-eighth of the former amount was injected intramuscularly into nine other cats, the consequence was always local, and sometimes general, tetanus. *Of this series, only four cats recovered.*

Some 3-5 days after the convulsive symptoms had disappeared, *an additional nerve trauma was inflicted on the animals of both series*: in some cases

---

[1] Unpublished manuscript.

bile was injected into the right or left sciatic nerve, and the nerve was then severed, in other cases drops of bile were introduced into the upper cervical ganglion. For almost all the animals, both forms of operation proved fatal. Some of them even died in the hours immediately following the operation, others lived for 2-6 days. In this experiment, it was found that the convulsive phenomena, which had disappeared some days previously, *suffered a relapse that took on an even more pronounced form than originally*. Here also it was noticed that touching produced a pronounced increase of the rigidity of the tail, hind extremities and vertebral column, twitching of the spinal muscles, etc.

Normal animals easily tolerate an injection of bile into the sciatic nerve. The consequence in their case takes the form of tissue dystrophy developing after a comparatively long period. We have performed operations of this kind so often that there was no necessity of repeating them specially in this case. As far as injection of bile into the upper cervical ganglion of normal cats is concerned, we made a series of control experiments. Of five cats, three died on the sixth or seventh day, two remained alive. *Not one of the animals exhibited convulsive symptoms*. In all of them, only coughing and general weakness was observed.

Weighing up these data, we have to recognise that a nerve trauma, applied to various regions of the nervous system of an animal that has only just recovered from tetanus, *is actually capable in some cases of restoring the previous picture of the disease in all its details*.

Thus, we find a repetition here of the phenomenon which we have already repeatedly encountered in investigating the processes combined in this book under the general name of nervous dystrophy. If traces of a previously existing irritation are retained within the nerve network, then a new, even accidental, action may evoke a reaction corresponding in form to the primary irritation.

We cannot, of course, count on restoring the original picture by means of a second blow in all experiments without exception. The second blow can evoke the reaction interesting us *only as long as the latter has not been finally extinguished*. Consequently, it is necessary here to take into account the basic factor of time, which, however, is not fully at the disposal of the investigator.

We have seen that *not only the result of the reaction but also its whole course may be re-established*. This means that the nervous process, developing in time and consisting of an intricate complex of successively developing stages, is contained in the nervous system as such *in the form of a ready-prepared mechanism*. The external agent is merely necessary to supply sufficient force to start the reaction. Subsequently, this agent can be completely neutralised or removed but the process will nevertheless proceed to its natural con-clusion.

In the above-described data, attention is attracted by the fact of local symptoms being transferred from the region of the segment immediately irritated to the opposite end of the central nervous system. This fact has not yet been made the subject of investigation in the pathogenesis of tetanus.

Up to now three forms of the development and course of tetanus have been known.

Usually, the disease begins with the nerve segment corresponding to the place of injection of toxin. From here the process gradually spreads to the spinal cord and brain. This form is observed in dogs, cats, rabbits, guinea-pigs, mice and some other animals.

In man and in horses, a second form occurs, in which tetanus begins at once with so-called general phenomena, omitting the local stage.

Finally a third form, described by Roux, can be obtained only under ar-tificial conditions, when tetanus toxin is introduced directly into the central nervous system. This form is known by the name of cerebral tetanus.

The features that we observed on injecting the toxin into the *corpus vitreum* of the cat *do not come under any of the above-mentioned categories.* This caused us to devote more detailed study to the tetanus syndrome in cats on injection of the toxin into various organs of the body.

The aim in view was to test the influence exerted by the *place of primary injection of the toxin on the form of the disease and successive development of its symptoms.*

Various types of experiment were performed by my collaborators Drs. I. P. Bobkov, A. L. Fenelonov, M. O. Ossipov and S. I. Lebedinskaya. The observations of Lebedinskaya and Ossipov [1] showed that, on unilateral injection of the toxin into the muscles of the knee the *first local symptom was frequently caudal tetanus.* The tail was rigid and sharply bent to the side in which the toxin had been injected. Even when the disease involves both halves of the nerve segment, the tail still remains bent asymmetrically.

On suboccipital injection of toxin, the first local symptoms are again exhibited in the tail and hind extremities. It might be thought that the nervous system of the tail is especially sensitive to the action of tetanus toxin. This aroused a natural desire to find out how the tetanus would develop if the tail itself was selected as the place for injection of toxin.

The result obtained was unexpected. *On subcutaneous injection of toxin in the distal portion of the tail, rigor frequently commenced in the hind ex-tremities.* Only afterwards did the tail become involved in the process. If a

[1] Unpublished manuscript.

small dose of toxin is taken (but one sufficient for producing the disease on injection into the tissues of other parts of the body), and is injected subcutaneously in the distal portion of the tail, it is quite possible that no symptoms at all will be obtained. It is interesting to note that in some cases such animals died fairly rapidly, but without developing either local or general tetanus symptoms. In these cases, the toxin apparently evoked some new form of reaction not typical of the disease.

I should like to call to mind here some experiments of my collaborators Doinikov, Suslov and Zhabotinsky, which were described above in the chapter on the generalisation of dystrophic phenomena. On the application of chemical trauma to the sciatic nerve, the most pronounced morphological changes are observed in the nerve elements of the corresponding segment. From here the affection spreads upwards along the spinal cord, *more or less uniformly diminishing in intensity*. An entirely different picture is obtained if one of the nerves of the brachial plexus is selected for the application of the trauma. Uniformity is here replaced by discontinuity. The process suddenly passes from the cervical into the caudal part of the spinal cord, *leaving intact its thoracic portion*. An analysis of the causes of this lack of correspondence led us to recognise differences in the course of the process of irritation itself. The irritating agent was the initiator of all the phenomena but played no part subsequently.

Similar data were also obtained in investigating tetanus symptoms. It is impossible to explain the strange anarchy prevailing here *if one starts out merely from conceptions of the movement of toxin in the nervous system*.

We were finally convinced of this by the material of my collaborators Bobkov and Fenelonov.[1] In testing the influence of the place of injection on the general picture of the disease, among other experiments we introduced the toxin into the upper cervical sympathetic ganglion. When this is performed on cats, *a remarkable picture of sagittal tetanus* almost regularly develops. The disease begins with the cervical muscles, as a result of which the head is turned to the side corresponding to the place of injection. This is followed by tetanus of the fore and hind extremities of the same side and also by muscle rigor of the same half of the trunk.

If the toxin is injected on the left side, the body of the animal will also be bent towards the left, while the left fore and hind extremities are sometimes stretched out like sticks. At the *same time, the right extremities remain flexible and retain almost their normal mobility*.

In some cases, the general picture appears in a pronounced form, in others it is more weakly expressed. Usually, the transition of the process to the op-

[1] Unpublished manuscript.

posite side of the nervous system is retarded, and the process itself rarely attains a considerable degree on that side, since the animal dies before this can happen.

In other experiments with cats, the toxin was injected either into the *m. sterno-cleido-mastoideus* or subcutaneously into the lateral part of the neck. In some cases, a sagittal form of tetanus was also observed here, but it was not pronounced.

Here again we recall our old experiments, the object of which was to study the morphological consequences of chemical trauma of various nerve structures. We observed then that changes in the ganglia of the sympathetic chain in rabbits after unilateral chemical trauma of the sciatic nerve (by croton oil) *spread mainly on the same side as that of the nerve subjected to trauma*. The analysis of the causes of this process also led us to deny that the irritating agent itself took part in it.

If we now compare the various forms of generalisation of the tetanus process, we shall have to divide them into two categories—frontal and sagittal. Both of them can take place in animals of the same species. Thus, on injection of toxin into the muscles of the hind extremities, cats usually experience the frontal form of the development of the disease. The first symptom here will be local tetanus, at the beginning in one, and afterwards in the other, hind extremity, followed by rigor of the vertebral column and fore extremities, opisthotonus, etc. The same cat, if inoculated in the upper cervical ganglion, develops sagittal tetanus. The cause of the difference indicated lies solely in *the choice of the point of primary irritation*. During the first period at any rate, it determines the course of the process of irritation within the network of the nervous system.

It would be a difficult task indeed to attempt an explanation of the phenomena described from the point of view of the movement of the toxin within the central nervous system, and to define the paths and forces of this movement!

Hence, *the process of generalisation of tetanus symptoms throughout the central nervous system can be independent of the presence of toxin within the reacting elements*. In that case, what proofs are there that the primary local symptoms themselves are necessarily connected with the toxin which, by moving along the nerve trunk, reaches the corresponding cells of the spinal cord and affects them?

This conception is based on the well-established fact that tetanus toxin moves along the nerve and penetrates into the brain-stem. Nevertheless, this fact alone is not sufficient. We have seen that absolutely indifferent substances are also capable of entering the nerve trunk and moving along it to the central nervous system. There must be some additional proofs for attaching special significance to this process.

Such proofs actually exist. The most important of them are the well known experiments of Meyer and Ransom. These authors introduced tetanus toxin subcutaneously into one of the extremities of a rabbit, simultaneously injecting a small quantity of anti-toxin into the corresponding nerve; in these conditions the tetanus symptoms were either absent or were retarded in comparison with the control. The conclusion was drawn that tetanus will not result if a barrier is established on the path of the movement towards the spinal cord, neutralising only that portion of the toxin which has penetrated into the nerve trunk.

We repeated the above-described experiments, and fully confirmed them. By this time, however, we had already become well acquainted with the significance of the act of operation itself. In introducing anti-toxin, *i.e.*, a serum, a complex mixture of foreign proteins, the authors aimed at establishing a "specific" barrier for the toxin; *they did not take into account that at the same time they subjected the nerve to trauma.* By so doing, they barred the road to all processes taking place along the nerve, and not only to the toxin alone. As a result of the operation, both the morphological and physiological substratum was altered. It is not surprising that in consequence the normal course of the tetanus process is destroyed. As a matter of fact, severing the corresponding nerve, as is well known, quite certainly prevents the development of tetanus.

Consequently, we considered it necessary to perform a new series of experiments. From a formal point of view, they were intended to repeat the conditions of the experiment of Meyer and Ransom. But, *instead of specific serum for barring the nerve path, we employed normal serum* (experiments of my collaborators V. M. Aristovsky and A. V. Ponomarev [1]).

The observations were made on rabbits. In various combinations, in one animal or several, with single or double controls, the sciatic nerve was barred by a small quantity of diluted anti-toxin or normal serum. Not only was there no difference in the results, but frequently tetanus developed later and was less pronounced in these extremities when normal serum formed the barrier than when specific serum was employed.

In order to settle the question finally, we decided to repeat the experiments in, so to say, a grotesque form, and *to bar the path for tetanus toxin by tetanus toxin itself.*

As controls, analogous experiments were made with anti-toxin and normal serum.

[1] Unpublished manuscript.

The toxin used for forming the barrier was diluted several times with physiological solution. The volume and mode of introduction into the nerve of all the substances mentioned was always the same.

As was to be expected, *the consequences of using toxin were the same as for both sera*. In some cases an even more pronounced effect was obtained by using toxin. Consequently, the act itself of introducing a foreign substance into the nerve, whatever the nature of the substance, plays a fundamental role in the process under consideration.

In another series of experiments, carried out on dogs by my collaborator S. I. Lebedinskaya, the toxin was sometimes injected into the sciatic nerve, at other times into the muscles of the knee. In two cases, this experiment was performed on one and the same animal.

Out of six experiments, only once did the process begin simultaneously in the experimental and the control animal. In the remainder, local phenomena were markedly retarded on the side of injection of toxin into the nerve as compared with injection into the muscles. This occurred both in experiments with different animals and on the same animal. A still greater difference was noted in respect of the time of transition from local to general tetanus and of the duration of the whole disease. After intramuscular injection of toxin, the disease took a more rapid and severe course. It must be added that the dose used in both forms of experiment was almost the same. In any case, toxin in this quantity is not capable of penetrating into the spaces of the nerve trunk from the peripheral tissues either under laboratory or spontaneous conditions. Moreover, a certain amount of it flows back through the puncture from the portion of the nerve that is swollen after the injection. Consequently, the cause of the disease here may be not only the toxin inside the nerve trunk, but also that part of it which enters into contact with the nerve endings inside the tissue.

Above, we reached the conclusion that the presence of toxin within the central nervous system is not indispensable for the generalisation of tetanus symptoms. Now, the same *must be repeated in regard to local tetanus*; in the course of our work, we gradually went further and further from the elements of the central nervous system, until *only a few nerve structures within the tissues* remained for us to deal with. We now concentrated our attention on these.

Thus, the question of tetanus was formulated as the question of a specific form of nerve irritation, which arises in the region of the nerve receptors and which is transferred from there to the centre, subsequently becoming manifested in the form of a ready-prepared complex reaction.

If this is the case we may expect that by separating the nerve endings from the more centrally situated parts of the nervous system, *or even by merely making them unexcitable during the time of encounter with the toxin, we ought to prevent the development of tetanus.*

The prophylactic value of severing the nerve concerned was known long ago in the pathogenesis of local tetanus. Unfortunately, this form of experiment does not furnish any proof in this case, since at the same time it interrupts the path for the movement of toxin. However, the task can be easily fulfilled by adding an anæsthetic to the toxin, in particular novocaine. The only drawback was the possibility that novocaine would have a direct effect on the toxin by neutralising it; hence my collaborator S. I. Lebedinskaya began her experiments by testing this question.

Standard doses of the toxin in our possession were established and several different mixtures of it with novocaine were prepared. They were dialysed at room temperature under conditions which did not allow access of any more water into the prepared mixture. Dialysis was continued until it was impossible to detect even traces of novocaine in the water. Following this, a test was made of the action of the dialysed toxin on dogs and rabbits specially selected in pairs, and a comparison made with the same doses of the original preparation. It was found that *the toxin had not changed in the least during its contact with novocaine.* The experimental animals became ill and died more or less simultaneously with their controls—sometimes a little earlier, sometimes a little later. We drew the conclusion that novocaine and tetanus toxin are indifferent to one another and do not enter into any kind of mutual reaction.

Then we passed to the basic experiments, also on dogs and rabbits. One animal of each pair received a subcutaneous injection into the knee of a definite quantity of tetanus toxin, the other—the same dose of toxin mixed with novocaine. The volume of liquid injected was the same in both cases. Since our aim was to study the genesis particularly of local tetanus symptoms, the doses of toxin used were kept within the limits of one MLD or less.

The results took the following form. *In more than half the cases, the animals that were given a mixture of toxin and novocaine did not become ill,* while all their controls exhibited the full syndrome of local, and often also general, tetanus with the fatal outcome inevitable in such cases. In another part of the experiments, the development of local tetanus symptoms in the experimental group of animals was retarded two or even three times in comparison with the controls. Finally, in a certain number, the difference was inconspicuous, but this occurred either on using an increased dose of toxin or on decreasing the percentage content of novocaine.

It is easy to understand the reason why increasing the dose of toxin also results in wiping out the difference between the experiment and the control.

In studying tetanus under laboratory conditions the whole of the required quantity of toxin is injected at once. Within a few minutes, the subcutaneous swelling at the place of injection disappears, the toxin being absorbed into the drainage system of the organism and passing into the general blood circulation, where, as is well known, its action is considerably weakened. Only a small portion of the toxin remains at the place where it was introduced. If, at this time, the structures subjected to irritation lose their capacity of reacting owing to anæsthesia, a further quantity of the toxin will be washed away. At the moment when normal nerve conditions are re-established, *the quantity of toxin on the spot will be less than the minimum necessary, and tetanus will not result.*

There is no doubt that it is precisely the threshold dose of the irritating agent that matters here, since not all the tetanus toxin is drained away from the place of introduction. It is easy to convince oneself of this by performing experiments with the same or an even greater percentage of novocaine, but increasing the dose of toxin. In that case, the reaction of the experimental animals will only be retarded, and even retardation will not always occur.

Tetanus toxin is a colloid and is taken up by the local tissue elements more energetically than crystalline substances. *The larger the dose introduced, the larger will be the remainder.* After a short period, the novocaine will be washed away and the phenomena of anæsthesia will pass off, but the quantity of toxin remaining at the point of introduction will be sufficient to produce irritation and call forth the corresponding reaction.

In a series of further experiments, we replaced novocaine by other anæsthetics—cocaine and quinine. The results obtained were fundamentally similar to those already described.

One further question remains to be examined, *viz.,* whether the addition of novocaine does not prevent the penetration of tetanus toxin into the nerve, and whether, perhaps, it may not be possible to explain in this way the retardation and even prevention of tetanus symptoms.

This supposition was tested and not confirmed.

We introduced a mixture of toxin with 5 per cent solution of novocaine into the leg muscles of a dog or rabbit and killed the animals after various periods. An emulsion was prepared from pieces of the corresponding sciatic nerve, taken at various levels, and introduced subcutaneously into white mice. *All the mice developed tetanus.* Consequently, the toxin did not lose its capacity of entering the nerve and moving along it, owing to the addition of an anæsthetic. Since, in spite of this, the disease is averted by anæsthetics, it is clear that *it does not owe its origin to that part of the toxin which penetrates into the nerve trunk.*

The logical conclusion is *that tetanus toxin does spread along the nerve trunk, but that this spreading does not play any essential role in the pathogenesis of either local or general tetanus.*

The complex reaction which we know under the name of tetanus is produced *as soon as the toxin encounters the peripheral nerve endings.*

It has its cycle of development, which is constant for the given animal, where each succeeding link is determined by the preceding one, and where variations depend on physiological differences in the nerve structures which were the starting points of the process.

It does not follow from this that the penetration of toxin along the nerve into the central nervous system is to be considered as an entirely indifferent action. We are very well aware how easy it is to produce tetanus by subarachnoid injection of the toxin. But it is a fact that there are a sufficient number of receptor nerve-endings in the submembranous spaces of the spinal cord and brain, capable of beginning the reaction under the influence of irritation. *Direct irritation of the nerve cells by the toxin penetrating into them is not at all indispensable in this case.*

Consequently, the cause of tetanus is tetanus toxin. But this does not mean that the tetanus toxin is directly responsible for all the tetanus phenomena from beginning to end.

This explains, at last, a strange fact which has long been a fundamental perplexity in the pathogenesis of tetanus. The fact is this: we have at our disposal very few sera whose specific properties cannot be doubted. Among these, two are pre-eminent—anti-diphtheria serum and anti-tetanus serum. By various technical devices, the concentration of anti-bodies in them has now been raised to a high figure. Nevertheless, *anti-tetanus serum does not exert any curative effect.* Its employment is of great significance, but *only in prophylaxis, i.e.,* in conditions which are in no way different from reactions *in vitro*; the specific serum simply neutralises the toxin, converting the irritating agent into an indifferent substance. Thereby the very possibility of irritation is prevented.

Even if, in the human clinic, it is possible to note from time to time a useful effect from subarachnoid injections, there always remains a doubt as to what precisely is the cause—*whether the specific properties of the serum or the act of operation.* Under laboratory conditions, however, when the disease follows the introduction of a definite dose of toxin, the appearance of the first local symptoms of tetanus is, as a rule, a sign of inevitable death, whatever the amount of serum afterwards injected, and whatever the manner of its introduction. In experiments with "pumping" also, we did not obtain any positive effect.

An interesting series of clinical observations were made by us some time ago in connection with five cases of pronounced spontaneous tetanus in human beings. Intra-lumbar injection of serum was made after preliminary extraction of the maximum quantity of cerebro-spinal fluid. The withdrawal of the fluid was carried out gradually, the amount withdrawn being from 40 to 110 c.c. The operation was repeated every 1-2 days until the appearance of marked signs of improvement (3-5 times in all). At the same time the serum was introduced into the blood. *In all these cases, the tetanus symptoms gradually disappeared.* In a sixth case, in which cerebro-spinal fluid was not obtained on puncture (*punctio sicca*) and the serum was introduced without preliminary emptying of the membranous sac, we did not obtain any effect and the patient succumbed. Later, these experiments were repeated with success in the clinic of Professor Y. Y. Janelidze.

This seemed quite all right at first; but certain observations made by us in the course of these experiments shook our confidence: in many cases the tetanus symptoms, after becoming weaker some hours after introduction of the serum, were later renewed with the same intensity as before, subsiding again after a second operation.

It is impossible to explain this if one starts out from the idea of a reaction between specific anti-bodies. If the weakening in the intensity of the tetanus was connected with the neutralisation of the toxin, where could the new portion of the latter come from to produce a renewal of the process? The amount of serum used by us so much exceeded the maximum possible content of toxin in the organism, that even if we had introduced an enormous additional dose of toxin, it would not have made itself manifest. Under the conditions of our action, the anti-toxin was present in excess in both the blood and the brain. This, however, did not prevent the renewal of the process in its original dimensions. *It is clear that the anti-toxin played no part here.* The reaction was merely a response to the operational interference, to an extra- or counter-irritation. This altered the conditions within the nerve network and created for a time being a new nerve battlefield which hindered the development of the process previously existing.

Lack of faith in the curative properties of anti-tetanus serum has already caused the clinic to return to the methods of symptomatic treatment. Thus, we see again employment of narcosis, which at any rate guarantees the patient a temporary alleviation of suffering; trial is made of magnesium, intra-lumbar injections of novocaine and even of solutions of carbolic acid (Synn Suvansa). It was found that novocaine and carbolic acid have an undoubted curative effect. True, this effect is not present in all cases; *it is, nevertheless, considerably more constant than that of specific anti-toxin.* Of course, the specific anti-toxin, introduced subarachnoidally, can neutralise the toxin that has made its way along the nerve trunk from the place of its formation. In this way, the intensity of the additional irritation may be, and will be, somewhat decreased. However, this does not abolish those tetanus symptoms which have already developed.

The sole conclusion to be drawn is that *serum treatment of tetanus is not specific since the cause of the disease changes with the development of the process.* On the other hand, influences which the clinic puts in the category of symptomatic influences now acquire the right to be termed causal. Serum does not exhibit any curative action in tetanus because the process, even during the period of incubation, loses those properties which immunology includes in the sphere of specific reactions.

The problem of the absence of curative properties in the serum is not the sole perplexity in the pathogenesis of tetanus. Indeed, such perplexities are rather numerous, but I do not consider it necessary to enumerate them all in view of the fact that it is not our task to study tetanus as a special pathological form. I shall only mention certain features which may be of use in elucidating questions with which we are more directly concerned.

A strange and unexplained fact is the *exceptional sensitiveness of horses to tetanus toxin.* It is not only relatively but even absolutely greater than that of the guinea-pig, although the latter is itself accounted one of the most sensitive animals. No assistance can be obtained here from consideration of weight relations.

This is another proof that tetanus cannot be explained as the pure result of the direct contact of each of the reacting elements with the toxin, since if it were so, the effect should depend on weight relations of toxin and substratum. Only the conception of this process as a specific and complex form of nerve reaction, *where the threshold of irritation is determined by the sensitivity of the reacting substratum,* is capable of introducing the necessary clarity.

Another fact, too, becomes comprehensible, one which has been noted in the clinic more than once and which is evidence that operating tetanus patients is useless: in those cases where the indubitable source of the whole process is removed (*e.g.*, by amputation), the tetanus symptoms *not only do not subside but are often sharply intensified.*

If the toxin, after penetrating into the central nervous system through the spaces in the nerve trunk, also participates in the development of the process, it is only as an auxiliary factor; we may, of course, take this factor into account, but *in practice it is useless to do so,* since the process is not brought to a standstill even when the toxin is removed from the nerve cells. In one of the earlier chapters of this book, devoted to the role of the cerebro-spinal fluid in the pathogenesis of tetanus, I brought forward data testifying to the considerable retardation in the development of the pathological process in animals from which the cerebro-spinal fluid had been periodically extracted. In our description there, we linked it up with questions of circulation, with the fact that removal of the fluid creates a mechanical obstacle to the spreading of the toxin. *These experimental results can now be given another interpretation as well.* The extraction of large quantities of cerebro-spinal fluid must be regarded also as a direct action on the nervous system, initiating a chain of additional irritations. This results in a temporary alteration of the mutual relations of the various parts of the nervous system. *Now when the state of the nervous system is changed, the process serving as an indicator will also develop in a new way.*

Here, not for the first time, we encounter a contradiction. Additional irritation in some cases intensifies the existing process, in other cases it weakens or even extinguishes it. However, strange as this fact may appear, it is undeniable; consequently, the only thing to do is to recognise it.

The cause lies in the fact that the substratum acted on is the nervous system, all elements of which are connected with one another in labile combinations. Only if the irritation arising in this network is weak is it extinguished without spreading far. Unusual forms of irritation, such as pathology has to deal with, spread over considerable nerve areas and produce a temporary transformation of intra-nerve relations far beyond the limits of immediate contact with the irritating agent. The response to irritation is here always complex, *the reaction always proceeds not along one path but along several different paths and is therefore manifested in various forms and degrees.* Depending on the individual conformation of the given nervous network, the strength of the irritation, the time and a number of other factors, one part or another of the reaction acquires preponderant importance and, obscuring the other parts, determines the external form of the process. Hence, difference in response is not due to the reaction proceeding from the very beginning in different and even opposite directions.

The degree of irritation plays a large part here. As a result of our observations, we found that the greater it is, the more rapid is its effect in intensifying the process already existing, or which previously existed and has still not disappeared.

I have in my possession the results of a series of experiments which may serve as partial evidence that the toxin, on penetrating into the region of the central nervous system, does not remain indifferent (experiments of my collaborator A. V. Ponomarev[1]).

A. V. Ponomarev. *Arkh. Biol. Nauk*, Vol. 28, No. 1, 1928.

Equal doses of tetanus toxin were introduced at the same time into the muscles of the left leg in two dogs of like weight and growth. Afterwards one of them was placed in a cell with a low ceiling and for the most part remained there lying down. The other, immediately after the injection of toxin, was harnessed to a cart loaded with stones, which it drew for 2-3 hours. In some of the experiments, we made the dog draw the load again after an interval of 12-15 hours. The result showed that *local tetanus developed earlier in the dog that had drawn the cart than in the control*. The difference was considerable. It often reached 20-26 hours. It is true that even in specially selected animals the time of appearance of the first symptoms does not always coincide. In the above-described experiments, however, it was shown in all cases, and the chief thing is that it proved to be proportional to the period during which the dog had been working.

A further interesting phenomenon was noted in these experiments. In the dog which had drawn the cart, general tetanus developed simultaneously with or immediately after the local symptoms. Trism, rigor of the vertebral column, etc., appeared almost immediately after the exhibition of the first local symptoms. We had cases where at the moment when the control animal became ill, the experimental dog had already perished or was on the point of death.

Experiments, described in another chapter of this book, have demonstrated that muscular work promotes an accelerated movement of the lymph (and of substances included in it) along the nerve trunk. It would seem that the immediate appearance of symptoms of general tetanus in our dogs is to be connected with this fact. But here again a doubt arises. Work performed by the muscles in the region of the nerve segment irritated by the toxin is also *supplementary work* for the corresponding nerve elements, and we know now the role of additional irritation in the pathogenesis of tetanus.

In any case, *this question is only of academic interest*. Whether the toxin penetrates into the region of the central nervous system or not, the basic features of the process are not altered.

Before the contemporary view of the pathogenesis of tetanus obtained confirmation and general recognition, there were isolated expressions of opinion shifting the centre of gravity of the process to the nerve periphery (Goldscheider, 1894; Courmont and Doyon, 1899). Few now even remember the existence of these views, which were crushed under the weight of the so-called "ocular" proofs provided by the new theory. The latter, as we have just seen, has also not been equal to the demands made on it, and we have returned to the starting point. Of course, this position cannot satisfy us either, since it takes into account only the reflex mechanism of origin of local tetanus and is quite powerless to solve the problem of the generalisation of tetanus symptoms. The objections raised by Ransom and Meyer (1903) were along this line. The authors pointed out that apart from the electric current, contemporary science does not know any means which, originating from one point, could alter the excitability of the whole nerve arc. They regarded this as an additional obstacle for recognising "dynamic spreading" through the nervous system of changes produced at the periphery. Such recognition, they said, would mean "coming into contradiction with all contemporary experiments."[1]

Paraphrasing the words of Hegel, we could reply here: "So much the worse for the experiments." Facts, and especially facts taken from the biological sphere, do not always have an independent significance outside the system created by them. Transference of the material from one system into another, with the aim of testing the latter, is only possible provided the material has an objective value confirmed in all directions. However, in the vast majority of cases each of our facts is only a fragment of a phenomenon.

The reference of various writers to the absence of appropriate data in contemporary science has not signified the actual absence of such data in nature, as indeed is proved by this book. We have adduced a sufficiently large amount of varied material putting beyond question precisely the "dynamic spreading" of irritation from the region of the terminal nerve apparatus at the periphery to the whole complex nerve network.

With this I shall bring to a close the examination of material dealing with tetanus as a special pathological form.

Our work has pursued a different aim. Even in the very beginning of this chapter, in elucidating the role of the nervous component in the origin of tar neoplasms in rabbits, I formulated two preliminary propositions:

1. The specific quality of an irritating agent is its capacity to evoke an unusual form of nerve irritation, bringing definite nerve mechanisms into action. This is expressed at the periphery by a number of functional and structural disturbances, developing successively according to a constant plan.

2. The nervous system has the property, during a certain period of time, which is sometimes quite long, of preserving traces of such irritation without any alteration of the characteristic features of the latter.

We are now able to confirm both these propositions. The specific quality of tetanus toxin is its capacity to evoke a characteristic and constant form of complex nerve reaction merely through irritation of the peripheral nerve apparatus.

---

[1] It is strange that they forgot here the well-known experiment of Türck on the stimulation by acid of a paw of a decapitated frog, as a result of which a very complex and completely co-ordinated reaction is obtained, consisting of a number of links.

Passing to an estimate of the nature of this irritation, we must mention the following points.

1. It cannot be referred to one of the known categories, such as tactile, nocuous, thermal, etc.

2. Its characteristic incubational period has a duration which is not met with among other, more or less simple, nerve reactions.

3. Arising at one point and progressively intensifying, the process involves a number of parts of the nervous system in a definite sequence, putting them in a state in which life is impossible.

4. The usual and constant form of this process can be altered only in part and only in the first stages, for instance, by the transference of the point of primary irritation from one nerve region to another.

5. Removal of the irritating agent is able to hold up the generalisation of the irritation only at the very beginning. If the process has reached a certain stage—removal of the irritating agent cannot arrest it.

6. Disappearance of the external symptoms of the process is not always evidence of its complete liquidation. Traces of the former special irritation remain in the nervous system for some time. In many cases, if a new action, even an ordinary trauma, is brought to bear on the nervous system, it can restore the process in its typical form.

Even a hasty glance at these six points enables one to recognise that they embody all the characteristic features of that other group of processes, already described many times in the pages of this book. However specific tetanus may seem in regard to many of its characters, it has a very close resemblance to what we have grouped together under the name nervous dystrophy.

This difference is that the non-specific influences giving rise to nervous dystrophy can be of very diverse nature. The variations here are connected only with the degree of irritation and with the place where the process starts. It was this fact which gave us the very idea of the existence of standard forms of nervous dystrophy. It must not be forgotten, however, that *this idea is a relative one.* If it was possible to produce tetanus, not only by tetanus toxin, but by a whole series of other substances and methods, we would also include tetanus in the group of standard reactions. The only thing that really appears specific is the course of the process in those cases where the illness, beginning with local symptoms, passes through a sequence of stages. Human beings and horses usually begin at once with the symptoms of general tetanus. *In this form, the process can easily be reproduced artificially* by employing various influences; this has repeatedly been demonstrated in the first part of this book, devoted to the study of convulsive states.

Hence, a specific reaction is also a group reaction; only the number of external influences known to be capable of producing it is comparatively very small.

The same holds for diphtheria also. Nobody will doubt, I think, that diphtheria is a specific process. Now, why exactly do we call it specific?

Two aspects of the matter must be distinguished here: the first is the external manifestation of the process; the second is the immuno-biological reactions.

A description was given above of the experiments of my collaborators Nikitin and Ponomarev,[1] who studied the effect of introducing diphtheria toxin into the central nervous system of guinea-pigs. The animals had previously been given intravenous injections of enormous doses of specific antitoxin. This did not save them from death, which usually occurred during the first twenty-four hours. On dissection, characteristic changes of the suprarenal glands and cardiac ganglia were discovered in these animals, although *under the conditions indicated not a single molecule of toxin could have reached either the suprarenal glands or the heart*. It is clear that these changes under ordinary circumstances also do not depend on contact between the toxin and the elements of the organs themselves, and that the producing agent consists in processes of a nervous nature. Nevertheless, the above-mentioned changes in the cardiac ganglia, and especially in the suprarenals, are regarded as *typical precisely of diphtheria*.

In another investigation, also previously mentioned, of my collaborator G. F. Ivanov,[2] who studied the morphological consequence of stimulating the region of the *tuber cinereum* in dogs by means of the "glass sphere operation," it was noticed that in all cases where there was a violent development of dystrophic changes in the tissues, and the animals perished within the first 2-3 days, there were *severe changes of the suprarenals, with pronounced lipoidosis*. The cells of the cortical layer were almost entirely filled with fat, to the same, or an even much greater, degree than occurs in diphtheria.

The following is another series of experiments carried out by my collaborator I. A. Pigalev.[3] The question that was being tested was whether the mechanism of the origin of the diphtheria deposit is related to the mechanism which determines the development of local symptoms in tetanus. It was possible to suspect something of the sort, since we have seen, for instance, that sore throat in scarlatina was a process of a nervous nature, being the reflection of the nervous process in the peripheral tissues.

[1] N. N. Nikitin and A. V. Ponomarev. *Arkh. Biol. Nauk,* Vol. 30, No. 1, 1930; *Zeitschr. f. d. ges. exp. Med.,* Vol. 70, No. 3-4, 1930.
[2] G. F. Ivanov. *Zeitschr. f. d. ges. exp. Med.,* Vol. 74, Nos. 5, 6, 1930.
[3] I. A. Pigalev. *Arkh. Biol. Nauk,* Vol. 27, No. 4-5, 1927; *Zeitschr. f. d. ges. exp. Med.,* Vol. 63, Nos. 5, 6, 1928.

Gibier obtained "diphtherial" inflammation of the tissues in rabbits by introducing the toxin into the rectum by means of a tampon or an enema. This form was inconvenient for our purpose in view of the relative difficulty of operating on the nerve connections of the rectum. Consequently, we performed our experiments on the ear.

In two rabbits, an artificial ulcer was produced on the back of the ear in its distal half. For this purpose, an area of about 3-4 sq. cm. of the skin was prepared and cut away. It is necessary to be very careful in separating the skin from the underlying tissues since the layer between the skin and the cartilage is very thin. Subsequently (or previously) in one of the rabbits, the *n.n. auricularis, occipitalis* and *facialis* are severed outside the region of the ear—by a single cut in the neck. The vessels and their nervous system are left untouched. In the second rabbit, which served as a control, the nerves were not severed. A tampon, periodically moistened with diphtheria toxin during 24 hours, was sewn on the ulcer thus produced.

It was found that usually in less than 24 hours a whitish, strongly adhering deposit appears on the ear of the normal rabbits. The bottom and edges of the lesion develop a dirty "greasy" appearance. On removing the gauze of the bandage, the deposit is partially torn away from the surface of the lesion, as a result of which slight bleeding occurs at these places. On the second day, the above-described phenomena are intensified. On the third and fourth days, if the rabbit has not died, heavy suppuration takes place owing to ordinary dirt contamination and this interferes with further comparison.

In more than half of the rabbits in which the nerves were severed *the wound in the ear retained its fresh appearance for 24-48 hours*, but then also developed suppuration.

In some cases, the difference was not pronounced. It is interesting to note, that to obtain a marked difference it is necessary to sever the nerves shortly before the application of toxin to the wound. With a longer period between the two operations, the difference in the effect is gradually effaced. I have already more than once cited facts of this nature and given their explanation in describing other observations of a similar kind.

Thus, one and the same preparation of diphtheria toxin had a varying effect on the tissues, *depending on the integrity or alteration of the nerve conditions in the corresponding region.* We see here an undoubted resemblance to tetanus. The resemblance goes further. Thus, rabbits in which diphtheria toxin had been applied to the denervated wound surface outlived their controls as a rule by what is for diphtheria a very considerable period—up to 3-5 days.

As far as diphtheria in man is concerned, here also the syndrome in itself does not denote anything definite, much less categorical. The final decision of the question depends entirely on the bacteriological analysis. *A negative answer transfers the disease to the group of ordinary processes, in spite of the presence in the throat of deposits characteristic of diphtheria.*

It follows from all this that in diphtheria also we have no firm grounds for regarding local manifestations of the disease as the result of direct contact of the toxin with each of the elements that have suffered. On the contrary, there is every reason to think that the majority of these manifestations owe their origin to the changes which the toxin evokes within the network of the nervous system. The latter, too, does not change diffusely but in a more or less definite sequence, and this is the reason for the constancy of the order in which the external symptoms of the disease develop. In this case again, however, the constancy cannot be treated as a specificity, since here also the reaction has a group character.

We have, therefore, decided the first question, that of the nature of the external manifestations of the process in diphtheria.

The second question concerns the immuno-biological reactions in this disease.

Let us begin with the fact that anti-diphtheria serum exhibits its properties both *in vitro* and *in vivo*. Moreover, it has *not only a prophylactic but also a curative effect,* by which it would seem to be favourably distinguished from anti-tetanus serum.

However, is this distinction actually so very great? Let us take experiments on animals. As was shown above (Ponomarev's experiments[1]), it is easy to choose such relations of diphtheria toxin and anti-toxin that the latter does not save the rabbit in spite of the fact that it is injected only 45 minutes later and in a dose more than a hundred times exceeding that required for neutralising the dose of toxin. When we accompanied this by "pumping," *i.e.,* when *we created conditions for the penetration of the anti-toxin into the region of the central nervous system,* the rabbits usually survived. It sufficed, however, to increase the interval between the injection of toxin and anti-toxin by a few dozen minutes for "pumping" to lose its useful effect, so that the animals died.

Three years ago we again repeated these experiments, but we varied the time-intervals within much wider limits (experiments of my collaborator N. N. Nikitin).

The rabbits were divided into two groups. The toxin was injected intravenously in a dose of about one MLD, since we were interested in securing the longest possible duration of the process. In the first group, anti-toxin was

[1] A. V. Ponomarev. *Arkh. Biol. Nauk,* Vol. 28, No. 4, 1928; *Zeitschr. f. d. ges. exp. Med.,* Vol. 64, No. 1-2, 1929; *Compt. Rend. Soc. de Bio'.,* Vol. 97, 1927.

introduced into the blood after 10 hours, in the second group after 30-40 hours, all the animals subsequently undergoing "pumping."

The result proved to be the opposite of that observed in Ponomarev's experiments. The duration of life was greater in the rabbits subjected to "pumping" after a longer interval. The procedure which in Ponomarev's experiments was the indispensable condition for preservation or prolongation of life *now accelerated death.*

The penetration of the anti-toxin into the region of the central nervous system, whether after 10 or after 40 hours, was belated in both cases. But the fact that in the second group the familiar trauma caused by "pumping" was considerably delayed gave the rabbit 1-3 extra days of life. These traumatic consequences of the operation in Ponomarev's experiments were entirely concealed by the neutralisation of the toxin within the central nervous system. The trauma was the lesser evil. In Nikitin's experiments, the neutralisation of the toxin was already unnecessary, and therefore *the effect of the operation proved to be due merely to trauma.* But the usefulness of the act of "pumping" itself depended on creating in the nervous system conditions capable of hampering the course of the basic pathological process. In the case considered the result was different; as in many other experiments described in this book, the new trauma intensified the pathological process already existing in the nervous system.

In the human clinic, we see essentially the same thing. In the first place, is it not strange that up to now *no firm view has been taken of the serum as a really specific agent in the treatment of diphtheria.* E. Friedberger, in one of his articles has collected a considerable number of contradictions of various sorts relating to this subject. Analysing the statistics of mortality from diphtheria, he points out, for instance, that in the epidemic of 1885-88 in West Prussia, mortality from diphtheria fell to one-third as compared with previous years, in spite of the absence of serum treatment, while in 1926-27 it increased greatly in spite of widespread application of concentrated sera in large doses. The author also cites Bingel's statistics dealing with 937 cases of diphtheria observed by him in the epidemic of 1913-16, in which anti-diphtheria and normal serum was employed in an equal degree. The statistics of mortality in both groups were alike.

Friedberger does not connect the rise and fall of mortality from diphtheria with the general adoption of specific prophylaxis and therapy, explaining them by other laws governing the epidemics; nor does he consider it proved that the complex of injurious influences in diphtheria infection can be identified with diphtheria toxin. Other authors (Cruveiller, Roux, Kraus, etc.) point out that there is no parallelism between the anti-toxin content and the curative effect of the serum. Gottstein asserts that the theory that immunity to spontaneous diphtheria infection is assured by the presence of anti-toxin in the blood is "an inspiring but still unproved hypothesis" (cited by Friedberger). Finally, everyone is acquainted with cases of relapse of diphtheria *within a short period after recovery.* Without any more ado, they are regarded simply as cases of reinfection.

If we set aside the facts and conclusions mentioned above, and take only those propositions which enjoy general recognition, it will be found that in the human clinic the *basic criterion of the curative action of anti-diphtheria serum lies, not in the quantity of specific anti-bodies, but in the time factor.* Statistics show that the curative effect decreases in proportion to the delay of the moment of injection of the serum. In this matter, therefore, the data of the laboratory and the clinic coincide. The curative action of anti-diphtheria serum, exactly as in the case of anti-tetanus serum, *must be judged through the prism of time.*

We may, of course, adhere to the old meaning of the term "specificity," applying it to properties inherent in a given irritating agent. In that case, however, the process begun by the specific agent will have a right to be termed specific only as long as specific anti-bodies are capable of abolishing it. As soon as this neutralisation loses its influence on the course of the process, the latter must be included in the category of non-specific processes. However, this cannot be done for the reason that even when it has lost its connection with the irritating agent, the process still retains the characteristic features of its development. Consequently, *the concept "specificity," must be defined along other lines.*

An analysis of the data obtained during the study of tetanus enabled me to formulate my point of view on this subject. But the pathogenic kinship between tetanus and diphtheria is obvious. The difference depends on the nerve structures which, because of their sensitivity, are the first to enter into combination wth the toxin and thus begin the process.

It is well known that, to produce an effect, *it is advantageous to inject tetanus toxin into tissues (cellular tissue, muscles) rather than into the blood, while with diphtheria toxin the reverse is the case.* At the same time, our experiments with "pumping" showed that, under certain conditions, if the anti-toxin reaches the region of the central nervous system, it ensures the recovery of animals which otherwise are bound to die. It is clear from this that *in experimental diphtheria the receptors of the special form of irritation are to be found somewhere in the spinal cord or brain.* Other nerve mechanisms, not the same as in tetanus, become involved in the pathological process.

Whatever the difference in details between spontaneous human diphtheria and the process artificially evoked by the toxin, it does not play any part in deciding the question from the point of view of principle.

Diphtheria in man can also be divided easily into two periods. They are both connected with processes of a nervous nature.

At the outset, the toxin is the irritating agent. It produces pathological changes in the nervous system, which in the first period have a functional character. This indicates that the pathological process is maintained only from the focus where the nerve elements are directly irritated by the toxin, *but the latter has not yet managed to inflict irreparable damage on them.* The removal of the irritating agent is here removal of the irritation and specific serum will certainly give a positive effect.

The second period begins with a change in the causes of the process, *i.e.*, from the moment *when the damaged nerve elements themselves become the source of irritation.*

The time of the transition of diphtheria from one period to the other must not be calculated in a formal fashion. Both individual peculiarities and epidemiological factors, in the broad socio-biological interpretation of the word, can shorten or lengthen it. It is highly probable that in many cases the second period begins almost simultaneously with the first, which explains failures in specific treatment, even though applied in good time and in heroic doses.

From the beginning of the second period, the course of the diphtheria process depends on the degree of injury inflicted on the nerve elements. Recovery is possible even here. The process gradually decreases, as we repeatedly observed in other forms of nervous dystrophy described above. *It can also suffer a relapse, i.e., suddenly repeat the entire syndrome of disease which had come to an end not so long before*, thereby giving rise to various perplexities and queries as to the cause of re-infection. Finally, it may take a gradually progressing course and kill the animal within a shorter or longer period.

Apparently, the nerve apparatus of the heart as a rule becomes involved during the development of this process within the nerve network, and consequently death ensues before the process itself passes into one of the standard forms of generalised dystrophy. However, in our animals which perished at later periods, after 20-30 days from injection of the toxin, it was always possible to observe some of the signs characteristic of extensive dystrophy—emaciation, loss of hair, inflammatory changes of the mucous membrane of the mouth and nose, hæmorrhages in internal organs, etc.

The production of large-scale derangements by minimal doses of toxin has always seemed puzzling. A special theory was even created to explain it, in which toxins were included among the enzymes. Whether it is correct or not, the fact remains that *this theory is not necessary for understanding the processes in a complex organism.*

In concluding this chapter, I wish to reiterate that the employment of serum in the second period of diphtheria is useless. Here we are confronted by the same phenomenon as in tetanus, since the prophylactic action of specific sera can be separated from the curative action only on the basis of practical considerations. *There is no difference in principle between these two conceptions*; the characteristic symptoms of disease are already observable in the first period of diphtheria, while the same period in tetanus proceeds without external symptoms. If in the future some characteristic is found by which the diagnosis of tetanus can be accelerated, even if by only a few hours, *there is no doubt that we shall come to recognise curative properties also in the case of anti-tetanus serum.*

The view put forward by us is new not only in a formal sense, but in essence, since *it is not explicable from the data which physiology has at its disposal.* Nevertheless, I consider it necessary to adhere to this view.

Essentially, there is only one obstacle to its recognition—the present *state of the question regarding the quality of excitation.* The opinion held by the majority is that the state of excitation conducted along the nerve in either direction is always alike, that it does not bear any individual marks.

What we have observed in the experiments with tetanus toxin raises very acute doubts in this respect.

There is no doubt that here some special kind of irritation was passed on to the centre, serving as the originator of a complex reaction with a definite cycle of development. It was established that the character of this reaction is *determined at the moment when the toxin comes into contact with the peripheral nerve apparatus.* The participation of other nerve parts is conditioned by this process. Consequently, even from the very beginning *some special or, figuratively speaking, "tetanus form" of excitation* passes along the nerve trunk.

It must be mentioned that recently the question of the quality of excitation has perceptibly lost the calm which marked its consideration at the time when the "all or nothing" principle was formulated. As early as 1892, Professor N. E. Vedensky secured data capable of shaking the sanctified views on this subject. Subsequently, in the laboratory of Professor A. A. Ukhtomsky, who developed the theory of dominants, many new facts were obtained providing evidence that "the nerve is an apparatus not only unusually labile . . . but an apparatus of varying lability, designed for faithful reproduction of diverse forms and rhythms of excitation." Professor A. A. Ukhtomsky's school defends this proposition against the theory of the uniformity of nerve impulses and against the "all or nothing" principle. Views closely allied to this were enunciated by Garten, who spoke of the presence of "inherent rhythms" of excitation in different tissues, and also by Lapicque and Piéron.

In 1923, a new work of Paul Weiss appeared, containing data of his experiments on the transplantation of extremities and isolated muscles in amphibians. The facts communicated by him at first aroused perplexity, but on testing they were completely confirmed. The basic phenomenon was as follows. A particular muscle is transplanted from one animal to another. In its new place a nerve branch is directed to it from the nearest nerve. By this means, connection is gradually established between the muscle and the central nervous system. When this has taken place, the muscle begins to contract, *but in an absolutely different way from what might have been anticipated*: the contraction of the transplanted muscle now takes place simultaneously with that of the same muscles in the new host. Thus, when *m. gastrocnemius* is transplanted into a fore extremity and connected with one of the nerves of the brachial plexus, it will contract, not at the same time as the muscles of the fore extremities, but when the *m. gastrocnemius* of the new host contracts.

The experiment can be made in several variations, but these do not introduce anything substantially new. To explain this phenomenon, Weiss proposed the "resonance theory," envisaging mutual interaction of the stations of despatch and destination, the latter playing the chief part for *it has to "answer the call," whatever the route—direct or roundabout—by which the given wave of excitation spreads*. It is clear that this is possible only on the assumption of qualitative differences in the character of the process which proceeds along the nerve and is termed excitation.

The facts that I put forward, without being identical with those just mentioned, must be referred to the same category of phenomena.

CHAPTER XX
GENERAL REVIEW

THE data set out in this chapter, like those in the chapters devoted to acute and chronic inflammation, can be applied to the interpretation of the pathogenesis of a number of other infectional processes.

We have already seen that time is one of the basic factors to be taken into account in assessing the curative properties of specific sera. But this only holds good *where we are not mistaken in the indicator, i.e.*, when the process gets its name from the cause actually producing it. Unfortunately this is not always so. As previously shown, in the experiments of my collaborators A. T. Dolinskaya and D. S. Chetvertak, we obtained an isolated affection of the kidney by staphylococcus in the form of so-called carbuncle; but the cause of the process was a drop of formalin introduced into the ovary three weeks beforehand. *Luckily for our analysis, we knew about this*; if the same experiment had been performed by nature, the deceptive obviousness would have made us regard precisely the staphylococcus as the cause of all the symptoms.

There is absolutely no doubt that such facts are widely encountered in the human clinic. *A disease gets its name not from the cause, but from one of the numerous consequences*, and often enough from that one which in the whole course of the process is, perhaps, less culpable than the rest. We have already had to dwell on this in describing our clinical experiments on the subject of cerebro-spinal meningitis.

It is well known that while recognising meningitis to be an infectious disease, we have almost no grounds for regarding it as contagious. Rare cases of family meningitis are no evidence, since we find here that besides infection a large number of other conditions also coincide. Contact with meningococcus is not sufficient by itself for the disease to develop. Some other process takes place in advance, preparing the situation in which the interaction of the macro-organism and micro-organism will subsequently take place. Now, if that is the case, what practical use do we get from our knowledge of the meningococcus? Does it help us to explain anything?

In having recourse to specific (serum) treatment of meningitis, we expect to do away with the microbe. But the latter itself appears only as the consequence of another cause. To abolish the microbe and to leave the conditions in force which made it pathogenic—such a formulation can hardly satisfy anyone, the more so, since the task of removing the microbe is far from simple to fulfil.

Specific reactions merely deprive the microbe of its capacity of being an irritating agent, they neutralise the microbe, converting it into a saprophyte. They by no means always destroy it physically. It is precisely this that has given rise to the fear of bacteria-carriers and the constant precautions for sterilisation in the case of patients recovering from scarlatina, diphtheria, typhus, etc.

Almost thirty years have passed since the first proposals for serum treatment of meningitis (Kolle and Wassermann). The period has been sufficient both for perfecting the original preparation and for clearing up the question of its actual value. In point of fact, however, even now we have not gone outside the sphere of primitive experiment. Every year we try new sera, prepared by means of new, merely accidental, antigens, and every year, after a short period of rapture, we have to regret the shattering of our illusions.

At times, the desire to obtain at all costs a specific effect from the use of serum in meningitis puts physicians in a definitely false position. For instance, I know of cases where children 3-6 years old have been given as many as five to nine injections of serum during 4-8 weeks. During this period some of the patients received injections amounting to 600-900 c.c. of serum. Their recovery was accounted a triumph of specific therapy, in spite of the fact that the favourable turning point in the process began after the sixth or ninth injection. It may be asked, why were the first injections a failure? Why did the *n*th portion of serum preparation, which up till then had been indifferent, suddenly acquire properties of specific action both on the disease and on the microbe?

Doubts of this sort are, apparently, finding their way also into the clinic; at any rate, the behaviour of medical practitioners is sufficiently clear evidence of such doubts. Without renouncing serum, and alongside of it, the clinic makes the most energetic use of all other forms of therapeutic operations in treating meningitis. It is practically impossible to find clear cases among its material. In spite of this, in its general conclusions the clinic is bound by tradition. If the favourable turning point of the disease coincides in time with one of the numerous injections of serum, then the effect is ascribed precisely to the latter and accounted specific. Hope springs up anew, work is concentrated on the search for the necessary microbe and the most subtle differentiation of its properties, new sera are prepared and new series of clinical tests are performed.

The laboratory supports the clinic with all its force. By means of controlled experiments it proves that, on mixing virulent meningococcus with various doses of specific serum, it is not able to produce meningitis in rabbits even on suboccipital or intra-cerebral inoculation. Such, for instance, were the recent experiments of Professor P. F. Zdrodovsky and his collaborators. These experiments are undoubtedly interesting, but they only prove that it is possible to produce meningitis in the rabbit by immediate injection of the virus into the region of the central nervous system and that *in such cases* even minimal quantities of anti-meningococcus serum actually have a specific effect. These facts, however, only make it more incomprehensible why the same serum, employed in enormous doses, proves to be useless in spontaneous meningitis of human beings, in spite of the fact that it is injected directly into the region affected.

The fact that it is possible to produce meningitis in rabbits in the experiment with intra-cerebral injection of meningococcus, has no precise significance. Infection under the same conditions by many other species of micro-organisms results in the same process, and even with much greater constancy. It is not surprising that specific sera will have an effect in such cases, since *the microbe here is made the actual initiator of the process.* But, the effect is obtained only during the first period, when the serum is injected either together with the microbe or in the hours immediately following infection.

The process confronting us in spontaneous human meningitis may be entirely different. When the kidney lies in the path of development of the dystrophic process evoked by irritating the nerve apparatus of the ovary or testicle, *it is the first organ to be affected by tuberculosis.* If the same process arises in another place, *it remains healthy to the end.* We know from the human clinic that simultaneous tuberculosis of the testicle and kidney is met with quite frequently, but not at all invariably. In our experiments, however, injection of the virus into the testicle gave 100 per cent of affected kidneys. It is clear that *tuberculosis of the testicle, developing spontaneously, is distinct from the same process artificially produced.* They may be externally closely related, but essentially they are different. In the first case, the virus is the *indicator* of one form of pathological state, in the second it is the *initiator* of another.

The nervous system in itself is both centre and periphery. Bio-chemical processes taking place in it are subject to the same nerve regulation as in the liver, heart, skeletal muscles, etc. The creation of temporary or permanent pathological nerve combinations results in the development of pathological processes in various organs, including those in the nervous system itself. Here, as in other places also, the *dystrophic process possesses qualitative peculiarities.* The latter, as we have seen, depend both on the place of origin of the process and on the character of the primary irritation. As a result, the process is in some cases evoked by meningococcus, in others by tuberculosis bacilli, and in still others by degenerative phenomena, etc. Immuno-biological reactions are not for a moment capable of altering anything in the origin and development of processes of this category. The most we can expect here is the elimination of the additional irritation by the removal of the microbe; *but it is precisely this that immunity does not guarantee*. The microbe perishes in the normal tissues, even in the immediate vicinity of the pathologically altered parts where it is able to maintain itself, as long as this vicinity retains its normal biochemical, and hence functional, state. If the first changes, which were the cause of the tissue dystrophy, prove to be temporary and gradually pass away, then the tissue alterations also disappear and the microbe disappears along with them. No special form of immunity is required for this.

We know very well that appropriately prepared serum cannot help having specific properties. In cases where it does not produce any effect in the organism, is this not a proof that the reactions mentioned do not play any part in the given process? It is difficult to renounce habitual and long-established views and especially to make up one's mind to choose a new line of behaviour. But this choice has already been made unconsciously; the preparation of sera against diphtheria and tetanus is a task undertaken by every institute working in the sphere of immunology. The production of other sera proceeds without any plan, according to the inclinations of individual workers, accidentally acquiring or losing interest in a particular question.

The time has come to make a revaluation of the whole situation from the very beginning. What we have observed makes doubt legitimate, and we venture to deny that recovery from cerebro-spinal meningitis is the result of immuno-biological reactions. Even when anti-meningococcus serum gives an apparently clear therapeutic effect, the latter may depend not on the specific properties of the serum but on the additional irritation which proves useful in the given case by causing the necessary transformation of the state of the organism.

The fact that cerebro-spinal meningitis often occurs epidemically cannot alter the matter. Acquaintance with the microbe—*the undoubted initiator of many forms of individual and mass diseases*—was a great advance in the investigation of the pathology of infection; herein consists the magnificent service rendered by Pasteur. But at the same time it has artificially simplified reality, making it possible to unite processes between which there is only an external resemblance, on the strength of a single, and often accidental, characteristic.

We know from the data of the epidemiology of cholera that it is preceded, accompanied and followed by so-called cholera-like diseases. Externally, these are in no way different from cholera (diarrhœa, vomiting, convulsions, coldness of the extremities, lowered pulse, etc.); but the cholera microbe cannot be discovered in the patients' organism. *Consequently, the external form of the disease here is not necessarily connected with the cholera vibrio.* The whole of this complex reaction must be referred to the category of group reactions; it has a definite composition of successively developing parts, and can be set in motion by the influence of other agents.

In the chapter on standard forms of nervous dystrophy I described our experiments on so-called "predisposition." *The latter proved to be a temporary or permanent alteration of the configuration of a given nervous system* in which separate points of pathological excitation have appeared. If, during periods of cholera epidemics, the whole complex of cholera symptoms is exhibited without participation of the corresponding microbe, it means that numbers of persons, usually living in one locality and often in similar social circumstances, are subjected simultaneously to the influence of similar but unusual irritations, creating a definite form of "predisposition" in the organism. The additional irritation (in our terminology, the second "blow") *transforms the hidden state of predisposition into a clearly revealed process.* It is probable that not every irritation is capable of acting as this "second blow," and that the cholera vibrio has a certain pre-eminence in this respect, for statistics show that its action does actually result in an aggravation of the process. But it is still more probable that the cholera vibrio is not the sole pathognomonic factor of cholera, just as cholera as a whole cannot be registered as a single "nosological unit." The activity of the microbe in this case becomes merely *the activity of a catalysing agent.*

Can the cholera microbe produce the typical syndrome of the disease in the healthy organism? I am, of course, speaking here of human beings, as the vibrio is in general not pathogenic for the majority of animals.

Curiously enough, it is difficult to settle this question. Cases of laboratory infection do not give a definite answer, since, firstly, there are very few such cases, and, secondly, the results obtained are contradictory. Best known is the experiment made in I. I. Mechnikov's laboratory. Several of his collaborators administered to themselves *per os* a definite quantity of pure culture of cholera vibrio. One of them quickly became ill with symptoms of acute gastro-enteritis, the rest remained healthy. Thus, we have no data for deciding in what precise way the microbe acted here—whether it was the actual initiator of the process, or only facilitated its more rapid appearance.

It does not follow from this that the cholera vibrio is in general innocuous, and that the danger of its presence, for instance, in water reservoirs, is exaggerated, since both its properties as a catalysing agent and its capacity to add something that aggravates the basic process are reflected in the statistics of cholera sickness and mortality. But in pathology, *i.e.*, in the theory of the origin and formation of diseases, it is necessary to dethrone it, or, more correctly, *to assess it at its real value*; otherwise we shall not find our way out of the mental blind-alley into which pathology has been driven by the accumulation of contradictions.

What has been said does not put meningitis, cholera or cholera-like diseases in a special, isolated position. We have no doubt, for instance, that infection plays an even smaller role in the epidemiology of grippe. Indeed, the common inflammatory type of affection of the oral and nasal cavities, lungs and gastro-intestinal tract (pulmonary intestinal form of grippe) *is the most standard of all the forms of nervous dystrophy which we have observed in our experiments*. It is not surprising that in this strange infection there are no signs of immunity, and relapse is possible even within a few days after recovery. It is precisely inclination to relapses that characterises processes of a neuro-dystrophic type and it is precisely in such processes that this phenomenon is entirely comprehensible. Cases of family grippe are easily explained by the uniformity of constitution and similarity of conditions of life and environment. Finally, the epidemiology of grippe includes forms of its spreading which are incompatible with the idea of infection. Thus, in one year, grippe starting from Berlin spreads for some reason to Paris, while in the following year it changes its direction by 180° and from Berlin moves to Moscow. The theory of infection does not answer these questions, consequently the solution must be sought in other spheres.

The old Russian term *"povetrye"* [1] has been replaced by the term "epidemic." Nevertheless, the old term still contains a particle of truth. Our experiments showed that bacterial, chemical and physical agents were alike capable of beginning dystrophic processes within the network of the nervous system; in their further course, these processes did not remain indefinite but, on the contrary, easily took on particular qualitative forms. In the huge complex of influences comprised in the words climate, season, meteorological conditions, etc., the analysis of the significance of the separate parts and their combinations is far from complete. It is more than probable that many of them do not act, as is usually supposed, in a general way, "undermining the resistance of the organism" (?), but in a particular way, *producing a definite form of transformation in the nervous system of animals of the same species*.

Returning to the basic subject of our exposition, I raise the question: Does all this imply that cerebro-spinal meningitis, cholera and certain other epidemic diseases do not belong to the category of specific processes? No, it does

[1] This old, popular term has its root in the word *Veter*, wind.—*Ed.*

not; these diseases are undoubtedly specific, but specificity must, as was mentioned more than once, *be assessed by quite other means than were previously used.*

The infectional process obtains its definite form and cyclical course *as a result of the constancy of the nerve mechanism underlying it.*

The microbe discovered in the foci of the affected parts can participate *in three aspects.* Either it is the producing agent, *i.e.,* the actual initiator of the process (as in plague, glanders, anthrax, etc.); or it acts as a specific catalysing agent, *i.e.,* it facilitates the occurrence of a process already prepared for beforehand by the action of other agents; or, finally, it merely makes its appearance in tissues the biological condition of which has been altered in a direction that is favourable precisely for this microbe and no other. In the last case, it is only an indicator of the process already present.

The microbe as initiator may subsequently become also the indicator of the pathological state evoked by it. This is seen most clearly in the case of syphilis.

In studying the pathogenesis of syphilis, it is necessary to bear in mind two absolutely distinct processes which *coincide in time* and therefore appear inseparable. Actually, however, they are fused only for a moment and only at the very beginning.

Both these processes begin from the moment of infection.

The first consists in the spirochæte penetrating into the tissues and from here into the circulatory system, and by this means being conveyed throughout the organism, multiplying and becoming fixed in certain, more or less definite places. It has been established that this distribution of the spirochæte takes place rapidly, in the course of a few hours. As an antigen, the spirochæte calls forth the reactions of immunity.

In gradually rendering the spirochæte harmless, in depriving it of its property as an irritant, the organism does not kill it. It lives on peaceful terms with it, as it lives with the bacilli of tuberculosis and many other pathogenic and non-pathogenic microbes. *As a result, we have spirochætosis; but from spirochætosis to syphilis is still a long way.*

The second process, the beginning of which coincides with that of the first, is the irritation of the nerve elements in the tissues at the place of infection.

To obtain sclerosis in rabbits, it is essential to make the inoculation in the skin tissue. The significance of this circumstance has already been repeatedly emphasised by me in analysing the genesis of a number of other processes. *It is precisely here, in the region of the peripheral nerve apparatus, that the process which subsequently gets the name of syphilis has its inception.* At this point, the spirochæte irritates the organism not merely as an antigen. The reaction which it evokes here has nothing to do with immunity reactions. By entering into intimate association with the nerve apparatus, it becomes a specific nerve irritant, it operates the starting lever of the fatal mechanism already known to us; once this mechanism is started, it continues like clock-work, and the process develops step by step, gradually involving the whole organism. If, at the moment of infection, the spirochæte penetrates only into the circulatory system while the nerve apparatus at the periphery for some reason remains untouched, syphilis will not develop, the matter will not go beyond spirochætosis and we obtain a "nuller."

The capacity of the spirochæte to be a nerve irritant and its antigenic function are connected with another. From the moment of the final attainment of immunity, a new infection by syphilis, in the sense of a repetition of its whole syndrome, is impossible, but a new spirochætemia may occur, a new generation of the spirochæte can easily settle in the immune organism, as was shown long ago by Kolle's experiments. It is clear that the organism does not prevent new spirochætes from settling in its tissues, but it will not react to this by the development of a special reaction. On the other hand, during the first period, while immunity has not yet been attained, the spirochæte not only preserves its property as an irritant of the nerve cell, but each new irritation inflicted on the latter encounters a soil already prepared by the action of the primary irritant. The rapidity of the response is now increased, *i.e.*, the incubational period becomes shorter.

Since the spirochæte is a very weak irritating agent, it is only after a long period (3-4 weeks) that it brings the nerve cell into a condition which is reflected in the corresponding peripheral tissues in the form of sclerosis. During the whole preceding incubational period, the spirochæte was not able to multiply in this focus. On the contrary, *it can be readily presumed that the focus even becomes sterile within a certain period after infection, like the sterile tissues of the dog before the development in them of dystrophic symptoms terminating in a trophic ulcer.* At the moment when sclerosis develops, the spirochæte makes its appearance there as a secondary inhabitant and multiplies. It settles only within the area where the physico-chemical and biological conditions are changed in such a way as to allow of its entry. Whether it adds anything itself which facilitates the maintenance of sclerosis is unknown; probably its presence is of no special significance. As soon as the characteristic dystrophic phenomena in the given region begin to diminish, the sclerosis disappears of itself, and with it also the spirochæte. The tissues once more become sterile.

There can only be one conclusion from this: *the connection between the spirochæte and sclerosis is not one-sided.* The mutual dependence is obvious here. If the spirochæte brings about the sclerosis, the latter, in its turn, creates the conditions for the appearance of the spirochæte.

The irritation caused by the spirochæte at any point of the nerve network does not die out but passes into the characteristic form of a remittent process. Thus, when sclerosis has appeared, it rapidly attains a definite or, more correctly, *marginal size,* beyond which it does not spread and, after persisting for a short time, it vanishes, quite apart from whether treatment is applied or not. A pause then ensues, followed by a roseolous rash, then again a pause, and so on, through a series of new local foci and new pauses. The result is a *definite cycle of periods of affection and free intervals.* This alone ought to turn attention in the direction of the nervous system for which a rhythmic form of activity is characteristic.

Affecting at the outset only the skin and mucous membranes, the process gradually becomes generalised throughout the tissues and organs but preserves its specific features both in the sense of having a "favourite" localisation, and as regards the character of the tissue changes. *The qualitative peculiarities of the original irritation merge, therefore, into the definite form of a progressively developing neuro-dystrophic process.*

The spirochæte is undoubtedly a weak irritating agent, which is the reason why the original reaction to it is delayed by 3-4 weeks. But we have already more than once seen that when the remote consequences of certain forms of nerve trauma are taken into consideration, *the weakness of the irritating agent proves to be the source of its strength.* The terrible devastation which is sometimes wrought in the organism by syphilis during the later stages is connected precisely with this fact.

To cure syphilis means to arrest the progress of the neuro-dystrophic process within the nervous system. Then the spirochæte will disappear of itself, just as it disappears from the sclerosis without any treatment during the "regressive development" of the latter, as a result of changes in the state of the tissues in this region.

As regards tuberculosis, the matter is more complicated.

I have already pointed out the usual diversity of the tuberculosis syndrome in man, in contrast with its stereotyped character in laboratory infection of animals (rabbits, guinea-pigs). This, together with a number of other facts, described in the chapter on chronic inflammation, led us to take the view that many forms registered in the clinic under the name of tuberculosis have, in point of fact, *no right to this designation.*

In the clinical sense, persons develop tuberculosis who are immune to it. We are not confronted here with the virus acting as an antigen, except perhaps in some cases where children are concerned. In the human clinic, therefore, the tuberculosis bacilli *are only very rarely the initiators of the disease*. Of course, the tubercle, as a local tissue reaction, is specifically connected with the irritating agent, but this is not sufficient for characterising the whole process.

On the other hand, in experimental tuberculosis produced by infecting healthy laboratory animals, the virus *is the initiator of the disease*, and being a specific irritating agent it consequently gives rise to a constant form of response. Deviations depend almost exclusively on the strength of the irritating agent and on the place where the process begins. As a result, *we obtain here in principle the same form of reaction as in tetanus.*

In cases of spontaneous tuberculosis, it is futile to increase immunity by the introduction of live or dead virus or specific anti-bodies. In our experiments on the infection of various places of the gastro-intestinal canal of rabbits with tuberculosis, we saw that *in one and the same* animal, *in one and the same* system of organs, the microbes behave differently at two almost *neighbouring places*. In one place, they produce generalisation of the process beyond the limits of the injection; in the other, they perish, sometimes so rapidly that it is not even possible to discover the spot. No attributes of the microbe, neither its resistance to acids, nor its waxy coverings, save it from annihilation. It is clear that the role of the waxy covering of the tuberculosis bacillus as an absolute factor in its resistive capacity *is a legend which it is time to cast into oblivion.*

Artificial immunisation can only safeguard against active tuberculosis, and does not save from passive tuberculosis, where the microbe only initiates another process. *The danger of tuberculosis is the danger of those forms of dystrophy with which the microbe becomes associated secondarily.* Everything that is capable of intensifying the dystrophy increases both the volume and the extent of tuberculosis even if the same means raises specific immunity to the highest level.

In the case of syphilis, we saw that the antigenic properties of the spirochæte and its capacity of being a nerve irritant are connected; on the attainment of immunity, a new inoculation of virus does not produce any visible reaction. *This does not happen in tuberculosis.* Immunity does not deprive the antigen of its property of being a nerve irritant, and tuberculin may easily intensify the already existing dystrophic process. Instead of the old foci being eliminated, new ones are formed, for the existence of immunity does not affect the capacity of the microbe to live in the tissues of the immune animal. At the present time, the clinic has witnessed so many failures from the application of specific therapy in tuberculosis that it has been almost entirely given up. Only in eye practice is tuberculin still sometimes employed as a means of treatment. But if tuberculin is useful only in the case of tuberculosis of the eye, *then the solution of this riddle must be sought not in tuberculosis, but in the eye.*

To sum up, the best treatment of tuberculosis consists in rest, suitable food and climate—that is to say, means which are equally effective in a large number of other chronic diseases that have outwardly nothing in common with tuberculosis.

The pathogenesis of tuberculosis could easily be subjected to more detailed analysis. The same thing could be done in regard to the pathogenesis of a number of other infections not mentioned in our exposition. However, I shall refrain from doing so, for such an analysis would anticipate experimental work that has yet to be done. The propositions advanced here concerning the nature of specific reactions in pathology aim not only at giving a new form of interpretation to these processes but, above all, at converting the problem under discussion into a subject for concrete work.

Up to the present day, this could not be done, for the term "specificity" has been understood as indicating a regularity of a very limited order, as a phenomenon *"sui generis,"* signalising, as it were, the impossibility of further analysis. *To call a process "specific" has meant, in essence, only to register it.*

This procedure is admissible in regard to biological processes, since we judge of the specific qualities of an agent by the reactions of the substratum on which it acts, *i.e.*, by the reactions of a complicated system of exactly regulated parts. Either we must give up recognising the history of development altogether, or, if we take it into account, we must draw the appropriate conclusions. How is it possible to assume that living protoplasm has retained its capacity for progressive development in spite of the infinite diversity of forms of resistance to which it has been subjected in the course of millions of years, finally giving rise to man, and that it has, nevertheless, remained dependent on innumerable specific agents ready at every moment to cause it to exhibit afresh some sort of unprecedented properties?

Invading this system from outside, the foreign agent evokes a reaction in elements which are not independent at any moment of their existence. Each forms part of manifold and definite working units, and the latter in their turn, are linked with one another by a system of connections. Physiological stimuli bring definite mechanisms into action for a definite period. Subsequently the process dies away or is automatically transferred to another region, for the order in which new links of the whole system are included is already predetermined in the function itself.

How otherwise could a complex organism arise?

We find closely similar relations in pathology. The difference consists in the unusual character of the irritation and the points at which it arises. It is natural that under these conditions the functioning of physiological mechanisms will undergo pronounced alteration, but by no means in an anarchic fashion. The process has *its own order, its own plan*, and, as we have repeatedly seen, this plan is consistent and strictly defined. Between its inception and its complete dying out, the process passes successively through several stages, the symptoms appear in a definite cycle allowing the registration of separate diseases and their systematisation. However, the individuality or specificity of the processes is not absolute. We are aware how long a time elapsed before the old concept of "fever" was differentiated into various forms of typhus—abdominal, exanthematic and remittent, how difficult it is even now to diagnose certain pathological forms, and on what minute details a correct decision rests.

The same applies to the separate symptoms. Let us take the rash of measles and scarlatina. These could be accounted strictly specific reactions, were it not for cases of so-called idiosyncrasy, where the same irritating agent produces in different subjects, different kinds of rash; in one case, the scarlatina type, in the other—that of measles. Every day, the clinic encounters such facts in various spheres of its work.

Hence, there are no genuine specific reactions connected with only one specific irritating agent. They all belong to the category of group reactions, only *the number of producing agents in each group is different.*

Our task was to elucidate the basic mechanisms common to all diseases; and the reader has seen that the results of each of our experiments invariably turned our attention to the nervous system. The same happened in regard to the question of specific reactions. *The quality of the irritating agent proved to be its capacity to evoke in the nervous system the cyclical development of a definite process, the basic laws of which are closely akin* to the laws of the phenomena united in this book under the name of neuro-dystrophic processes.

A specific irritating agent does not evoke only one form of reaction within the network of the nervous system. Ordinary nerve trauma is always added to the special irritation. The special form of the dystrophic process is accompanied by the standard form, and can even be entirely obscured by the latter; or, on the other hand, the standard form may begin to appear a long time after the special one has been eliminated. *Herein lies the danger of those specific methods of treatment which are commonly used in clinical practice.*

More than once, isolated voices of physicians have been raised in warning against the seductions of inoculations and of so-called diagnostic tests (the reactions of Pirquet, Shick, Dick, etc.), which are widely used in schools and children's clinics. Such voices have not been heeded as they should have been, since they only pointed out isolated facts and could not explain them.

Indeed they met with numerous objections on the part of those who held the view that skin inoculation tests are harmless on the ground that in the vast majority *of cases such operations are not followed by any immediate harm.*

We see now that these arguments are inadequate. It is only possible to speak of the harmlessness of specific reactions, in cases where the producing agent actually possesses only specific properties; but such cases are practically impossible. *The other process develops slowly and creeps in unnoticed.* Its consequences belong to another category of phenomena and we are not accustomed to connect them causally with the primary specific agent. The facts adduced in this book settle this definitely, and to shrink from the solution of the problem thus raised would be consciously (and, perhaps, criminally) to close one's eyes to reality. The process may break out after many weeks or months and be manifested in an unexpected form, being, nevertheless, *causally connected with an operation about which both doctor and patient have ceased to think.*

Of course, the consequences mentioned are neither inevitable nor necessarily ruinous. The danger in this respect should not be exaggerated; but it must also not be underestimated, especially in cases where the trauma is inflicted more than once on *young animals.*

A characteristic feature of neuro-dystrophic processes is their capacity to leave behind in the network of the nervous system hidden traces which subsequently become sources of additional pathological stimuli, giving rise to new pathological foci. It is   precisely by this means that the process spreads through all parts of the network. The repetition of an irritation from outside not only gives rise to a new process but may cause the revival of an old one that was to all appearance wholly extinguished. Such is the basis of our experiments with a "second blow" which served as material for our concept of "predisposition"—a concept which the physicians have never attempted to explain and which previously was given the name of *"locus minoris resistentiæ."*

Our subsequent study of neuro-dystrophic processes showed that the question of the strength and weakness of the irritating agent is not so simple as it was believed to be, and that it depends on the combination of many conditions, since an irritating agent *may be weak with one state of the nervous system, and strong with another.* Finally, it was established that in a number of cases we can speak of the strength or weakness of an irritating agent only in relation to reactions following shortly after the irritation; whereas in estimating the results right to the end, including the remote consequences, *the concepts of strength or weakness may change places.* The appearance of new foci of irritation transforms the network of the nervous system. New pathological combinations gradually extend the disturbance and lead to symptoms of general dystrophy. In the final analysis this is old age. In many of our experiments, we have repeatedly observed aging as one of the consequences.

On two or three occasions these observations presented a special interest. *The most pronounced effect was* obtained with young dogs, which at the age of 6 to 8 months were subjected to a nerve trauma in the form of prolonged "weak" irritation, *e.g.,* the injection of brain emulsion in one of the sciatic nerves, with, or even without subsequent severance of the nerve. The animals continued to live in the laboratory and did not undergo any new operations. If in the period following, the neuro-dystrophic process thus begun does not lead to any severe consequences of the type described above, the animal recovers quite rapidly and for a long period appears to be healthy. In other cases, emaciation and dryness of the skin gradually develop, the hair thins and loses its lustre, bald spots appear in places, the muzzle becomes gray, the eyes frequently suppurate and water, the teeth are covered with deposit and decay, the gait is disorganised, the behaviour alters, etc. Within 1-1½ years, we have all the signs of old age, as if the animal had already outlived the usual span of life of its species (12-14 years).

Such a result, of course, is not obtained in all cases, since *the process of generalisation of the dystrophic symptoms proceeds at various rates;* however, it is met with in a sufficiently large number of experiments. Having artificially created a *single* point of pathological excitation in the nervous system of a young animal, we then left it in peace; *but this active point served as the stimulus for the progressive development of new foci.* In such conditions, even the weak irritations of everyday life, which are ineffective in a healthy animal, evoke an unusual reaction of the pathologically changed nervous system and participate in the further advance of the process.

From this point of view there is no difference between the "immortality" of the amœba and the "mortality" of the higher animals. *In principle, both the one and the other are "immortal,"* but advancing along the scale of perfection, the higher animals lose the possibility of making use of this property, since under complicated conditions of life there is no environment which would guarantee them from the accident of an unusual irritation. *It is sufficient that this should happen only once.* The system of cumulative relations itself will do the rest. As a result, the least scratch or prick is capable of being a stimulus for senescence. The effect is enhanced if the scratch is accompanied by chemical irritation, especially from a substance of a protein nature which has the property of evoking special forms of irritation.

One of the greatest specialists in hygiene has remarked that the art of prolonging life consists in learning not to shorten it. The more complex civilised life becomes, the more do new factors arise, the biological advantage or harmfulness of which cannot be immediately assessed. It would be sad if medicine itself, which is called upon to preserve the life of individuals and of society as a whole, were to create damage of this nature. Consequently, the clinic, and especially the children's clinic, should accurately estimate the real need for skin tests and all sorts of inoculations, and become quite clear as to the reality of their harmlessness; otherwise, the so-called *"achievements of science" may easily be converted into one of the methods of crippling humanity.*

This question becomes especially acute owing to the fact that the existing methods of active immunisation of human beings are not unanimously accepted. In this field, we have more hopes than achievements.

Even the interpretation itself of the results of mass inoculations is strangely contradictory and ambiguous. One frequently reads or hears that even if active immunisation does not lower the percentage of cases of disease among those inoculated, still it alleviates the form and course of the process. Supposing this to be true, where does specific immunity come in? *The form of the given pathological process may be light or severe, but, once it has begun, this means there is no immunity.*

Under spontaneous conditions of infection, let us say of scarlatina, the organism cannot all at once come under the influence of a quantity of virus which neutralises the whole amount of anti-bodies present; therefore, the animal cannot become ill. If all the anti-bodies were neutralised the organism would lose its immunity, and the alleviation of the form of the pathological process would become incomprehensible.

The abdominal typhus clinic, more often than any other, is confronted with relapses *beginning almost immediately after recovery; in these relapses, the syndrome repeats the whole cycle of the disease just terminated.* If the recovery was due solely to the development of specific immunity (as is generally accepted), then why such a sudden loss of this immunity?

Two years ago, one of my friends, Professor B., developed abdominal typhus in the classical form which is now comparatively rarely met with. From the third week onwards, the bladder had to be emptied daily by a catheter. Even when the temperature had returned to normal and other symptoms had disappeared this operation had to be continued. As a result, the patient developed a slight cystitis, following which the typhus syndrome reappeared in the previous classical form and again lasted exactly three weeks. *The disease reproduced in the most precise fashion the whole course of the process that had only just come to an end.*

I shall refrain from any categorical judgment as to the causes of the above-described relapse, but I cannot avoid the suspicion that it was caused by the second "blow" to the nervous system, in which the process taking place had not yet been fully extinguished. Careful study of analogous cases, which are not rare in the typhus clinic, would, of course, make it possible to obtain a more exact idea in regard to this subject. At the present moment, however, we are interested in a different matter.

If, even in the exceptional conditions of immunisation created by overcoming the disease, there is no guarantee against immediate heavy relapses, then it is clear that the severity of the process is not connected with so-called immunity reactions, and that the *effect of inoculations mentioned above does not depend on specific anti-bodies alone*. The repeated action of the specific agent in small doses trains the nervous system in increasing its resistance to the given form of irritation and perhaps also to a number of other irritations of a similar kind. Simultaneously, however, another neuro-dystrophic process can arise and we can never say in advance whether it will disappear without leaving any trace.

Statistics show apparently that by active immunisation to abdominal typhus, we actually neutralise this irritating agent, rendering it indifferent. The subject does not develop typhus, or overcomes it easily. But this effect cannot be called absolutely positive if it is obtained by a procedure which creates a focus of pathological excitation *capable later of acting as the source of another pathological process*. If this is the case, we must estimate the application of specific antigens for the purpose of obtaining specific immunity *as an inevitable but temporary working stage*.

In the prophylaxis of infection, our task is to ensure such a state of the macro-organism that at the moment of its encounter with the micro-organism the nervous system should not be involved in the process, *and both ordinary and specific irritation should prove too weak to evoke the disease*. Up to the present, this goal was attained by decreasing the strength of the irritating agent; but the same task may be achieved in another way: increasing the resistive capacity of the macro-organism by training its nervous system ought to give the same effect to an even much greater extent. Hence it becomes the task of the investigator to establish the concrete conditions in which this training is not accompanied by harm in other respects.

This chapter cannot be concluded without mentioning incubation. This question has been raised more than once in this book, and it remains for me merely to summarise the results.

The incubational or latent period of a process is a widespread biological phenomenon, but in the theory of infection and immunity it attracts special attention. Up to now many regard it as a period of "concealed struggle" between the micro-organism on the one hand, and the macro-organism on the other. This point of view is unsatisfactory, *for it gives no answer to the question as to the form of the* mutual relations of micro-organism and macro-organism during incubation.

The whole conception is a verbal echo of well-known, biological ideas arising from the theory of evolution.. There is, of course, a particle of truth in it, provided that the valuation is made on a historical scale and is evidence merely *of the evolution of the properties of the complex organism.* The complex organism, as is well known, is capable of elaborating various kinds of adaptions to the conditions of its environment. These include reactions to antigen. The differentiation of this capacity of the organism is remarkably subtle. It is evident, therefore, that *it is an old, excellently constructed function, in no way inferior to secretion of saliva, circulation of the blood, etc.* The encounter between the micro-organism and macro-organism is the impulse evoking this function, just as bread placed in the mouth evokes secretion of saliva. In both cases the quality and quantity of the response corresponds to the character of the agent evoking it.

But where does disease come in here? What we have been speaking of is a normal or *physiological function,* directed towards active maintenance of the equilibrium between the organism and its environment.

Disease, as we have seen, is something entirely different. Its manifestations *go outside the limits of physiology,* they are not necessary to the organism. Moreover, the first external signs of disease sometimes begin a long time after the foreign agent has been acting. *By this time the reactions to the antigen may already be present.* We know, for instance, that in the climax of abdominal typhus Wiedal's reaction is a trustworthy indication for diagnosis. Consequently, by that time the macro-organism already responds actively and specifically to the micro-organism. Nevertheless, it has still to pass through a series of pathological changes during a period of at least two more weeks and, moreover, without any guarantee of a favourable outcome. *Hence, struggle is not disease, and disease is not struggle.* We have here two categories of absolutely distinct phenomena. Coinciding in time, they actually intermingle their features but *do not fuse them.* Incubation occurs in both groups, but it also is a distinct process in each, both in time and in essentials. Pathology can be interested only in that one of them which represents the introduction to the disease, *i.e.,* belongs to the pathological symptoms.

Three facts established by us serve to decide the question of incubation.

In the first place, our experiments have shown that the latent period of action lasting some days, weeks or even months is not a special property of substances of a protein nature, and still less of definite micro-organisms; *this property may be shared by many other substances* since the cause of the phenomenon depends only on the organism that undergoes irritation.

In the second place, it was found from the same experiments that incubation is a typical feature of neuro-dystrophic processes.

Finally, the third fact was established during the study of specific reactions, a number of features compelling us to include them in a special group of processes allied in type to nervous dystrophy. Hence, we have come to regard incubation as the time during which the irritation arising from one or several nerve points draws other parts of the nervous system into the process and brings about temporary or permanent functional changes in them.

If that is the case, then *not only the initial but also the second and third symptoms of the disease have their incubational period.* Incubation lasts from the moment of irritation until death or recovery; the disease itself is considerably shorter since we are accustomed to measure it only from the time when external symptoms are found. In essentials, *incubation is the disease itself* and not a latent state of some other process, for the external symptoms are already a secondary feature.

It follows from this, that if there are elements of mutual interaction in the encounter between the foreign agent and the reacting organism, then the whole action is in accordance with purely physiological laws. The pathological processes arising simultaneously proceed independently. The task of medicine consists in finding means of actively interfering in their course

The first attempts at work in this direction form the subject of the last part of this book.

CONCLUSION

CHAPTER XXI
BASIC PROPOSITIONS

THIS book cannot have a conclusion.

I have more than once had occasion to mention that although the question of the role of the nervous system in pathological processes was first raised a long time ago, it has not lost its novelty even today. The reason lies in the fact that *this question has always been analysed as a special aspect of the study of separate pathological forms.* The nervous system was regarded as a supplementary factor, introducing some extra features into the intricate complex of symptoms of a particular disease. Leaving out of account certain attempts (including the old investigations of Samuel and the recent work of Ricker) it can be said *that no real appraisal of the nervous factor has ever been made from the point of view of general pathology.*

At the beginning our work also had a sporadic character, passing from one subject to another according to the logic of the experiment itself. Subsequently, when the need for systematising the materials became clearly defined, we discovered also the inadequacy, or more correctly, the simple absence, of the necessary basic principles.

From that moment, the conditions of our work took another form: *what had previously been the subject of our work we converted into its method.*

Instead of investigating tetanus or tuberculosis, we conducted our work by means of tetanus or by means of tuberculosis, etc., with the aim of making a comparative study of the nerve mechanism of processes which often externally had nothing in common with one another. Naturally, under the new conditions many details were elucidated relating also to the processes themselves taken as indicators, but this now became a secondary problem, a by-product, as it were, of the basic output.

In setting to work, we, like everyone else, regarded neuro-trophic disturbances as a special form of reaction of the organism, forming the subject matter of a special chapter of pathology. The further our analysis of the subject advanced, the more necessary it became to enlarge the circle of phenomena where the nervous component is the fundamental part of the process determining the outcome of the disease and the fate of the animal. I am not speaking here of various forms of vascular derangements, the nervous nature of which is sufficiently clear at the present time. Our work has shown that various destructive changes, acute and chronic inflammation, neoplasms, and even trauma, are closely connected with processes of a nervous character. At the present moment, we are in a position to assert that *neuro-dystrophic processes are not confined to a limited sphere, that they enter into the composition of all pathological processes without exception, are not separable from them, and, consequently, do not constitute and cannot constitute a separate chapter in pathology.*

In order to make clear the position adopted by us, it is necessary to turn to the history of the subject.

The time is still quite recent when the existence of a trophic function of the nervous system was *only a matter for debate.* The controversy arose in the middle of the nineteenth century and has persisted to our day. All will remember it; there is now no necessity to resuscitate its whole history, since the embittered disputes have gradually died down and we have, at last, the right to speak of the trophic role of the nervous system without fearing to encounter objections at every step.

The question at issue was first raised by pathology and the clinic. It is natural that, before recognising the fact, physiology and morphology demanded proofs. *Morphology demanded a definite substratum in the form of a "trophic nerve cell," while physiology insisted that the process should be shown at work in those conditions of technique in which it had confidence.* This was the chief cause why the question was held back for many years. The process *was hardly susceptible of appreciation* under the usual conditions of physiological investigation; hence, its very existence was doubted. Since, at the same time, it was impossible to deny the existence of a whole series of characteristic phenomena, attempts were made to explain them by the facts of the past. This gave rise to the "vaso-motor theory" of neuro-trophic influences; this theory has persisted to our day and explains everything by "the play of the vessels" and by the quantitative variations in the nutrition of the tissues, and the drainage of products of metabolism. Other views on the subject were formed along the same lines.

The faith of the physicians in the authority of physiology made them share the same opinion. The controversy that flared up within the confines of the laboratory spread to the clinic. However, pathology and the clinic could not wholly disclaim their own observations and conclusions. Not all contemporary medicine has its origin in contemporary biology. Medicine is a much older system than scientific physiology; true, it has joined the route of physiology, renouncing many of its former theories and constructing new ones in contact with the more exact sciences, but it cannot cancel its past altogether, and in this it is right.

Contemporary physiology studies fragments of processes under suitable and artificially created conditions—whereas medicine is occupied with life in the totality of its simple and complex manifestations, including all those exceptional combinations which only nature knows how to produce. *Contemporary physiology, is still practically an analytical science—medicine has at all times been interested only in synthesis*, defending its right day by day to pursue its propositions to the end and to use them for practical purposes. *This is the basic and inevitable feature of medicine*; for medicine cannot be guided merely by the approbation of laboratory research, and it often maintains an independent attitude.

Such a rupture took place between the laboratory and the clinic in regard to the question of neuro-trophic processes, and the clinic has continued to collect and systematise the relevant material in its own way. An important part was played here by the experience of the World War, 1914-18. It became evident that the consequences of nerve traumata are by no means restricted merely to anæsthesia, pain, paralysis or vaso-motor disturbances. A lively interest was once again awakened in neuro-trophic phenomena. This attracted the attention of research laboratories, and proofs were at last obtained capable of convincing the old physiology of the existence of the direct influence of the nervous system on bio-chemical processes in the tissues; these proofs were reinforced by the study of the nerve aspect of so-called vegetative processes. The foundations for this were laid even before the World War, but it reached its full development only during recent years.

It should be noted, by the way, that the proofs now discovered by physiology *were necessary for physiology itself*. The recognition of the existence of trophic processes by physiology had come too late; as far as the clinic is concerned, the matter was already beyond dispute. Some years ago, when we began our systematic work in this field, the data published by us still produced the impression of something unusual, in spite of the fact that the propositions to which these data were related could have been known even for decades.

The subject must be considered to date from the experiments of Magendie (1824). On injuring intra-cranial portions of the trigeminus nerve in rabbits, he noticed the resulting development of eye disease in the form of ceratitis. These experiments were repeated by Samuel, Meissner, Schiff, Kirchner and others.

Their data made it possible to establish that, as a result of injury to, or irritation of, the intra-cranial portions of the trigeminus nerve in rabbits, conjunctivitis and ceratitis, sometimes even penetration of the cornea, is exhibited on the side of the trauma. At the time, a controversy developed around these experiments, and this has only recently begun to die down. *The subject of the discussion was not the fact itself, but its interpretation.* Some considered the inflammatory changes in the eye as the direct consequence of the nerve trauma and saw in them the manifestation of a special "trophic function" of the nervous system. Others sought an explanation simply in the loss of sensitivity of the eye, resulting in an increased percentage of accidental lesions. In proof, experiments were performed providing evidence that the disease could be prevented in the operated rabbits if the eyes were protected from external influences. Meissner and Schiff showed that this is not quite correct. By injuring only part of the Gasserian ganglion they *preserved the sensitivity of the eye and nevertheless obtained the development of ceratitis and ulcers of the corneal membrane.* Berthold noted that on stimulation of the Gasserian ganglion in rabbits, changes took place not only in the cornea, but also in the middle ear, *i.e.,* in a region the alteration of which cannot be due to post-operational damage from without.

Samuel carried out a large number of experiments of various kinds with the aim of proving the existence of the trophic function of the nervous system. This provided him with material for elaborating a special theory expounded in his book, *"Die trophischen Nerven"* (1860). He gives a detailed analysis of the experimental and clinical data in his possession and not only arrives at the conclusion that there exists in the organism a special "trophic nervous system," but he even gives a general plan of its distribution and functioning. This theory did not receive general recognition and for a long time served only as a subject for criticism. However, the author did not remain alone. Very soon, Charcot categorically pronounced in favour of the connection of certain chronic local changes with the disturbance of some sort of special function of the nervous system. The same point of view was put forward by Duplay and Morat (1873), Erb, etc.

After the American Civil War, the work of W. Mitchell, Morehouse and Keen appeared, devoted to an examination of the pathological consequences of nerve trauma. The development of dystrophic phenomena in the tissues after injury to the nerves was regarded by them as a peculiar form of nerve reaction.

Following the discovery of the secretory nerves (Ludwig, 1851), Heidenhain undertook a detailed analysis of the nervous aspect of the secretory process. In a series of experiments, he elucidated the significance of various forms of innervation in this process and arrived at the conclusion of *the existence here of trophic influences of the nervous system, and even of the presence of trophic fibres in the composition of the sympathetic nerves.*

At about the same time the classical experiment of Claude Bernard with "sugar puncture" became widely known. The phenomenon observed by him has up to the present time not received a final appraisal, although it has been the subject of ardent research for sixty years, but there is no doubt that the question of the active participation of the nervous system in the processes of metabolic regulation was thereby definitely raised.

In 1884, the dissertation of V. I. Razumovsky appeared, dealing with atrophic processes in bones after severance of the nerves.

In 1885, I. P. Pavlov published his research on the nerves augmenting the beats of the heart. Together with the data of Claude Bernard and Heidenhain this research must be regarded as the basic experimental material of physiology in this sphere. The earlier observations were based on facts belonging to the sphere of pathology.

Later, a certain decrease of interest in the subject becomes apparent. Individual researches appear sporadically. The greater part of them are clinical and hardly deal with the theoretical aspects of the question.

Among the experimental clinical investigations of this period (1901-06) we must mention the works of Spiess, who succeeded in showing the influence of anæsthesia upon the course of certain local pathological processes (acute and chronic inflammation, neoplasms). At the time his observations did not attract the attention they deserved. Under the influence of Virchow and his school, the opinion was maintained that the nervous system plays no essential part in such processes. It was considered that a final negative answer had been given to the question.

The pathological consequences of nerve traumata were explained either by the loss of functions or by local alteration of vascular reactions.

Since the beginning of the present century, the joint efforts of physiology and morphology have laid the foundations for a systematic study of the sympathetic nervous system. The principles of its differentiation and distribution were established and it was found that together with certain other nerve structures it enters into the composition of the vegetative nervous system.

The starting point in the development of this knowledge was provided by the observations of Gaskell, but the basis of contemporary views here was laid by Langley, Sherrington, and others. The most important feature of these works was the discovery of vegetative centres (more correctly of vegetative regions) in the spinal cord and brain. *The sympathetic nervous system was found to be included in the central nervous system and fused with it morphologically and functionally* to such an extent that it became simply impossible to speak of any exact boundaries between them. In the last resort, this made it necessary to separate under the name of the vegetative nervous system a special functional group, consisting of central portions, the sympathetic chain and the nerve structures within the organs at the periphery.

Very soon, the clinic also developed a new department of surgery, *viz.*, the surgery of the vegetative nervous system. Of the works in this sphere, one must mention the researches of Leriche and his collaborators, who successfully employed operation on the sympathetic nervous system in the treatment of chronic ulcers.

The abundance and diversity of the materials on nerve trauma, obtained during the last World War, revived the memory of past experiences and resuscitated ideas which had been buried since the end of the past century. As a result, *four directions of work became clearly marked out.*

One proceeded from the observations of Samuel, Charcot and other clinicians; the second began with the experiments of Claude Bernard; the third owes its foundation to the researches of Ludwig, Heidenhain and I. P. Pavlov; while the fourth arose from the experiments of Loewi.

Samuel's ideas found a response mainly in the clinic. In various places, simultaneously and independently of one another, physicians once more began to study the nature of the trophic consequences of nerve injuries. The work of some tended to be concerned with operations on the sympathetic ganglia and paths (Leriche, Mathey-Cornat); others concentrated their attention on parts of the central nervous system.

Among the leading workers in the second direction one must mention Molotkov, Shamov, and Brüning. A. G. Molotkov collected material which finally determined the part played by the centripetal end of a damaged spinal nerve in the development of trophic disturbances at the periphery. Severing the nerve above or below the place of injury (neuroma), he observed the consequences of each of these operations. It was found that severing the nerve below the neuroma usually caused no change in the development of chronic ulcers and other trophic affections of the lower extremities. The same operation, if carried out above the point mentioned, healed these diseases—sometimes in a remarkably short period. Similar observations were made by Brüning, Shamov, Polyenov, A. S. Vishnevsky, and later by others as well. Shamov, as a result of his clinical data, comes to the conclusion that the arcs of those reflexes which participate in peripheral trophic disturbances (trophic ulcers in particular) include both central and sympathetic nervous elements. Similar conclusions were arrived at by Brüning, Hahn and Polyenov. In his subsequent researches, Molotkov considerably enlarges the group of pathological processes in which the nerve factor plays a decisive role. A number of theoretical works in the field of pathology (one must mention here Ricker, and a number of Russian investigators, Davidovsky, Abrikosov, Burdenko,

Mogilnitsky, Weil, etc.) helped to strengthen the view that the nervous system actively participates in the development of certain pathological processes.

The second direction of research began, as mentioned above, with the investigations of Claude Bernard. The purpose of these was to establish the role of the nervous system in general metabolism. We are indebted not only to the laboratory but also to the clinic for successes in this field. The clinic collected and systematised data concerning the pathology of the subcortical cerebral ganglia (*corpus striatum, hypothalamus, nuclei peduncularum cerebri*) The observations made in this connection were a direct impulse for a number of laboratory experiments in which clinical observation, physiology and morphology mutually supplemented one another. In this way, the conception of the role of the nervous system in the physiology and pathology of carbohydrate, salt, fat and protein metabolism was gradually created by the labour of many workers including Aschner, Karplus and Kreidl, Marinesco, Mohlant, Freund, Trendelenburg, MacLeod, Eckhard, Jungmann and Meyer, Levi, Dresel, Ascher, Kraus, and Zondek, Biedl, Cushing, Foerster and many others; among Russian authors—Burdenko, Mogilnitsky, Astanin, Pines, Alpern and their collaborators. Many of these works provide ground for thinking that the nervous system has a really direct influence on the course of physico-chemical processes in the organism.

The third series of researches, begun by the works of Ludwig, Heidenhain and I. P. Pavlov, studied the influence of the nervous system on local tissue metabolism by means of physiological technique.

Among the works of this group, Babkin's researches must be mentioned. Using the method of conditioned reflexes he has succeeded in showing that, in spite of severing the sympathetic nerves of the salivary gland, the composition of the saliva continues to vary with various forms of conditioned stimuli, *i.e.*, remains as before, dependent on the unconditioned reflex for which the given conditioned stimulus is the signal. Alpern and his collaborators have developed in detail Heidenhain's experiments on the direct influence of nerves on the composition of saliva. In 1922, Magnus-Alsleben and P. Hoffmann published simultaneously their researches on the influence of the sympathetic nervous system on the vital staining of the striated muscles of frogs. They also came to the conclusion that the sympathetic system has a direct influence on this process. Later (1930-31), Bykov showed that it is possible to elaborate conditioned reflexes influencing the processes of oxidation in the tissues.

In 1913, Boecke published his observations on the sympathetic innervation of the skeletal muscles—a problem which had been discussed earlier by Perroncito. Boecke showed the presence in striated muscle of sympathetic elements connected with muscle fibres and not with the blood vessels. Before him (1895), D. A. Timofeyev had followed sympathetic fibres into the interior of the Pacinian corpuscles. Boecke's researches served as the starting point for a large number of works of other morphologists, some of whom confirmed, while others denied, Boecke's data. The same thing occurred among the physiologists. Thus, de Boer (1921) and Orbeli (1922) almost simultaneously came to the conclusion that the sympathetic nervous system exercises direct influence on the tonus of striated muscles. Analogous observations were made in N. A. Mislavsky's laboratory. Orbeli succeeded in demonstrating this process under various conditions of experimental physiological technique (Tonkikh, Ginetsinsky). A series of Orbeli's subsequent researches were devoted to the influence of the sympathetic nervous system on the work of the central nervous system (Streltsov). In spite of the very careful technique and the definite results, both series of experiments were subjected to adverse criticism as regards principle as well as technique (Beritov). In this criticism, the vaso-motor theory of trophism again appeared on the scene, the question being thus brought back to the starting point from which it had arisen in the past. Physiology, demanding purely "physiological proofs," found itself in a vicious circle.

In any case, not all physiologists approached this question from the customary point of view. Thus, I. P. Pavlov was one of the first physiologists who recognised the scientific validity of indicators taken from the pathological sphere. In 1922, he published an article devoted to the description of a number of severe pathological changes in various organs of dogs that had undergone operations on the gastro-intestinal tract.

He regards these processes of a dystrophic character as definitely due to the injury of nervous mechanisms.

There remains the fourth group of researches, which started with the well-known experiment of O. Loewi (1923). After stimulating various nerves of an isolated heart, he collected the issuing fluid and passed it through another heart. It was found that the fluid taken during the period of irritation of the vagi or the sympathetic nerves had the same effect on a normal heart as the immediate irritation of the same nerves. Consequently, *irritation of different nerves in the tissues of the heart leads to the formation of different substances.* The properties of each such substance correspond to the functional state of the given nerve (*Vagusstoff, Sympathicusstoff*). Subsequently, these data were considerably extended by the work of various investigators, including that of I. P. Razenkov and his collaborators, who showed the existence of the same phenomenon during the functioning of other organs, for instance the digestive glands. The facts obtained are not only evidence of the existence of the neuro-humoral regulation of physiological processes; *they once more confirm the thesis that the nervous system has a really direct influence on the chemical processes in the tissues.*

Since then, and especially in recent years, a large number of works have appeared dealing with the participation of the nervous system in tissue metabolism. These works relate to various branches of physiology, pathology and medical practice. I shall not describe them here, since they do not add anything essentially new to the question, and *only increase the quantity of material.* Moreover, this book does not aim at giving a full list of all the facts relating to this subject. The addition of one more case demonstrating the participation of the nervous system in physiological or pathological processes is of no consequence.

At the present stage of science, the basic tasks are:

1)   *To establish the forms of this participation;*

2)   *To obtain a concrete conception of the work of the corresponding nervous mechanisms.*

3)   *To determine the laws of a general and special character applying to processes of this nature.*

I have also deliberately avoided citing literature that is of significance only from the point of view of discussion. In summarising the results and giving an explanation of the causes that have so long prevented the recognition of the phenomena under consideration, what has to be taken into account is not separate factors *but the general conditions under which the study of the question proceeded.* At the present time, this can and should be done.

It is noteworthy that during the earliest period, the question of neurotrophic regulation as one of the forms of physico-chemical processes in the tissues was regarded quite calmly as something inevitable and self-evident. Some will remember, for instance, that as far back as 1874 Charcot made the following statement on this subject: *"Rien de mieux établi en pathologie, que l'existence de ces troubles trophiques consécutifs aux lésions de centres nerveux ou de nerfs."*[1]

It would seem that from the theoretical side also, the recognition of these propositions should not encounter any obstacles. Finally, the discovery of secretory nerves decided this same question in an absolutely simple fashion.

How is it possible to understand that, under the influence of a nerve stimulus, a gland cell passes from a state of rest into one of secretion, if this act is not looked upon as direct nerve influence on tissue metabolism? *The nerve is secretory only because it is trophic.* The one cannot exist without the

---

[1] "Nothing in pathology is better established than the existence of these trophic disturbances resulting from lesions of the nerve centres or nerves."

other. If we deny this, what suffers is by no means the conception of trophic nerves, but that of secretory nerves. Motor, receptor and secretory nerve functions were noted as functions *sui generis*, and recognised without any struggle, although the essence of the phenomena taking place here still remains unknown. The theory of trophic nerve functions aroused a storm of opposition, although *we cannot conceive of any biological processes without changes in matter.*

The cause of the struggle that arose did not lie, therefore, in facts or direct contradictions. *The basic cause lay in the question being raised from the very beginning as a question of a special and completely new nervous function, distinct from those previously known.* According to the accepted physiological view, all forms of nervous activity are connected with a definite morphological substratum specially designed for this purpose. The same demand was put forward now also and did not receive any formal satisfaction.

The history of the theory of the trophic functions of nerves is therefore divided into two parts: *the history of the subject itself and the history of misunderstandings.*

As already mentioned, the basic misunderstanding lay in regarding the trophic function as a special function distinct from those previously known. Even considerations of a general character ought to have shown that this was improbable. In a complex organism, the nervous component enters into the composition of every process without exception. The concept of an organ, of its structure and function, takes this into account, since an attempt to change the nerve conditions of an organ may easily lead to the loss of the organ itself.

As long as a given tissue is in a normal condition, the neuro-trophic processes in it remain invisible precisely because they determine the state of normality. Any change beyond the usual limits is a signal of the transition to pathology. This is why pathology and the clinic are so far ahead of physiology in this question. Physiology, claiming to study the normal state, for a long time had no suitable means of approach to the phenomena mentioned. The inertia resulting from what had been useful in the past prevented a review of the basic propositions of physiology itself, and *instead of revising its own methods, the failure was ascribed to the subject under investigation.*

The second misunderstanding in the history of the theory of neuro-trophism is the demand that *direct nervous influences on metabolism should be definitely demonstrated in "resting" tissues.*

A strange term! It is supposed to separate reactions that are the consequence of the activity itself from those that form part of the complex of causes of the activity. But, surely, every tissue change, at whatever time it is manifested and however it finds expression, is already evidence that the tissue is not in a state of rest.

Nevertheless, much effort was expended in vain in the endeavour to satisfy the above-mentioned demand. It can hardly be said that these efforts added anything essentially new to the sum of knowledge already obtained. It suffices to recall the well-known experiments of Heidenhain on the question of the secretion of salivary glands. They led him to recognise trophic nerves on the basis of precisely those changes that take place in a "resting" gland, outside the period of its secretion, under the influence of nerve stimulation. The convincingness of his data is in no way inferior to that of all the results of the further treatment of these data at the hands of later investigators.

Hence, the question of the direct influence of the nervous system on the course of physico-chemical processes in the organism was even at that time decided positively, not merely for tissues the functional state of which was easily distinguishable from the state of rest (glands), but also for others where this difference is not pronounced. These include fasciæ, tendons, bones, etc., the peculiar forms of affection of the bones in *tabes dorsalis*, severe local destruction of various tissues in syringomyelia, and, further, such diseases as *myositis ossificans*, where bone develops in the place of muscle tissue, left no doubt of their nervous nature. They could not be explained either by simple atrophy from disuse or by vascular derangements.

On looking for the cause of the demand that the phenomena of neuro-trophism should be demonstrated in "resting" tissue, one sees that it also is based on the question of an indicator. Facts which are convincing within the bounds of one science are not considered as proof by another. Hence, the origin of disagreements and an atmosphere of distrust and uneasiness.

Finally, there is yet another question. This concerns the direction taken at the present time by the *theory of the vegetative nervous system.*

It is interesting that its right to independent existence was recognised without any struggle. The chief obstacle confronting the trophic nervous system was easily overcome by the vegetative nervous system, because from the outset it satisfied morphology by presenting a material substratum. This, by itself, not only strengthened the position of the new theory, but *led to an exaggerated conception of the isolated nature of vegetative nerve functions, isolated as they were in a special system.* This was a reflection of tradition, an act of obeisance to the old theory of localisation, understood in a narrow and purely formal manner. It is here that criticism ought to begin its work.

Numerous researches, for which the works of Gaskell and Langley were the starting point, have enabled the sympathetic paths to be traced within the central nervous system and separate stages of them, or vegetative centres, to be established. These investigations are closely bound up with others, the starting point of which must be considered the "sugar puncture" of Claude Bernard. Fundamentally, this work is of a purely analytical character. It consists in excluding from the nervous system particular regions connected with processes regulating metabolism. These regions or centres were graded and systematised. However, in order to get a clear idea of the whole combination, it is necessary to assess the actual significance of each component, *to define exactly what must be understood by the term "nerve centre."*

In the vast majority of cases, we are confronted here by a finally fixed, *summary function.* It is something like the short formula of a few symbols which forms the culmination of a mathematical calculation that may have occupied many weeks. *The use of the formula is justified in suitable cases, but it does not give any idea of the process that created it.* If, in analysing a complex nerve reaction, the whole preliminary path is not taken into account, then the nerve centre which carries out the completing portion is also only a *fragment of the process.* We recognise as a nerve centre any group of elements, the direct irritation of which results in a definite action at the periphery (in general, movement). But with these elements, others are connected, and with these, in their turn, still others. And everywhere, direct irritation brings in new parts. *In a complex physiological action, each of these links, whether permanent or accidental, is a nerve centre.* Thus, a nerve cell of the intestinal canal can be a centre for epilepsy. Consequently, the vegetative nervous system is not more independent than, let us say, the pyramidal system and others. *The name "vegetative nervous system" merely unites a certain number of working functions belonging to those lower centres that are called upon to realise the last stages of the process.*

It does not follow from this that we deny the theory of localisation altogether. We desire only that the concepts in this field should finally be made more precise. The differentiation of the nervous system, and the aggregation of nerve elements of the same designation into ganglia or centres, are facts that cannot be doubted. *But this does not mean at all that a particular nervous function proceeds within special elements from beginning to end.*

From the very moment of its origin, the question of neuro-trophism was analysed from the general to the particular. When a series of misunderstandings assailed the question, the method also suffered. As regards neuro-trophism, this was manifested by fear of synthesis and distrust in it. In place of general laws, special ones were put forward, and these were connected, moreover, with special nerve regions. *The fact that vegetative functions were ascribed to the sympathetic nervous system can have useful consequences only for analytic work; for synthetic work it is of no use.* Along this line it is possible to enlarge the conception of the special physiology of separate sympathetic structures and of their complexes; but, at the same time, it can strengthen an incorrect conception of the generalisation of trophic nerve functions, enclosing it in the sphere of definite morphological associations.

As a result of several years of work, my collaborators and I have become convinced that *in studying processes of this nature the traditional subdivision of the nervous system into central, peripheral, sympathetic, etc., has no justification.* Many examples in this book have shown that from any nerve point it is easy to bring into action nerve mechanisms, the functioning of which terminates at the periphery in changes of a bio-physico-chemical character. Let us suppose that the final part of the process is realised in all cases by a particular portion of the so-called vegetative nervous system. Is that really sufficient cause for isolating the whole process in a special group? Much greater justification exists for the thesis that *any nerve point, not excluding peripheral nerve structures, can become the originator of neuro-dystrophic processes serving as the temporary or permanent nerve centre of these processes.*

The vegetative nervous system is only a special case of those forms of physiological relationships which were previously known under the name of neuro-trophism. No special characteristics were included in this new conception. *The clinic approached the question synthetically, while theory approached it analytically.* But it is customary to repose more trust in the data of laboratory experiments in science than in the observations made in the clinic. An idea of the clinic is recognised as scientific when it is supported by the laboratory, and the latter, rather naively, reckons the age of the idea precisely from this point.

The circumstance that the physiologist or histologist of the present day is not able to isolate a "trophic nerve cell" has ceased to be an objection and has lost its force as a refutation. *The form of the decision of this question we can calmly leave to the future.* Numerous clinical observations and absolutely direct experiments have shown that *the nerve form of regulating physico-chemical phenomena in the complex organism does exist.* The process has both a general significance for the whole organism and a special one for each separate organ.

It would seem that this is all that is required.

Another reason why research activity in the direction mentioned can be carried on independently of the recognition of special trophic nerve elements lies in the fact that *there are no non-trophic nerve elements in the organism, i.e., elements that have neither direct nor indirect connection with metabolism.* In actual work the question that has to be put is not that of the trophic nervous system as such, but of the *nervous component of processes* which are very diverse in external form.

It was pointed out above that whenever our procedure affected the nervous aspect of any phenomenon, this resulted in changes not only in the nerve portion concerned but in the whole intricate complex.

Gradually two basic facts were established. The first is that many pathological processes, the cause of which had been regarded as absolutely foreign to nervous influences, have been found to be in reality *entirely dependent on the latter* for their origin.

The second thesis concerns all the processes not belonging to the first group. To whatever chapter of pathology they belong, however complicated their composition and however variable their course, *the nervous component remains from beginning to end the factor that determines their general state.* It, as it were, unites the separate elements into a whole, it forms the cement, any change in which inevitably alters the appearance of the process in all its other parts. It is impossible to separate it from the remaining elements of the complex process. *Apart from memory, we do not know of a single nervous function which can be realised by itself, without change in the state of some other organ. It is clear from this that the external manifestations of nervous processes in a complex organism must be just as diverse as in general all the manifestations of life.* Under the conditions mentioned, an appraisal of the role of the nervous component of pathological processes presents innumerable difficulties.

This is the reason why this book cannot have a conclusion.

The varied material, obtained as the result of a considerable number of experiments, connected by unity of aim, allows us, however, to attempt to give some formulations and generalisations.

Without mentioning details. I shall formulate some of the propositions which years of research have convinced us are trustworthy.

1. The forms of nervous activity known to us—motor, receptor and secretory—are manifested by changes in the state of various parts of the organism and are *inevitably connected with changes in matter*. Hence, nervous influences on the course of bio-physical and bio-chemical processes in the tissues (neuro-trophic influences) are not a form of physiological relation new in principle; they are not a characteristic, and still less a unique, nervous function.

2. Direct irritation of definite nerve structures may give rise to bio-chemical changes in the blood and organs without these being accompanied at the same time by any other easily noticeable reaction. This gives rise to the conception of the independence of the nervous functions of metabolism. In

point of fact, this is merely a series of preparatory changes indispensable for the subsequent development of a chain of reactions. *Whenever the function under consideration is actually manifested independently, out of contact with other physiological processes, this means that it has already become pathological.*

3. In relation to processes of a neuro-trophic character, the theory of localisation has only a relative application. The grouping of functionally united morphological elements does undoubtedly take place; *this, however, determines not the whole process but only its separate links.* Taken by themselves, these links have no independent character and do not constitute a whole. Moreover, they can be brought into action by the most diverse energy sources, which in this way are temporarily included in the chain of nervous centres of the given process. Consequently, the trophic nervous function as such has no exact localisation. The morphological groups of elements performing this function are scattered throughout the whole complex nervous system, consisting of central, peripheral and sympathetic parts.

4. Each of these structures is linked by simple and complex connections, not only with other nervous mechanisms, but also with tissue elements at the periphery, *and performs its function in association with them.* Hence, there cannot be any form of interference in neuro-trophic processes which does not affect other functions at the same time.

5. The alteration of the nervous part of any process at a given place and time is the sum-total of a series of other processes, one of the links of the continuously changing combinations which are built up within the nervous system. A special combination exists in so far as it is connected with the general combination and is derived from the latter, which itself is the mobile sum of all the special parts. *It is obvious from this that the irritation of any point of the complex network of the nervous system can evoke changes not only in the adjacent parts but also in remote regions of the organism.*

6. These changes consist in transformations of the internal nerve conditions, gradually developing and later becoming extinguished. Their influence upon various forms of nervous activity is by no means uniform. In the general physiological complex, there exist nerve combinations of varying constancy, depending on the constancy of function and the functioning periods of the separate systems. *Since a pathological nerve combination is always a new combination, interference in its course can be achieved more easily than in cases where we are confronted by a stable physiological process.*

7. The stability of combinations of a pathological type is also very diverse and depends on a number of factors. They owe their origin to the action of some irritating agent. *But the strength of the irritating agent is the degree of irritation.* The disturbances occasioned can be transient or permanent. If ir-

reversible changes (even at only one point) arise in the nerve network as the result of local irritation, the process is not confined merely to loss of a particular function or part of a function. *Besides traces of former damage, we shall have here a focus of new pathological excitations, drawing other, healthy parts into the process.* A temporary, pathological nerve combination becomes constant and acquires the same stability in relation to influences acting on it as the nerve combinations underlying normal physiological processes. *From this time onwards, new irritations, impinging on the altered nervous system, will frequently be reflected in its damaged areas by an intensification of the pathological excitation which is already taking place there.*

8. This is the reason why, when we attempt to interfere in the pathological re-grouping of the internal nerve combinations, we frequently obtain at the outset a certain intensification of existing pathological symptoms. *The old combination is destroyed by our treatment not directly, but only because new ones are created.* This naturally requires time. The operation itself, however, is always and under all circumstances an ordinary nerve trauma in a greater or lesser degree. The result of it is rapidly seen, especially in the case of elements which are already irritated at the given moment.

9. In consequence of this, even under precisely equalised experimental conditions, we cannot always obtain an identical effect. To foresee the direction which the process will take, it is necessary to know in advance the history of every individual nervous system, *to have a record of its personal characteristics.* Here, therefore, importance attaches, not only to the character of the process taken as indicator, or to the form of the procedure chosen, but also to the individual course of development of the irritation within the nervous system itself. This makes it comprehensible why the external influences to which a given animal is subjected do not result in predisposition, for instance, to all infections. *Predisposition is created by definite combinations of internal nervous relations and not merely an "undermining of the general state."*

10. As proved by a number of investigations carried out by us, the locus of inception of the neuro-dystrophic process determines for some time the form of its development. The quality of the irritation applied, which is connected with the production of so-called "specific reactions," is of even greater significance. All these things, taken together, produce a great diversity in the external manifestations of dystrophic processes. *It is natural that not every means, even if unconditionally active, i.e., capable of producing a transformation of the internal nervous conditions, is reflected in the same way in the course and fate of various pathological reactions.*

11. If the irritation exceeds a certain limiting strength, then, no matter how the process began and whatever it was that originally evoked it, it be-

comes generalised throughout the nervous system and usually acquires a standard course of development. It then becomes almost impossible to arrest it, and it culminates in general dystrophy and death.

12. Hence, we obtain the rule that *only weak degrees of irritation can have a useful significance; strong ones inevitably do damage.* In appraising various forms of operation, it is necessary to take this fact into account in the first place.

The propositions here laid down do not claim to be a final solution of the question of the nature of the reactions under consideration. However, they are sufficient to throw light on the direction taken by our experimental work in the clinic.

When speaking above of the youthfulness of contemporary medicine, I had in view, of course, only the science of medicine. Medicine in general is one of the most ancient systems. It must be frankly admitted that *contemporary medicine does not owe its successes in the sphere of treatment to science alone.* Scores of its methods and procedures rest on empiricism and even on chance. Only in the sphere of infection, of mechanical therapy and of hygiene are its achievements connected with a really scientific analysis of the phenomena. For the rest, anarchy prevails, here and there corrected by separate facts and partial comparisons. *We have an infinite number of medical theories, but we have not had, and do not have, a theory of medicine, a theory capable of embracing all the data and directing them into channels where they can be most actively utilised.*

However, medicine cannot wait. In its theories the aims of the future must be combined with the tasks of the present day. That is why it is, perhaps, one of the first of the biological sciences to start looking for a way out of the position in which biology finds itself as a whole.

However elementary a biological phenomenon may seem outwardly, it always presents a certain complexity, it always consists of a number of simpler elements. The difficulty of analysis and subsequent synthesis lies precisely in the fact that all the parts are connected here in a mobile fashion, *i.e.*, they are continually altering with time. In these circumstances, the endeavour to get a knowledge of the whole body by determining its constituent parts proves to be hopeless, for *as soon as one element is excluded the remainder immediately enter among themselves into a qualitatively new form of relationship.* The same holds good also of the reverse, *i.e.*, the attempt to reproduce the original combination.

The position of medicine, aiming at actively interfering in the course of pathological processes and directing them in a channel determined on beforehand, seems to have been rendered extremely difficult. Nevertheless, we know that medicine does treat, and frequently even treats very well, diseases about which it not only does not know everything but hardly knows anything at all. Such, for instance, are rheumatism, many skin diseases, nervous diseases, so-called "constitutional" illnesses, etc.

What is the point here? *It is clear that exact knowledge of all the details is not indispensable for useful interference in the course of a pathological process.* It suffices sometimes to comprehend accurately the basic condition, the "leading link," and by grasping it to manipulate the whole chain. This opens up the prospect of a scientific approach to medical practice; *it is precisely this that gives rise to the need, experienced by all, for the creation of a unitary theory of medicine.*

From the time of mystical schools and of *"Naturphilosophie,"* only one attempt has been made to formulate such a theory, *viz.*, Virchow's cellular-pathology. But here, also, the only general idea was the independence of cell reactions, which *in practice led, not to the unification, but to the dispersion of medical views.* Consequently, also, the searches for the leading link, on which medicine would like to concentrate its attention, can by no means always be regarded as searches in the proper meaning of the word. Frequently, they were merely windfalls. The big pharmaceutical works in Europe and America organise their activity approximately in this way. Their chemists and technicians sometimes have to prepare hundreds of unnecessary preparations so that medicine might select one of them. The necessary link is, therefore, searched for at random, and only later the work begins of explaining the mechanism of the action of this link in each separate case.

It is obvious that medicine will not quickly attain its aim by proceeding thus from special case to special case. As long as the nature of all pathological processes without exception is not united by some general characteristic, as long as the method of dividing diseases according to their differences is not supplemented by the method of uniting them according to their resemblances, we shall not have a theory of medicine, i.e., we shall have no hope of putting an end once for all to the anarchic form of the development of medicine as a science, and of passing to planned and systematic work.

The new direction in pathology, that can arise from a study of the role of the nervous component of pathological processes, endeavours to fulfil both tasks necessary for the creation of a theory of medicine. *It gives a concrete conception of the leading link, and it establishes the principle of the integration of all the innumerable separate pathological forms into a single system.*

In order to realise the idea of the "leading link" in medical practice, it is necessary first of all to emancipate oneself from certain customary forms of approach to the concept of therapeutical interference. The latter, as everyone knows, pursues the aim of abolishing pathological phenomena in the organism. In this way, a conception of disease is inevitably created *as of an irruption of something foreign which must, and actually can, be expelled.* This kind of conception is produced by the "causal method" of estimating pathological states, regarding the process as the collision, and subsequently the prolonged interaction, of two factors.

We have seen that this view will not bear criticism. The act itself of collision between the organism and the foreign agent in the majority of cases escapes observation and appraisal. Consequently, in practice, we only very rarely have to deal with a period of interaction between two factors, since they very rapidly become fused into one. *We obtain, not a disease in the organism, but a new organism,* distinguished from the original one by a number of constant or accidental features. If diphtheria, neoplasms, nephritis, diabetes, etc., were to preserve from beginning to end an active connection with the individual cause that produced them, *there could, of course, be no talk of any leading link in medicine.*

The inclusion of a certain number of additional factors in the existing normal system *transforms the latter* and adapts it to new conditions of activity. But from that moment on, *the additional factor not only determines the general state of the system, but itself depends on the system.*

Actions exerted secondarily on this new system will inevitably have their reflection also on the factors which originally changed it. As a result of interference, conditions may be created in which the pathologically constructed combination *is not removed but disintegrated.* This takes place precisely because the disease is not something foreign to the organism but becomes part of it, combined with all the rest into a single whole.

With such a formulation of the problem, the idea of the "leading link" becomes converted into a concrete task, consisting in finding, studying and utilising a number of means capable of creating temporary regroupings of the relations in a complex organism. Weighing up the entire mass of data described in this book, it is clear that we must seek for such a form of interference among the actions influencing the nervous system.

Of the means used by the clinic for putting an end to pathological processes of a neuro-trophic character, the first, in point of time, were operations aiming at removal of the damaged nerve elements or interruption of the paths of "pathological reflexes." *At the outset of our work, we also judged the task in this way; however, we were compelled subsequently to change our attitude to the subject.*

Closer analysis showed the untruth of a proposition which even now enjoys general recognition. It is widely considered that the method of irritation and the reverse method of exclusion are the basis for the study of all departments of nervous physiology. The former method takes account of newly arising phenomena, while the latter makes it possible to note the defects in, or even the absence of, entire functions. I shall not take it upon myself to judge how far this view is actually justified in relation to other departments of physiology, but it has proved inapplicable in *the sphere of the study of the nervous component of pathological processes*. In point of fact, we cannot exclude anything here, and whatever the external appearance of our procedure, it can never be a subtraction, for it *always adds something new to what existed before*. Indeed, we even found that both irritation and exclusion of one and the same nerve structure was often expressed by absolutely identical consequences at the periphery. It became clear that neither means acted by itself, *but only commenced some third process for which either served merely as the historical starting point*. Severance and excision of nerve structures can, as is well-known, produce a therapeutic effect, *i.e.*, temporarily abolish dystrophic phenomena in the tissues. But the mechanism of action here is different, and is not what it is officially accounted to be.

Hence a formal account alone does not suffice for understanding the favourable effect of the operations mentioned. By removing one of the purely external manifestations of the disease at the periphery, these procedures are capable of extending the complex of its causes at the centre. As a result, we get a relapse, and usually in an even more severe form, or even a generalisation of the dystrophic phenomena with all its consequences. And we witness that the most authoritative representatives of this comparatively new branch of surgery (Leriche and others) in summarising their "achievements" are already sounding the alarm and openly calling for renunciation of all operations which are associated with more or less considerable nerve trauma.

In our experimental work, we renounced this long ago and clearly explained the cause of the contradictions created. *It became evident that the usefulness of operating on the nervous system is often due to the very act of interference itself, and not to its form, while the harm, on the other hand, depends on its form and is associated with excessive trauma.*

During recent years, we have made it our aim to study a number of different irritations, not connected with anatomical derangements of the nervous system, but capable of producing at least temporary transformation of the mutual relations of its separate parts. Various forms of skin irritations were tested, a special form of brain massage, termed by us "pumping," was invented, etc.

I shall describe here some of the experimental clinical observations belonging to this sphere.

CHAPTER XXII

PARKINSON'S DISEASE

OUR first experimental work in the clinic goes back to the time when we were studying the genesis of convulsive processes. In the early part of this book, I pointed out that we attempted to use the conception of "neuro-toxins" to explain certain of the data obtained by us at that time. The scientific history of this conception is as follows.

At the beginning of the present century, the theory of cyto-toxins was evolved in I. I. Mechnikov's laboratory. It was based on the experiments of Bordet, who was the first to obtain hæmolysins, and F. Y. Chistovich, the discoverer of precipitins. Shortly afterwards, a number of other cell toxins of biological origin were reported, including neuro-toxins (Delezenne, Centanni, Enriquez and Sicard). Among Russian scientists, an important investigation on the subject of neuro-toxins was made by V. K. Khoroshko. As early as 1912, he found it possible to take a positive view of the role of neuro-toxins in the genesis of a number of pathological nervous processes, in particular epilepsy. We were inclined to support this standpoint, since we considered that on the disintegration of a frozen portion of the cerebral cortex some irritating substance is formed which enters into combination with nerve elements and acts as a nerve poison. We regarded this substance as an "auto-neuro-toxin," and we attempted to use it for active and passive immunisation, many circumstances co-operating to suggest this possibility. We observed, for instance, that repeated slight freezing of small portions of the cerebral cortex in dogs frequently enabled them to tolerate comparatively easily subsequent freezing in what was usually a fatal dose. We were inclined to look on this as active immunisation of the animal to "auto-neuro-toxin." But subsequently it was found that a certain proportion of normal animals also fail to become ill, whatever the form of freezing applied. We killed such animals at the end of various periods, and we always found that the disintegration of the cortical substance in the frozen portion proceeds just as energetically as in the cortical substance of dogs that had died after fatal epilepsy. A special blow was delivered to our conception of the role of neuro-toxins in this process when it became clear that "fatal" freezing of the cortex at the usual spot, if carried out under narcosis but without morphine, practically loses all effect. Finally, our observations showed that *we have no firm grounds for recognising qualitative differences between separate forms of epilepsy*. Suppose that, after freezing the cortex, neuro-toxins and the products of disintegration of nerve tissue in general do play a part in the development of epilepsy. How, in that case, are the above-described forms of reflex epilepsy to be connected with neuro-toxin? As we have seen, these forms of reflex epilepsy are in no way to be distinguished from those observed as a result of freezing the cortex and which also frequently prove fatal.

Gradually, other grounds for our previous views also began to be under-mined. We passed from experiments on active immunisation of dogs to pas-sive immunisation. At the beginning, results were obtained here which seemed to encourage confidence in the correctness of the line adopted. However, here also contradictions subsequently revealed themselves. For experiments on pas-sive immunisation, we used the blood of dogs that had twice undergone cortical freezing in a fatal dose and had remained alive. Serum was prepared from their blood in the usual way. We injected this serum *subarachnoidally* into normal dogs on one or several occasions. After a certain period, the animals under-went the freezing operation in a fatal dose with the employment of morphine, as a result of which many of them remained alive, while some of them did not even show convulsive symptoms or only to a weak extent.

When the corresponding experiments were transferred to the human clinic, here also in some cases so-called "promising" results were obtained. After repeated subarachnoid injection of even small quantities (0.2-0.5 c.c.) of the serum prepared by the method mentioned into some patients who had suffered from daily attacks, the latter temporarily disappeared altogether, or their number was noticeably diminished. Improvement was noted both during a short and a comparatively long period. However, it was found later that re-peated subarachnoid injection of normal horse serum into a healthy dog could alleviate the convulsive syndrome obtained after freezing a portion of the cor-tex. Hence, it became clear that if the serum of dogs "immunised" to freezing had any action, the effect depended *on the introduction itself of foreign sub-stances into the region of the central nervous system*. The irritation resulted in a transformation of internal nerve conditions obstructing the development of the convulsive syndrome.

Proceeding further along these lines, it was easy to mark out a number of problems for laboratory and clinical experiment.

As early as 1926, simultaneously with the experiments on the effect of the serum from our dogs on epilepsy, by agreement with Professor M. P. Nikitin we performed some similar experiments in the nerve clinic of the Len-ingrad Medical Institute, on patients suffering from Parkinson's disease. Here also, in cases that had not gone too far we obtained a definite, if inconstant, therapeutic effect. Our observations were then temporarily interrupted, but later on they were renewed (experiments of my collaborator Z. A. Malinovsky [1]).

Parkinsonism, like every complex nervous reaction, requires for its realisation the presence of a definite background against which the process takes place. Changing this background ought to deflect the process in a favourable or unfavourable direction. As pointed out above, we obtained changes of this kind by subarachnoid injection of foreign substances, the effect depending only slightly on the quantity of substance introduced. All that had to be done was to select a suitable agent which would inflict a minimum of incidental damage to the organism. *We adopted the blood of the patient himself.* In the Institute for Surgical Neuro-Pathology in Leningrad were collected rather more than twenty cases of Parkinson's disease. They included both comparatively fresh and old forms.

At various intervals of time, each of the patients received subarachnoid injections of blood taken from the veins of the patient himself. At the outset we used large and even very large quantities, from 5.0-20.0 c.c. Subsequently, we changed to small doses of 0.3-1.0 c.c. *The effect was thereby hardly influenced.* The main thing was not the dose injected, but *the place of injection.* Injection by suboccipital puncture had a more rapid and more prolonged effect than lumbar injection. Before injection, a corresponding quantity of cerebrospinal fluid was withdrawn. Moreover, in a number of cases this was combined with the method of "pumping."

An undoubted therapeutic effect was obtained in two-thirds of all the cases. Flow of saliva decreased and sometimes ceased, the face lost its lifeless appearance, the movements ceased to be fettered, the characteristic stupor disappeared, there was an improvement of the gait and other motor acts, *e.g.*, speech. The patients, especially if young, became more disciplined, in some of them convulsive symptoms in the eye region disappeared or were greatly weakened, they began to read, to be interested in their surroundings and to take part in the general life of the ward. Three of the patients very soon took up their usual work, which they had been compelled to abandon. For several months, one of them took up sports. Almost all the patients became able to look after themselves. Many resumed their participation in household affairs.

The duration of the favourable effect of the operation described was not uniform and depended to a considerable extent on the age of the patient, as well as on the age of the illness. *Sooner or later, however, there was a gradual return of all the symptoms in the same form as before treatment.* A repetition

[1] Z. A. Malinovsky. *Arkh. Biol. Nauk,* Vol. 32, No. 5-6, 1932.

of the procedure described above again alleviated the disease and resulted in temporary disappearance of the symptoms. Sometimes the effect lasted only 2-4 weeks, in some cases it could be observed during 3 and even 5 months.

I shall not undertake to assess the therapeutical significance of the method described. What is undubitable in regard to the above-mentioned clinical experiment is that even such a complicated and stubborn process as Parkinsonism exhibits considerable perturbations in its development as a result of non-specific influences brought to bear on the nervous system. The duration of the effect, it is seen, was sometimes considerable. In any case it greatly exceeded the time during which the injected substance remained in the medullary region. This circumstance once more emphasised that *the nature of the substance introduced was hardly responsible for the effect obtained.*

A very interesting fact is the *inevitable restoration of the previous pathological symptoms in precisely the same form as before.* Consequently, throughout the period in which it was not visible, the process remained in a latent state. Other conditions which made the manifestation of the corresponding mechanisms possible were altered; but as soon as the old conditions were re-established the process was renewed in its former limits.

This explains many strange facts observed in the nerve clinic. Let us take, for instance, traumatic epilepsy with a bone defect in the cranium. The patient is operated on, the scars are removed and the defect is covered by a piece transplanted from the rib. The attacks cease. After some time they are renewed again, and often with even greater violence. A second operation is performed, the transplanted pieces of rib which have already become grafted, are cut out. The attacks disappear, again only for a certain time. A new transplantation is undertaken, and again the disease is checked. I do not know how long it is possible to go on repeating this, but such experiments have actually been made, and they are well known.

All these forms of operation aimed at removing the source of irritation and protecting the brain, but the favourable result was achieved both when the brain was given protection and when it was deprived of this protection, and in both cases the effect was a temporary one.

CHAPTER XXIII
RHEUMATISM

LATER on we had recourse to the method of "pumping." By now a large number of observations have been made on the changes produced by its aid in the course of various pathological processes. We shall begin with rheumatism.

The fact that dystrophic disturbances pass outside the limits of the segment primarily affected and become gradually generalised, and that the pathological changes frequently exhibit symmetry, turned our attention to this disease, the nature of which is still problematical. The disease has certain features of an infection, but it is not infectious, although it can occur epidemically. It can be included more readily than other disease in the concept of "catarrhal" disease. The significance of this point cannot be assessed with sufficient accuracy. *Usually its significance is denoted by the irresponsible term "predisposition."* We have seen that this concept conceals phenomena which are very close to those of a neuro-dystrophic type.

As in every disease which can be suspected of having an infectional character, here also interest has been concentrated on the infectional agent. To find this agent, searches are made everywhere; in the blood, in the secretions of the nasal cavity and upper respiratory paths and, finally, in the loci of greatest change—the joints, the cardiac muscle, the warty growths of the cardiac valves. Others expect to find it in an invisible filtrable virus with which some other microbe is merely associated. The only basis for this is that *rheumatism is a disease of infectional appearance, manifested by a number of local changes of an inflammatory character, without any signs of an external agent in the tissues.*

The clinical investigation of rheumatism and its pathological anatomy have already been well worked out. Since the work of Aschoff it has become known that rheumatism is a peculiar form of inflammation having its own cycle of development and a special morphological substratum. The researches of Talalayev, which have acquainted us with the metamorphosis of this substratum, have made it possible to divide the process into stages. Something quite different is obtained if rheumatism is approached from the point of view of its ætiology and pathogenesis. It is easy to demarcate these two concepts for any group of pathological processes except inflammation. *Here we cannot help approximating them, for the following reason.*

The cause of inflammation is considered to be the external damage; the inflammation itself is the reaction to the latter. When the external agent is found *all the remainder is regarded as explained.* If the external agent cannot be found, we continue our search, or we wait, and in that case we are even ready to postulate the existence of an invisible virus so as not to infringe the principle.

It is not surprising that in this connection the theory of rheumatism has had to pass through many diverse stages, since, in spite of exhaustive search, the microbe has not been found. The proposals put forward at different times by certain investigators (Rasenow, Menzer, Small, Schottmüller, Grätt, Fahr, etc.) did not satisfy others. *The theory of allergy was next brought to the assistance and toxin appeared on the scene in place of the microbe.*

The nature of this toxin also remained unknown since it also was a mere supposition. Nevertheless, the "allergic theory" of rheumatism, elaborated chiefly by Weintraud, Klinge, Strazhesko, etc., has now become almost more popular than any other.

We have never had any doubt of the fact that processes of a nervous nature underlie the large group of phenomena united by the term allergy. Confirmation of this can be found in almost all the material described previously. Here is another observation of this character.

My collaborators N. G. Kotov and B. N. Kotlyarenko, in investigating the genesis of certain skin reactions, came across the following fact: scarlatina developed in a child in whom the Dick reaction (scarlatina toxin) had been tested three weeks before on the skin of one forearm. The scarlatina rash was spread uniformly over the whole body of the patient except for the immediate vicinity of the place where the toxin had been injected. *This portion appeared as a pale spot against the general background of the rash.* At the same time, an especially strong rash developed at the symmetrically situated place of the other forearm, *in the form of a restricted island or red spot against the general background of the rash.* Becoming interested in this phenomenon, they devoted special attention to it and succeeded in observing it again in other cases. The degree to which it was expressed varied. In all such reactions, time plays an important part, but it is not in the power of the investigator to reproduce it (or other similar phenomena) experimentally, since this would entail experimenting on human beings.

These cases must be interpreted as being due to the fact that, in a single individual in the region of a particular nerve segment but on different sides of it, it is possible to observe simultaneously non-receptivity and enhanced receptivity to scarlatina toxin. Both these processes develop as a result of a single action of the antigen, applied at only one point of the cutaneal surface. *I do not think that the nervous character of these two processes requires any further proof.* What is interesting is merely that under the influence of the same interference, two reactions of opposite significance may arise simultaneously in a single nerve segment; *i.e.,* one and the same mechanism forms the basis of both hyperergic and anergic phenomena.

Therefore, in processes of a neuro-dystrophic character, the old conception of enhanced or diminished receptivity takes a concrete form. *The endeavour to attribute the cause of allergy to a toxin—whether of exogenous or endogenous origin is absolutely arbitrary.* We have seen that nervous dystrophy can be produced alike by physical, chemical or biological irritation applied to one point or another of the nervous system. The presence of an external agent in the inflammatory foci is not at all indispensable and, moreover, *proves nothing, since it can be accidental.*

We carried out our clinical experiments on the subject of rheumatism with the aid of the "pumping" method. Looking on rheumatism as a specific process of a nerve character, we had also to regard *sodium salicylate as a substance, the effect of whose action is only exhibited through the nervous system.* We made the supposition at the beginning that, by strengthening the penetration of this preparation into the region of the central nervous system by means of "pumping," we could perhaps obtain a better effect and in a shorter period of time. This view had to be given up. It has already been pointed out above several times that "pumping" itself must be regarded as a *special form of nerve irritation.* Once begun, this irritation gradually develops within the network of the nervous system, temporarily creating a new combination of relations inside it. The neuro-dystrophic process is also nothing but a labile combination of nerve relations, existing temporarily or permanently. It is clear that *under the new conditions it may lose its former character* and either disintegrate or, on the contrary, become intensified. As can be seen from what follows, it is precisely this that determines the effect obtained.

The appropriate experiments were performed in 1928-29 in the Obukhov Hospital by my collaborators M. A. Gorshkov and A. A. Babkova,[1] under the general supervision of Professor I. I. Grekov.

They began by selecting from the hospital records cases of rheumatic patients who had been treated in the hospital during the preceding two years. These were patients who had entered with acute symptoms of rheumatism; 127 were first cases, and 97 were relapses. All the patients had been treated

[1] M. A. Gorshkov and A. A. Babkova. *Vest. Khirurg. i Pogr. Obl.,* No. 47, 1929; *Zeitschr. f. d. ges. exp. Med.,* Vol. 67, Nos. 1, 2, 1929.

with sodium salicylate in a dose of 3.0-10.0 gm. per day, bandages, baths, salicylic dressings, etc. Many of them were given repeated intravenous injections of sodium salicylate. Of 127 cases, suffering from acute rheumatism for the first time, 48 per cent recovered, 46 per cent obtained some improvement, and 6 per cent were recorded as without improvement. Of the 97 patients with a repetition of acute rheumatism, 33 per cent were discharged as cured, 64 per cent as "improved," and 3 per cent as without improvement. On the average, the first signs of a clear turning point in the disease occurred from the twelfth to fifteenth day of treatment.

For the experiments with "pumping," we decided to use sodium salicylate internally, in a dose of 5.0 to 6.0 gm. per day, since this was the average dose administered to the above-mentioned 224 patients in this hospital.

In the great majority of cases, "pumping" was carried out only once. If the patient had not yet been given salicylate preparations or had ceased taking them owing to the absence of therapeutic effects, then sodium salicylate was prescribed on the day before the operation or on the day itself, as well as during the next 2 or 3 days. "Pumping" was performed by means of lumbar puncture, usually in a sitting position (it is interesting that in almost all cases of rheumatism there is increased subarachnoid pressure, which is sometimes very considerable).

For the operation, we used a 10.0 c.c. "Record" needle. The withdrawal and reinjection of the fluid was repeated from 8 to 40 times. The last portion of fluid was removed. The operation must not be carried out too slowly or too rapidly. Rapid extraction, especially during the second half of the operation, always produces headaches, which do not pass off until the evening and sometimes persist until the following day. In isolated cases, vomiting occurred.

In all, we had 100 patients with the polyarthritic form of rheumatism. Among them were 52 first cases of acute rheumatism, 33 repeated acute cases and 15 chronic cases. The list of those recorded as recovered includes only patients in whom tissue and temperature changes were abolished and who had no complaints.

In the group of first cases of acute rheumatism, *70 per cent completely recovered and in 30 per cent improvement was noted.* Of the latter, more than 50 per cent were discharged with the joints normal.

Of the repeated cases of acute rheumatism, *total recovery was noted in 73 per cent, improvement in 24 per cent, while 3 per cent remained without improvement.* Of the 24 per cent discharged as improved, 50 per cent also had objectively normal joints.

Of the cases of chronic rheumatism, recovery was noted in 4 cases out of 15, improvement in 9 cases, while 2 remained without improvement.

The first sign of clear improvement occurred in the majority of the patients, *not after 10-15 days, but within the first 10-24 hours.* This relates not only to improvement of the general state, decrease of pain or fall of temperature, *but also to such symptoms as reddening, swelling and stiffness of the joints.* In many cases these symptoms disappeared within 24-48 hours after "pumping." First signs of objective and subjective improvement within 10 hours after "pumping" were noted in 27 per cent of all cases, and within 48 hours in more than 80 per cent. Within 48 hours, objective changes had completely disappeared in 24 cases, and in 18 of these there were also no subjective complaints.

On entering the hospital, changes in the heart were noted among 53 per cent of the patients. Cardiac murmurs either persisted or gradually became weaker (in 21 per cent). Among 47 patients without affections of the cardiovascular system on entry, such changes were afterwards observed in only one case.

The above gives a summary of our observations. At present, this method has been tested in a number of hospitals in Leningrad and elsewhere, and the facts described have been confirmed by many workers. Professor Lenorsky and his collaborators, in employing the method of "pumping" in cases of rheumatism, carried out bio-chemical investigations at the same time, and thus considerably broadened the basis for the conception of rheumatism as a special form of neuro-dystrophy. The work of Professor Nikolayev has also provided many examples of this nature. We have obtained a definite impression that the method of "pumping," combined with sodium salicylate, constitutes one of the most hopeful forms of therapeutic treament in cases of acute rheumatism.

This view has been especially strengthened by cases of acute rheumatism *where prolonged treatment with even enormous doses of salicylic preparations not only did not produce any improvement but was accompanied by a deterioration of the general state and affection of a number of new joints.* More than forty such cases have already come under our observation. Intense salicylic treatment was applied during 2-6 weeks either without result or with evident progress of the disease.

Even here "pumping" had a rapid positive effect in the majority of cases. Very often, in patients who until then had lain immovable in bed, *within 15-30 hours the temperature fell, the pains vanished, as also redness and swelling of the joints, and the patient began to walk. Within 5 to 7 days, some of them felt themselves to have recovered and could be regarded as objectively healthy.*

We obtained very similar results in some cases of polyneuritis.

As regards chronic rheumatism, the effect of "pumping" consists fundamentally in abolishing the symptoms of deterioration which develop on the general background of the old damage. Cases where the morphological substratum was more deeply affected remained without alteration.

During the last few years, we have treated a number of cases of acute rheumatism by means of "pumping" alone, *without any salicylic treatment.* It is interesting that an undoubtedly therapeutic effect was obtained in these cases also, although it was somewhat weaker than where the two methods were combined. The precise cause of the greater efficacy of the combination of those two methods is made clear further on.

The data described provide grounds for thinking that both acute and chronic arthritic rheumatism are a reflection in the peripheral tissues of one of the forms of what we term neuro-dystrophic processes. The disease can be arrested even in acute cases, but traces of the former irritation may still be preserved. An appropriate irritation, again applied to the network of the nervous system, will evoke the excitation of the damaged parts, serving as a source of the same pathological irritation. *The result is a relapse of the disease.* If the nerve parts concerned have been altered to such an extent that they cannot be corrected, the process assumes a chronic form.

This makes it possible to understand the role played by the constitution in the development of rheumatism. Our experiments have shown that the locus of inception of the neuro-dystrophic process determines, at least as regards time, its further development. Moreover, in a number of experiments with the infliction of a second trauma to the nervous system, we were able to evoke the forms of the neuro-dystrophic process corresponding, not to the second, but to the first operation. At the present time my collaborators I. A. Pigalev, E. Y. Yelkina and V. N. Popov have succeeded in producing serious affections of the joints in rabbits, without subjecting *the bones themselves to immediate influence.* Everything depends on the choice of the nerve points that begin the reaction. Hence, whatever the source of the individual peculiarities of the nervous system in the particular animal—whether derived from inheritance or acquired during life—the character of the reaction depends on these conditions.

One further point remains to be dealt with.

The observations on the course of rheumatic processes enabled us to note some interesting peculiarities. Sometimes after "pumping," *the temperature which had reached 39-40°C., rapidly fell to normal, but for several days the joints still remained swollen, hot and extremely painful. In another group of cases, on the contrary, the swelling of the joints went down almost visibly,*

and all other local symptoms were also quickly abolished, while the temper-
ature still remained high for several days. Thus, we were confronted by a
peculiar dissociation of the symptoms of the disease.

In whatever light this phenomenon may be regarded, there is no doubt
that inflammatory changes of the joints and the temperature reactions *are not
immediately connected with one another.* The patient's fever is not due to the
number of inflammatory foci in the organism. If a connection is to be sought
between the two processes, *it cannot be a direct one.* It is necessary to go back
to the moment of the initial irritation which evoked the disease.

Developing within the nervous system, the process proceeds in more than
one direction and embraces various nerve parts, including those concerned
with temperature regulation. *Consequently, a number of separate parts are
responsible for the syndrome of rheumatism. Although the various symptoms
may arise, perhaps, from a single point, they develop not in succession but
parallel to one another.* Usually the abolition of one symptom coincides with
the abolition of all the others. Then the process disappears all at once. *But it
may also be disintegrated in such a way that for a certain period some of its
elements remain active.*

CHAPTER XXIV

TYPHUS EXANTHEMATICUS

THE question that has just been raised is of theoretical importance and requires, therefore, further investigation. For this purpose, we decided to test the phenomenon by means of another pathological process which externally has nothing in common with rheumatism. We selected spotted typhus as an example.

Its symptoms are various and can be registered objectively: fever, rash, enlargement of the spleen, clouding of consciousness, a definite cycle of development, etc. All these are combined in a standard syndrome, ensuring accurate diagnosis. The process apparently fuses all the separate symptoms into a single whole, and hence we are justified in regarding their disintegration as evidence of *the operation of laws of a genuinely general character*.

I entrusted this work to my collaborators V. S. Galkin and N. G. Kotov. The work was carried out in the Botkin Infectious Diseases Hospital in Leningrad. The plan and technical methods used in the research were similar to those employed in the work on rheumatism.

Naturally, this does not mean that we thought of curing typhus patients by means of sodium salicylate and "pumping." *If spotted typhus is distinguished from rheumatism by origin, syndrome and consequences, this itself indicates that the forms of active treatment and the course they must take cannot be absolutely identical in the two cases.* But the phenomenon of the dissociation of the symptoms of rheumatism could only arise in our experiments because the treatment applied did not have a specific character and was not aimed at the cause of the disease *but affected its mechanism.* If the separate symptoms of spotted typhus have the same form of interrelation, then we ought to obtain a corresponding effect here. *This was fully confirmed by our work.*

The clinical material consisted of 63 cases of spotted typhus taken as far as possible during the first week of the disease. Examination showed that in this epidemic the average duration of the disease was 14-16 days. In regard to severity, we had 4 cases of typhus in a light form, 34 cases of average severity, and 25 severe cases.

As in the case of rheumatism, sodium salicylate was introduced internally to the amount of 4.0-6.0 gm. per day, being employed on only 2 days—the day before "pumping" and the day of the operation itself. The operation was carried out by means of a lumbar puncture, the patient lying on his side, and consisted of 8-10 extractions and re-injections of the cerebro-spinal fluid. The last portion of fluid was removed. "Pumping" was usually carried out on the 5th-7th day, more rarely on the 8th-9th day of the illness.

As regards therapeutic effect, the patients could be divided into 4 groups.

1. In 7 cases, all symptoms of the disease disappeared immediately after the operation. The temperature fell critically to normal, the rash disappeared or paled considerably, the general weakness, headache, clouding of consciousness and delirium passed off. This effect occurred in both light and severe cases.

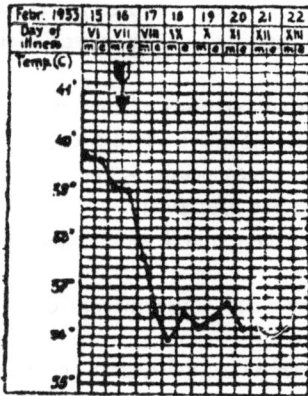

Fig. 12. *Typhus Exanthematicus.* Chart Showing Critical Fall of Temperature Immediately After "Pumping."

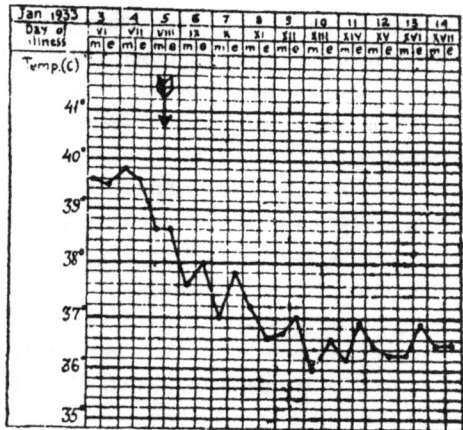

Fig. 13. *Typhus Exanthematicus.* Chart Showing Fall of Temperature in the Form of Lysis, After "Pumping."

2. In 8 cases, our action resulted in improvement and subsequent rapid recovery. The fall of temperature began on the second complete day after "pumping," the rash became paler even during the first day, and then delirium passed off and consciousness was regained. The whole process of the elimination of the pathological symptoms took 2-4 days.

3. In 16 cases, there was a pronounced improvement almost immediately following the operation. The temperature fell, the rash paled, the other symptoms diminished. However, in the following period the previous syn-

---

[1] The arrow in this and the following diagrams indicates the performance of "pumping."

drome was restored, though it did not last long. All these 16 cases belonged either to the severe or average category.

4. In 32 cases, the operation had no therapeutic effect, although here also the disappearance of one or other of the symptoms was noted on several occasions. Of these patients, 4 died, all of them with the severe form of the illness. Three of them died after 7, 8 and 14 days respectively from the time of operation, in one case after 2 days. The last patient suffered from double catarrhal pneumonia. After "pumping," the temperature fell from 40° to 38°C., but the state of the patient remained severe with unconsciousness, cyanosis and delirium. Post-mortem examination revealed, besides pneumonia symptoms, pronounced degeneration of the heart muscles.

In order to estimate the significance of each of the components of our operation, 24 control observations were made. In 12 cases "pumping" alone was employed and in 12 others only sodium salicylate in the above-mentioned dose. No effect was obtained in any of these cases.

Considering in detail the question of the mutual relations of the separate symptoms in spotted typhus, we can divide our material into several categories.

1. The temperature falls, the rash pales or even disappears, but consciousness is obscured, delirium increases, hallucinations are manifested.

2. The temperature falls but the rash, as also the general state and other symptoms, remain unchanged.

3. The temperature falls, delirium disappears, the consciousness clears, but the rash not only persists but is even intensified.

4. The temperature remains high but the rash pales, delirium disappears and the consciousness clears.

5. Only the rash disappears, all the rest remains as before. This phenomenon is met with most frequently of all (we obtained 14 cases of it).

The phenomena of the dissociation of the disease symptoms can sometimes be observed independently, without employing any external influence. The latter, however, provokes the reaction, causing it to appear more frequently and in a more pronounced form.

Two others of my collaborators, A. A. Babkova and A. A. Kanarevskaya,[1] carried out a number of experiments in the same hospital on the treatment of spotted typhus *by subarachnoid injection of serum from convalescents,* Similar experiments have already been made in the typhus clinic, but the results obtained are contradictory (Orticoni, Durend). It was not our aim in these experiments to reconcile the contradictions. We anticipated before beginning the work that the result would be indefinite. What we had in view was *to*

[1] A. A. Babkova and A. A. Kanarevskaya. *Arkh. Biol. Nauk*, Vol. 34, No. 5-6, 1933.

compare the effect of specific and non-specific influences exerted on the nervous system in this disease.

Observations were made on 22 patients (cases of extreme and average severity). In another group of patients, the same treatment was employed, but the serum from convalescents was inactivised by heating for one hour in a water bath at 56°C.

In these experiments a certain therapeutic effect was obtained in some cases, but it was almost always temporary. Moreover, it was *not possible to observe any difference in the effect of "active" and "inactivised" serum.* Consequently, the changes in the disease are not due to specific agencies. In these

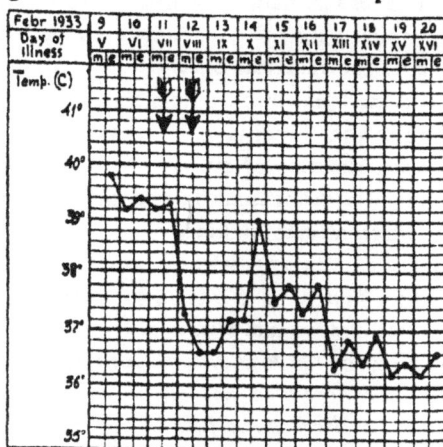

Fig. 14. *Typhus Exanthematicus.* Temporary
Remission of Temperature After "Pumping."

experiments, *we also observed dissociation of the disease symptoms,* approximately in the same form as in the experiments with sodium salicylate and "pumping."

Thus, the dissociation of the symptoms of a complex pathological syndrome, such as we observed in the experiments with rheumatism, was not accidental. *The separate symptoms of an illness are undoubtedly connected with one another, but the connection is historical, while the immediate causes of each of them differ and are independent of one another.* This once again emphasises the hopelessness of any idea of a "causal treatment" of infectious diseases, however attractive it may seem, because in many diseases the treatment is begun too late.

CHAPTER XXV

MALARIA

THE data obtained as a result of our observation of cases of rheumatism resistant to salicylate treatment, inevitably raised the question of malaria. In spite of the fact that the ætiology of all forms of this disease has been exhaustively studied, its pathogenesis remains obscure. Thus, the theory making the origin of malarial symptoms directly dependent on definite features in the cycle of development of the malarial plasmodium depicts the process in an excessively simplified form. Ideas of chronic malaria are based only on words almost from beginning to end. Finally, up to now we still do not know what exactly is the mechanism of action of quinine. Difficulty arises on account of cases of so-called quinine-resistant malaria and the fact that in cultures the plasmodium reacts indifferently to quinine.

We have seen in the experiments with rheumatism that sodium salicylate, *which had produced no effect for 2-6 weeks,* suddenly acquired this property within one day, solely because we had temporarily changed the reacting object by our operation affecting the nervous system. *Hence, activisation of the properties of sodium salicylate depended not on changing the disease-producing basis of rheumatism but on altering the field in which the reaction takes place.*

Consequently, we are justified in thinking that in the quinine-resistant cases of malaria also, it is not the plasmodium but the organism that is responsible.

Formulating the question in this way sufficed by itself to indicate the experimental task. A large number of my collaborators in Moscow, Leningrad and Samarkand took part in its fulfilment (Drs. Pigalev, Borodulin, Galkin, Ginsburg, Kostanyan, Averbuch, as well as Professor Zavodsky and his assistants, Novikov and Ponomarev). These investigations have not yet been fully completed, but it is already possible to summarise some of the results. For the most part, I shall base myself on the work carried out in Moscow in the Second Clinical Hospital (Head Physician, I. S. Kazanovich) by my collaborators V. S. Galkin, E. M. Ginsburg, R. G. Averbuch and V. A. Kostanyan, since the data obtained by them provide a basis for preliminary treatment.

In all, more than 50 patients were under observation; but in a number of cases the investigation cannot be regarded as completed in view of the short time since the commencement of the observations. Consequently, I shall include in this review only 33 cases of quinine-resistant malaria. *All the patients had been treated with quinine repeatedly during months and years, but without result.* The majority of them were inhabitants of malarial districts.

As regards the forms of the disease, there were 29 cases of *malaria tertiana*, 3 cases of chronic malaria and 3 cases of tropical malaria.

Our treatment was as follows. During the course of 48 hours, each patient received 0.25 gm. of quinine four times a day (1.0 gm.). On the third day, "pumping" was performed in the morning. On this day, the same dose of quinine was repeated, after which it was discontinued.

All the patients were under observation for 1-4 months after the "pumping" operation. It is interesting that in malaria the reaction of the patients to "pumping" was considerably greater than the same reaction in rheumatism (headache, sleeplessness, often vomiting, and sometimes agitation and even delirium). This must evidently be associated with the quinine and not with malaria, since "pumping" carried out in many other diseases did not produce this reaction. Moreover, on several occasions we tested the effect of "pumping" in malaria without giving quinine, and there were no such consequences. In severe cases, the above-described symptoms persist for about 48 hours, usually they last 20-24 hours.

In all the 27 patients with tertian malaria, *plasmodium vivax* was found in the blood. Some of the patients had attacks daily, others every other day or in groups lasting 5-6 days with short intervals. The general state of health was satisfactory only in two, in the rest there was depression sometimes reaching exhaustion. All were pale, many bilious, with dyspeptic symptoms: diarrhœa with mucus and blood, constipation. The majority suffered from headaches. They complained of feeling ill, quickly becoming tired, frequent vertigo, noise in the ears. Some of the patients had been pensioned off as invalids, others considered themselves incapacitated.

In only one case was the spleen found to be normal, in the remainder it was enlarged. It could easily be felt, sometimes attaining very large dimensions, *the anterior edge going down to the level of the navel.* In half the cases, the liver also was enlarged, but not strongly (1-3 fingers' breadth below the ribs). In the majority of the patients maximal resistance of the erythrocytes was observed, and decreased quantity of hæmoglobin. Anisocytosis, poikylocytosis and polychromatophilia occur.

In 16 cases out of 27, quinine treatment accompanied by "pumping" caused a sharp break in the course of the disease. The temperature fell to normal. The patients felt different; they became cheerful, regained the capacity to work and the majority put on weight. The amount of hæmoglobin also

increased. The maximum resistance of the erythrocytes fell. The spleen contracted to normal in 12 cases, and in 3 others it considerably decreased in size.
The contraction of the spleen began in the first days after "pumping" and continued progressively. These changes were controlled not only by percussion
and palpation, but also by drawings under X-rays. It is interesting that in 3 of
the 12 cases mentioned above, where the spleen returned to normal, it had
reached the navel line. The liver also diminished and ceased to be perceptible
on palpation.

The second group of patients suffering from tertian malaria consisted of
11 persons. The general characteristics of these cases coincided with those

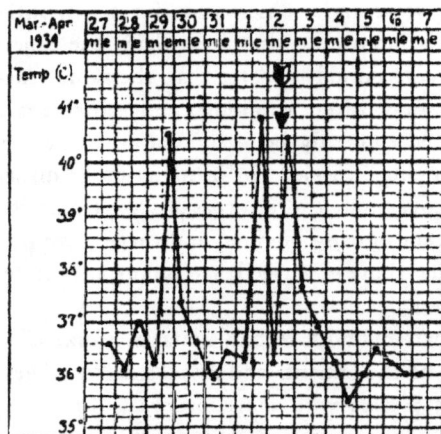

Fig. 15. Malaria. "Pumping" and Cessation
of Attacks

given for the preceding group. *"Pumping" here also removed some of the
symptoms and produced a regressive development in others.* After a certain
period, however, a relapse took place, in 5 cases after 16-30 days and in 6 cases
after 9-12 days. But the character of the disease had changed. The intervals
between the attacks grew longer. In one patient, in whom the attacks had
previously appeared in groups, with small intervals between them, the attacks
after "pumping" began to appear singly and with intervals of 2-4 weeks.
Another patient, who had suffered from fever every 1-2 days, had an interval
of 12 days after "pumping," followed by 2 attacks in succession, then an
interval of 20 days and 3 attacks, and so on. It is especially interesting to note
that quinine, which had previously lost its therapeutic quality for these patients,
now easily interrupted the attacks which appeared after the relapse. In this
group, the spleen and liver decreased in size in exactly the same way as in the

first group, but, sometimes, on renewal of the attacks, an enlargement of the spleen was again noted.

We had 3 cases of chronic malaria. *Plasmodium vivax* was present in the blood, as it had been also in the past, but at the moment of entering the hospital attacks had already ceased. Instead, there was a state of weakness, progressive exhaustion, continual headache, subfebrile temperature, shortness of breath, attacks of tachicardia, general illness, etc. The spleen was enlarged in all cases. Quinine treatment had long ago ceased to have any effect. The disease was of 20 years', 3 years' and 2 years' standing respectively. The effect of our operation was positive in 2 cases. In one of them, precisely the one in which malaria had existed for twenty years, the result must be considered excellent (the observations were carried on for 5 months). The patient himself

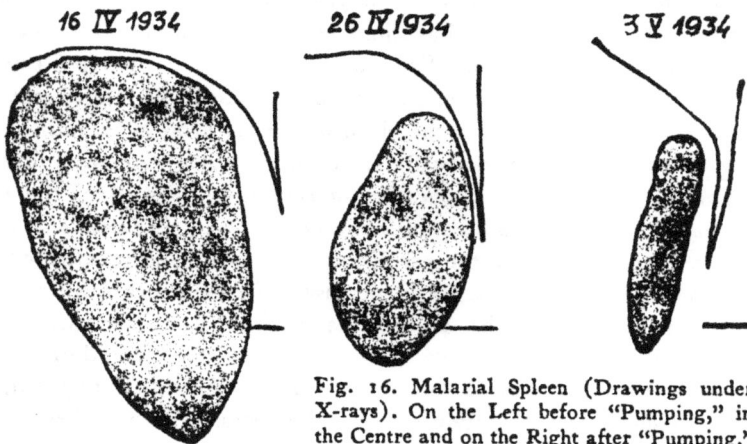

Fig. 16. Malarial Spleen (Drawings under X-rays). On the Left before "Pumping," in the Centre and on the Right after "Pumping."

considered that he was "regenerated." In both positive cases, the spleen contracted to normal and the maximum resistance of the erythrocytes was lowered. In the third case there was no effect.

Our observations included 3 cases of tropical malaria. All three patients were seriously ill. The age of the disease was 7, 5 and 3 months respectively. The rhythm of the attacks was irregular. They were daily or almost daily, with very short intermissions. Other symptoms were exhaustion, wax-like pallor, in one case heart weakness, œdemata, shortness of breath, enlarged spleen.

In 2 cases, quinine treatment accompanied by "pumping" had a therapeutic effect. *There were no attacks for two months.* The working capacity was restored, the patients felt well, the spleen returned to normal. In the third patient, the interruption of the disease was observed only during 17 days, during which period the general state noticeably improved and the spleen decreased in size. The attacks, on renewal, proceeded with less force and frequency than before.

Special interest attaches to cases of quinine-resistant malaria, *treated by "pumping" alone, without quinine or any kind of chemical therapy.* This work was carried out in Uzbekistan by Dr. I. L. Bank[1] and Professor P. A. Alisov, who is a consultant of my laboratory.

The material comprised 17 cases—5 men and 12 women. The duration of the disease was from 6 months to 3 years. *Treatment by quinine, given by various methods and in various doses, had produced no result.* Some of the patients had been given as many as 250 injections of quinine. In 11 cases the tropical form was noted, in 1 the tertian form, in 2 the quartan form, and in 3 a mixed form. Among the latter was a case combining tertian, quartan and tropical forms. Of 11 patients with the pure form of tropical fever who had been treated by "pumping" without quinine, the temperature fell to normal in 10 cases and did not rise again. The spleen returned to normal in 6 cases and considerably diminished in size in 4 cases. All the patients were then repeatedly investigated for plasmodium in the blood by the big drop method throughout a long period. This was periodically preceded by provocation with adrenalin, sometimes accompanied by application of cold to the region of the spleen. *In 10 cases out of 11, the parasites were absent from the blood and did not reappear.* In only one case the parasite remained and the temperature continued subfebrile with a tendency to increase. Of these patients, 8 were under observation for four months. During the whole time, the attacks were not renewed and the plasmodium did not appear in the blood. In all of them, the capacity to work was restored and the general state of health improved.

In the single case of tertian malaria, the parasite did not disappear, and all the other symptoms of the illness persisted. It is interesting to note that in the case in which tertian, quartan and tropical malaria were present simultaneously, after "pumping" only the parasite of the tropical and quartan forms disappeared from the blood, those of the tertian form remained. Although the spleen contracted from 5 to 1½ cm., the attacks of fever did not stop.

It is clear from this that the transformations in the organism which result from "pumping" must be classed among subtle reactions. The changes thus produced are very inconsiderable, nevertheless they are sufficient to destroy the conditions for the multiplication and perhaps for the existence of definite forms of plasmodium. At the same time, closely allied forms do not experience any difficulty in carrying out their vital functions.

The results of these experiments cannot be considered absolutely clear from the point of view of experimental technique, since the patients had been

---

[1] Unpublished manuscript.

previously treated with quinine, even though unsuccessfully. It is true that an interval of 2-3 weeks had been specially arranged between the last application of quinine and the operation of "pumping." Nevertheless, one cannot deny the possibility of traces of quinine having been retained in the organism. To remove any doubts in this respect, an analogous series of experiments were performed on patients suffering from Persian (recurrent) typhus, where this aspect had been taken into account from the beginning. The data obtained are described in the following chapter.

Let us pass now to an appraisal of what has been described. The effect obtained by us can be termed therapeutic. This, however, does not mean at all that we recommend precisely this method. There is no doubt that this method will have its place among the means for the treatment of malaria, in cases unsuccessfully treated by other methods. However, sooner or later, it may be replaced by another method, less complicated in technique and still more effective. This is only to be desired.

Our experiment has a different significance. It enables us to see deeper into the pathogenesis of malaria and reveals aspects of the process which had remained concealed. By a mechanical, unspecific means, applied to the nervous system, we succeeded in temporarily changing the nature of the organism. On the basis of what has been shown to be a very inconsiderable change, the pathological process nevertheless could not maintain itself. Consequently, its *temporary or permanent elimination was achieved as the result of another process, the source of which lay in the irritation of the nervous system.*

This is the fundamental significance of the observations described.

We are not casting any doubt, of course, on the infectional nature of malaria. *But we do very seriously doubt that each of its symptoms actually owes its origin to direct irritation by the antigen.* Neither the temperature, nor the spleen, nor the other elements of the disease can depend on the microbe or its toxins. If we are able to abolish these symptoms by a single application of an unspecific action on the nervous system, are we not justified in presuming that they have their roots in the same region? The microbe by its periodical multiplication undoubtedly inflicts an additional, and perhaps considerable, damage, supplementing the symptoms of the process. But the basic features of the latter are connected with a change in the properties of the affected organism.

We can now understand why dogs, rabbits, horses and many other animals do not develop malaria. Even insignificant changes in the functioning of the human nervous mechanism proved sufficient to make the pathological action of the plasmodium impossible. *It is clear that in an animal of another species the conditions preventing the development of malaria may be part of the natural and permanent properties of this animal.* This explains why precisely in the theory of infection the famous "Koch's triad" cannot be observed. We also obtain data for approaching the question of *the secret of the action of quinine in malaria, of salvarsan in syphilis and salicylic preparations in rheumatism. The substances mentioned have the properties of irritating agents producing a definite form of nervous irritation.* But the exhibition of these properties demands the existence of certain constant conditions. When these conditions are abolished, the substances lose the capacity to produce the required reaction. The irritating agent itself, of course, cannot acquire or lose anything. It is a simple, constant preparation. The change occurs in the organism, in the substratum which undergoes irritation. It acquires or loses the property of responding to irritation. *By re-establishing the necessary conditions through an additional counter-irritation, we restore these properties that it has lost.*

Ehrlich's idea of discovering or synthesising chemical substances with a specific action on particular pathogenic microbes has led to the discovery of only very few such means, and, even in their action, *specific tropism obviously plays no part. Therapia sterilisans magna* has not justified itself in practice precisely because the *underlying principle is incorrect.*

To bring this chapter to a conclusion, it remains to say a few words about fever. I have already given grounds for doubting that temperature is the immediate reaction of definite mechanisms to external damage.

The peculiar process with which we are concerned develops within the nervous system along different directions, but not anarchically. On involving regions connected with temperature regulation, *it communicates to them also its own special rhythm.* For many pathological forms, this rhythm is so characteristic that frequently one can determine by it the ætiology, course and outcome of the disease. Hence, fever constitutes one of the links of the whole picture; *a change from its typical form is, therefore, the signal of a deviation in the whole course of the process.* It is not surprising that the typical form of fever in each pathological process is considered a favourable feature. It is not far from this to the widely-spread opinion that fever is useful for the course of an infectional process. In point of fact a normal course of the fever merely testifies to a normal form of development of the process, but is by no means a condition determining its favourable outcome. Its significance as an indicator has been estimated correctly; but the conception of it as one of the forms of struggle of the organism against infection is far from being as firmly based as is customarily believed. The endeavour to retain a normal type of fever for diagnosis and prognosis can be understood, but to forbid interference in the course of temperature changes in the treatment of the disease is a quite arbitrary proceeding.

CHAPTER XXVI

PERSIAN (RECURRENT) TYPHUS

The results of our experiments with malaria made us desire to test the question on other processes in which the exciting agent is present in the blood during and between the attacks. My collaborator Professor P. A. Alisov, in charge of the Infectious Diseases Clinic in Samarkand, carried out a series of experiments on a disease of rare occurrence in our latitudes, *viz.*, Persian recurrent typhus.

In Uzbekistan, this disease, although not very widely spread, is endemic.

It is produced by a special species of spirochæte discovered in 1912 by the veterinary surgeon Yunkovsky. Nicolle and Anderson made a detailed study of a stock of the Turkestan parasite received from Professor Pavlovsky and gave it the name *Spirochæta sogdianum*. The carriers are apparently certain species of ticks occurring in Persia and Turkestan. The epidemic usually breaks out in spring, which is connected with the emergence of the ticks after the winter period.

The disease is characterised by its prolonged and stubborn character. It is true that the attacks do not reach the degree seen in European recurrent typhus, but there are many of them, the intervals between them being irregular, so that *the whole disease lasts 2½-3 months*. This finds marked expression in the general state of the patient, and frequently results in symptoms of exhaustion. As in European recurrent typhus, enlarged spleen, pain in the legs, and shivering are to be noted. The temperature reaches 38.5-39°C. The skin often takes on a yellowish colour. Sometimes the attack can take place without rise of temperature, being expressed then by general breakdown, rheumatic pains of the whole body, headache, etc. During the attacks, and sometimes between them, the spirochæte can be found in large quantity in the blood.

Contemporary medicine is powerless in treating this disease. Neither salvarsan nor any of the arsenic preparations allied to it, which have such decisive action in European recurrent typhus, produce the slightest effect in this case (Martsinovsky, Ruge, Kassirsky, Iren, etc.). Consequently, Professor Alisov *decided to employ here the method of "pumping" by itself, without any accompanying administration of drugs*. Together with his collaborator I. A. Ku-

373

sayev,[1] he carried out observations on 18 patients suffering from Persian typhus. The method of "pumping' was employed in the usual form, as already described by us several times. After it, the patient was kept in bed for some days. After "pumping," headache, a usual symptom of recurrent typhus, became intensified and lasted 1-2 days. After that it completely passed off.

In 11 cases out of 18, the patients could be regarded objectively and subjectively as healthy within 40 hours after "pumping." The temperature returned to normal, the spleen diminished in size and the spirochæte disappeared from the blood. A daily test for the spirochæte was carried out during 2-3 weeks, always with a negative result. All the patients were under observation

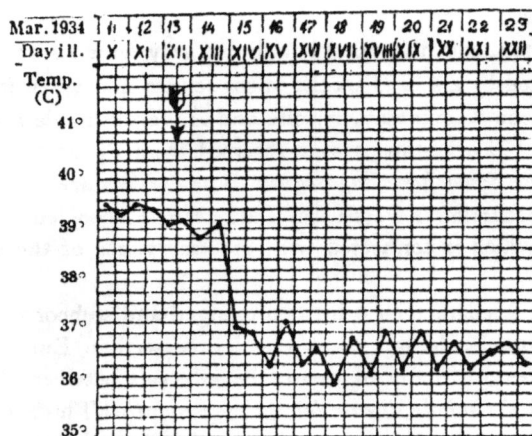

Fig. 17. Persian (Recurrent) Typhus. Recovery After
a Single "Pumping" Operation

for three months. Throughout this period none of them had any new attack of the disease. Of these 11 patients, 4 had been given "pumping" at the height of the first attack, 4 at the height of the second attack, 1 at the height of the third attack, 1 at the height of the fourth, and 1 during apyrexia after the second attack.

In a second group, consisting of 4 patients, "pumping" had to be employed twice, after which the attacks ceased, the spirochæte disappeared from the blood, and the other symptoms were abolished. All the patients remained under observation for 3 months and there was no renewal of the attacks.

A third group consisted of 2 patients, each of whom had one attack after

[1] Unpublished manuscript.

"pumping" had been carried out once. After that, the attacks ceased and the spirochæte finally vanished from the blood. These two patients were also under observation during 3 months.

The fourth group comprised only one patient, aged 12 years, who had whooping-cough as well as Persian typhus. A single "pumping" produced no effect.

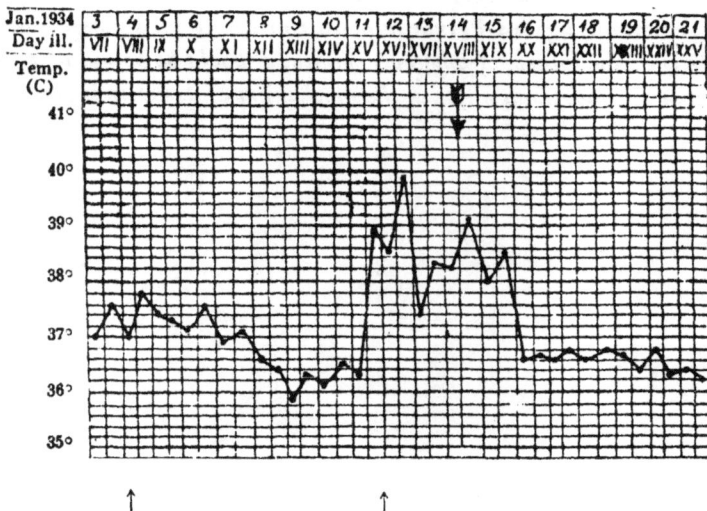

Fig. 18. Persian (Recurrent) Typhus. Recovery After "Pumping" Performed Twice. The Small Arrows Indicate Occurrence of Attacks

As a result, the investigators come to the conclusion that in Persian (recurrent) typhus, "pumping" without any administration of drugs represents the simplest and most hopeful treatment, not resulting in any unfavourable subsidiary effects. The temperature falls to normal within 40 hours. The spirochætes disappear from the blood within the same period. The general state of the patients shows a marked improvement.

The material described above supplements the data obtained in the work on malaria. Here also, in the majority of cases our action interrupted the disease without the employment of any other means to which the immediate effect on the exciting agent of the disease might have been ascribed. *If a temporary transformation alone of the nerve interrelations suffices for abolishing all the symptoms of an infectious disease, where must one look for the source of the development of these symptoms?*

The onset of the attacks, the rise of temperature, the enlargement of the spleen, etc., do not occur because the foreign agent penetrates the organism from outside or emerges from its refuge in the organism itself and spreads in it. Exactly the reverse is the case. The microbe makes its appearance because the organism makes this possible. A specific exciting agent produces an equally specific form of nerve irritation leading to a perfectly definite process. With this its role comes to an end. The reacting substratum is responsible for everything that follows.

Apart from what has been described above, we do not at present have any therapeutic means against Persian typhus. *But if any such means were to be found in the near future, of whatever nature, it would be bound to agree with our system of conceptions as far as the mechanism of its action is concerned.*

CHAPTER XXVII

ANÆSTHESIA AS AN IRRITATION

WE employed the method of "pumping," both by itself and in combination with other forms of treatment, in various illnesses. At the present time, I cannot yet give a report of this work, the available data being insufficient. There can be no doubt that the form of nerve irritation produced by this method must have certain definite features. As a result, *each form of nervous dystrophy, against which our action is directed, changes its course in its own fashion.* The effect obtained in the treatment of rheumatism cannot serve as an example for the treatment, let us say, of typhus. Among scattered clinical observations of this kind, we have facts on which both positive and negative conclusions can be based. An estimate of these data will be given when it has been possible to systematise them. At present, however, I shall pass on to an account of another series of our clinical experiments, in which our operation took the form of anæsthetising extensive nerve tracts.

At the beginning of the present century, Spiess applied the method of local anæsthesia in inflammatory processes and noted its therapeutic action, on the basis of which he elaborated a special theory. He considered that the initial factor in inflammation of the tissues was the "primary pain," the abolition of which by means of anæsthesia was favourably reflected on the subsequent course of the process. His doctrine did not find any response, owing to fears that injections would cause the basis of the infection to advance into neighbouring healthy regions and thus produce a further extension of the process *per continuitatem.*

The systematic researches of Professor A. V. Vishnevsky and his collaborators once more revived the question, not only of the permissibility, but of the advantage of applying local anæsthesia to the region of inflammatory foci. Working along these lines for a number of years, A. V. Vishnevsky elaborated his method of anæsthesia, called by him the method of "creeping infiltration."

He employed it with success not only in inflammation but also in the treatment of such diseases as trophic ulcers, gangrene of the extremities, *psoriasis vulgaris,* and some others. His aim was to cause an interruption of the paths of "pathological reflexes," with less trauma than in the usual forms of operation. Moreover, on the basis of observations on inflammatory processes, he regarded novocaine as a means exercising immediate curative action on the affected nerve elements.

At that time we estimated the curative effect even of direct interruption of the nerve paths, or of extirpation of the corresponding nerve structures, not only as a consequence of disconnection (*i.e.*, putting a stop to pathological irritation), but also as a factor promoting transformation of nerve interrelations, *i.e., as a factor of additional irritation.* It is easily comprehensible that this point of view acquired even greater significance in relation to local anæsthesia.

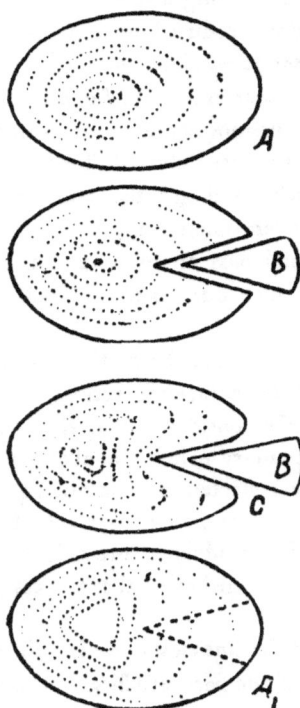

Fig. 19

A. V. Vishnevsky found that a temporary "block" in the paths of the "pathological reflex," although it lasted only a few dozen minutes, nevertheless gave a result that was not only not worse, but frequently even better than the usual bloody operative means. The therapeutic effect of such anæsthesia employed on a single occasion could sometimes be followed up for months and years. In particular cases, its useful effect progressively increased throughout this period.

Could there be a better proof than this that we are confronted here neither by the action of novocaine itself as a curative means, nor by simple anæsthetic disconnection, for a short period, of the periphery from the damaged elements of the centre?

In 1932, when I began the study of anæsthesia as a method of active interference in the course of pathological processes of various kinds, I adopted the following diagrammatic scheme as a starting point.

The nervous system (A) of a given animal is a completely closed network in which all the elements are connected with one another not only structurally but dynamically. Let us suppose that a certain portion (B) is temporarily separated from this labile network. The remaining portion will not simply be the system A minus B, since the elements will unite in new combinations. This process, beginning at one spot will progressively spread to neighbouring and remote nerve parts, before gradually dying out. We shall be faced, not with the system A minus B, but with a new system C—figuratively speaking, a new animal. If we now reconnect the temporarily separated portion B with the rest of the organism, we shall not get A again, because neither the original action of subtraction nor the subsequent addition follows the rules of simple arithmetic. Time plays a part. In both cases new combinations, new connections are created. On relinking the disconnected elements, the order of their inclusion will be different from the order of their separation. As a result, instead of the system A we shall get a system A_1. This, of course, will be closely related to A, and will, moreover, have a tendency to approximate to it, but it will not attain this in full measure, at least for some time.

In this respect the onset of anæsthesia and its cessation act alike. If, during anæsthesia, a nerve combination that formed part of the complex of conditions governing a pathological process was broken up, then it may happen that, even with the full restoration of the system A, the pathological process may not be renewed, *since other elements of the given complex system have no longer the original form of interrelation.* This would mean that the temporary curative effect has become permanent. It is possible to count on such an effect in practice mainly in pathological processes of an acute nature, in which the changes in the nerve elements have not yet attained the degree of irreparable disturbances. But in chronic processes also, a favourable turn may last as long as the process evoked by us is still going on in the nerve network, where it slowly spreads and gradually disappears.

Even *a priori* there would be reason to believe that any form of such temporary disconnection of nerve parts in any part of the organism would have a repercussion on a pathological nerve combination precisely because *the latter is always in a state of excitation.* But it is also clear that the place and form of operation, the degree of irritation and a number of other factors will determine the final result. Hence, *the same means may result in a positive effect in one group of processes and in a negative effect in another.*

The question here will be decided by experiment. Prolonged work in the laboratory has convinced us that, in beginning a new series of investigations, it is often advantageous to go from the complex to the simple, from the strong to the weak. Therefore, in commencing work on anæsthesia, we took an interest in Professor A. V. Vishnevsky's method, since his "creeping infiltration" makes it possible to involve really extensive nerve regions. Of the separate procedures, the one most worthy of attention from our point of view was the method of novocaine "blockade" of the lumbar section of the sympathetic chain. In the first place, according to the anatomical investigations of

A. A. Vishnevsky and N. F. Rupasov, this makes it possible for the novocaine solution to affect not only the lumbar ganglia of the sympathetic chain but partially also autonomous nerve structures such as the *flexus renalis, suprarenalis* and, in part, *solaris*. In the second place, A. V. Vishnevsky had already demonstrated the harmlessness of using this method in the human clinic and its usefulness in a number of pathological processes of a neuro-trophic character (gangrene, ulcers, etc.).

I communicated my views to Professor A. V. Vishnevsky and also to a number of our other clinicians and *proposed to them that they should widen the sphere of application of the method mentioned so as to go outside the limits of those processes which have direct, anatomically defined, nerve connections with the region selected for anæsthesia.* At the present time, we have already accumulated a considerable amount of clinical data by work in this direction.

The technique of anæsthetising the region of the kidney is described by A. V. Vishnevsky[1] as follows:

The patient is placed on his side, in the position for a kidney operation (a bolster is indispensable). An injection is made with a small hypodermic needle in the hollow between the twelfth rib and the long muscles of the spine. A long needle (10-12 cm.), attached to a large syringe (10.0-20.0 c.c.) is then introduced through the swelling produced. The direction of the needle is strictly perpendicular to the surface of the skin. Continuous injection of the solution precedes the forward movement of the needle. Penetrating through the muscular layers and the posterior folium of the renal fascia, the point of the needle reaches the interfascial space. This can be noted, during the injection, by the sudden cessation of resistance of the tissues and also by the fact that the novocaine solution begins to flow easily without effort. As a result, it is possible to introduce freely into an adult from 150-200 c.c. of a 0.25 per cent solution of novocaine, with the addition of two drops of adrenalin to each 100 c.c.

Besides the above, other forms of anæsthesia are also employed, for instance, in the region of the upper and lower sympathetic ganglia of the neck (vago-sympathetic blockade). In some cases, we resorted to anæsthesia of an entire extremity, *e.g.,* the thigh. The technique of this operation consists in circular, intra-cutaneous injection of a 0.25 per cent solution of novocaine. From here the subcutaneous tissue is infiltrated circularly by a large syringe. Afterwards, by means of deep punctures, the solution is introduced under the aponeuroses to the bone. This method is termed by A. V. Vishnevsky cir-

[1] A. V. Vishnevsky. *Arkh. Biol. Nauk,* Vol. 34. No. 4, 1933.

cular blockade of the extremity. It requires the injection of 200-250 c.c. of 0.25 per cent novocaine solution.

As regards technique, the most simple method is the lumbar blockade. It was one of the most suitable for our purpose, since it made it possible to anæsthetise an extensive complex nerve region. It is impossible, of course, to regard the consequences of temporary disconnection of various nerve regions by means of anæsthesia as completely identical in every case. *The most effective form of action for a particular process has to be discovered in practice.*

Some of our results from the use of this method will be found in the following chapters.

CHAPTER XXVIII

AFFECTIONS OF THE DIGESTIVE ORGANS

In the chapter dealing with standard forms of nervous dystrophy, I put forward a number of proofs that when this process becomes generalised it ceases to depend on the locus of its inception. *Actions on the tuber cinereum, sciatic nerve, upper cervical ganglion, cerebral cortex or abdominal sympathetic chain may give rise to the same affections in the peripheral tissues.* There is no doubt that these changes take place in all parts of the organism, but we find that they are most pronounced at certain definite and constant points. The latter include the eyes, especially the mucous and corneal membranes, the oral cavity, the cavities of the nose and middle ear, the lungs, the pyloric portion of the stomach, the duodenum, the region of transition from the small to the large intestine, and the rectum. It was natural to begin clinical experiments also with diseases localised in the above-described regions. Professor A. V. Vishnevsky together with his collaborators carried out extensive work in studying the influence of lumbar blockade on ulcerous affections of the stomach and duodenum. The research included several scores of cases of ulcer which were carefully followed up clinically both before and after the operation. The conclusion arrived at by the author is formulated as follows:

"In a large number of cases of ulcerous affection of the stomach and duodenum, the means employed by us produces a lasting curative effect, which finds both objective and subjective expression."

It is interesting that in a large proportion of the patients, certain of the disease symptoms, especially pains, were intensified immediately after the operation. This period lasts several days, after which the pains decrease and gradually pass off. In some cases, a repetition of the lumbar blockade was necessary. The operation had no effect in the case of old calloused ulcers.

In some cases, Professor R. A. Luriya succeeded in showing by means of X-rays that lumbar blockade results *not only in the disappearance of ulcerous symptoms but also in the cicatrisation of the ulcers themselves.* At the present time, I have in my possession several letters from physicians confirming that in the case of gastric ulcer the novocaine lumbar blockade frequently gives a rapid effect which is well maintained. Relapses do sometimes occur, but *this is natural in view of the character of the process itself.* The method is also interesting because it confirms our views of gastric and duodenal ulcer as processes of a nervous nature.

My collaborators I. A. Pigalev, A. A. Babkova and A. A. Kanarevskaya examined 45 cases of various diseases of the gastro-intestinal tract of a chronic character where the method of temporary disconnection of various nerve regions was employed.

The data obtained can be divided into three groups according to the efficacy of the operation; in 26 cases the effect was satisfactory, in 12 it was weak and in 7 nil. The first group consisted of patients in whom the pains and dyspeptic symptoms permanently decreased or even disappeared, whose general state, appetite and sleep improved, and who gained in weight. In the second group there was temporary improvement or the liquidation of only some of the symptoms.

Dr. I. A. Kramarov sent me some interesting data from Stalinogorsk in a letter dated June 9, 1934. He employed the method of lumbar blockade with novocaine in the case of 3 patients suffering from œsophagal cancer. In all 3, the contraction had reached such a degree as to allow only the passage of liquids. The œsophagal passage was so rapidly restored that on the fourth day the patients were transferred to an ordinary diet—bread, meat, etc. The general state improved and they put on weight. Unfortunately, I have no information of the further history and therefore it remains unknown how long the effect lasted or to what exactly it was due.

CHAPTER XXIX

AFFECTIONS OF THE CAVITIES OF THE MOUTH, NOSE AND MIDDLE EAR

At the present time, one of the most widespread pathological processes is alveolar pyorrhœa. In describing experimental data in one of the earlier chapters, I already gave grounds for considering that this disease belongs to the category of neuro-dystrophic processes. It remained to test this in the conditions of clinical experiment.

The work was carried out by my collaborators P. A. Glushkov and A. A. Vishnevsky.[1] The first observations relate to 25 patients. In all cases, all the features necessary for diagnosis were present. For a considerable time, both before and after the operation, no other form of treatment was employed. The operation consisted in lumbar blockade, using 120-190 c.c. of 0.25 per cent novocaine solution. The patients remained 3-4 days in the hospital, after which they came for inspection to the out-patients' department. Observations were made on three points: 1) the state of the mucous membrane of the oral cavity, and the gums, 2) purulent secretion from pockets at the necks of the teeth, 3) looseness of the teeth. In practically all cases a favourable effect was obtained in one degree or another. In five of them, a positive result was immediately noted. Included here was one patient suffering from papillomatosis of the mucous membrane of the mouth in the form of papillomata occurring singly and in whole groups. *These all disappeared within a few days after the operation.*

In the second group, *improvement was preceded by a short period in which the pathological symptoms increased.* Intensified hyperæmia, more abundant secretion of pus and further loosening of the teeth were noted here in the days immediately following the injection. After 2-10 days, this period was followed by improvement which was sometimes very marked. The hyperæmia disappeared or became weak and diffuse, the swelling of the mucous membrane and the amount of pus at the necks of the teeth diminished, the dentures became stronger and sometimes reached almost normal condition.

The third group comprises 7 cases where the reaction to the operation was inconsiderable. Here also, certain positive features were noted, *e.g.*,

[1] A. A. Vishnevsky and P. A. Glushkov. *Arkh. Biol. Nauk*, Vol. 34, No. 4, 1933.

disappearance of hyperæmia, diminution of secretion, but this was usually only a temporary phenomenon. The looseness of the teeth remained unchanged, since in the majority of cases atrophy of the edge of the socket had already taken place under the gum, and, consequently, strengthening of the teeth was mechanically impossible.

Relapses were noted in all three groups, sometimes after a few weeks, sometimes much later, but in some patients the effect lasted for about a year.

It is possible that the material described does not decide the question of the therapy of alveolar pyorrhœa, but it lays down the line along which further research ought to be directed.

Another of my collaborators, Professor D. A. Entin, also had many cases of alveolar pyorrhœa, papillomatosis of the oral cavity and simple and ulcerous stomatitis, where lumbar blockade proved useful even when all other curative means had failed to give any effect.

Two of my collaborators, A. A. Vishnevsky and I. A. Pigalev, at different times carried out observations on the effect of lumbar blockade on the development of scurvy. A positive effect was obtained in almost all cases. Sometimes the effect was exceptionally marked. Patients who had been compelled to remain in bed for many days owing to œdemata and hæmorrhages in the lower extremities not infrequently regained the power of independent movement within two days after the operation, depression was replaced by cheerfulness and the appetite restored. Very soon the œdema and hæmorrhage of the gums disappeared and subsequently the teeth also became stronger.

At the present time, hardly anyone doubts that scurvy develops on the basis of avitaminosis. It is evident, however, that the latter *cannot be considered the direct cause of the affections in the tissues*. The latter suffer secondarily. Avitaminosis only gives an impulse to the development of the neuro-dystrophic process, in exactly the same way as the glass sphere placed on the *tuber cinereum* of a dog.

We consider that noma, or watery cancer, is a disease of the oral cavity allied in nature both to alveolar pyorrhœa and to scurvy, though developing more acutely. I should like to recall that we observed several absolutely typical cases of noma in our dogs after the "sphere" operation. Sometimes the ulceration began to progress irresistibly, resulting in destruction of the epithelial, muscular and cutaneous parts of the cheek, and laying bare the bony parts of the jaw over a considerable area. On this account, I was very interested to receive a letter from Dr. S. P. Ponomarev at Starominsk in the Azov-Black Sea region. During the summer of 1934 he succeeded in collecting eight cases of noma at different stages of development which were successfully cured by novocaine lumbar blockade. His patients were demonstrated at the session of the Regional Surgical Society in Rostov-on-Don.

I have also received letters from physicians informing me of successful employment of lumbar blockade in several cases of disease of the accessory cavities of the nose and middle ear. In acute purulent inflammation of the middle ear, complicated by mastoiditis, the treatment sometimes interrupted the process and made surgical operation unnecessary.

CHAPTER XXX

AFFECTIONS OF THE EYE (CERATITIS)

I HAVE pointed out elsewhere that among the special symptoms of generalisation of neuro-dystrophic processes are included affection of the eye in the form of ceratitis.

In our laboratory, my collaborator Professor V. V. Chirkovsky[1] carried out systematic observations and experiments on this question. The results were summmarised in a special article. They can be formulated in the following statements.

1. In animals (dogs and rabbits) *by action on various nerve regions we succeeded in obtaining* affections of the cornea in the form of ceratitis of different types—ranging from restricted, superficial to deep-seated, purulent and extensive ceratitis. Among these regions, one must mention above all the Gasserian ganglion, the peripheral portions and even comparatively fine branches of the trigeminus nerve, the *ganglion ciliare, tuber cinereum,* upper cervical ganglion, lumbar-sacral region of the sympathetic chain, and in special cases—the brachial plexus, sciatic nerve and even places of the cerebral cortex selected at random.

2. The largest percentage of cases of the above-described alteration of the corneal membrane is obtained as a result of injury to nerve parts in the immediate periphery of the eye, including the upper cervical ganglion and *tuber cinereum.*

3. Where *unilateral* injury to one of the above-mentioned nerve structures resulted in ceratitis, *we frequently observed that the latter developed in both eyes. It is of interest that in a certain percentage of cases, ceratitis developed immediately on the contralateral side.*

4. Work with a comparatively large amount of material showed that whatever the nerve structure selected for injury, *the development of ceratitis does not invariably follow.*

5. We consider that this circumstance, taken in combination with the other facts enumerated above, is categorical proof that the ceratitis was not a direct consequence of injury to the given nerve structure, *i.e., that none of these nerve structures can be regarded as a* special trophic centre for the corneal membrane of the eye.

[1] V. V. Chirkovsky. *Arkh. Biol. Nauk,* Vol. 34, No. 4, 1933.

6. It follows from this that all the forms of operation undertaken by us served merely as *impulses for the commencement of a complex nervous process in which ceratitis was one of the links*. That the process actually arises in this way is evident from the exceptional diversity of the incubational period; in some cases we obtained an effect within a few hours after the operation, in other cases only after several months.

At the time that the experiments were transferred to clinical conditions, we were already aware that it is *by no means always essential to apply our action to the innervation of the affected organ*. Such a form of action could even be of harm, intensifying the irritation already existing in a definite group of nerve structures. It is more advantageous *to apply the action to nerve regions not primarily connected with the affected organ*. Moreover, our experiments were of a general character and had the aim of establishing exactly how changes of the relations in remote parts of the nerve network would be reflected in the given process.

The work on this subject was carried out in the First Eye Clinic of the Leningrad Medical Institute by Professor V. V. Chirkovsky and his collaborators I. E. Barbel, A. A. Vishnevsky, L. A. Dymshits and R. K. Mikhaelyan.[1] The chief point on which our interest was concentrated was *to obtain an effect in ceratitis of varying ætiology by means of an identical form of action.*

For observing the course of the process, we used the method of bio-microscopy as well as the usual methods of clinical analysis. Changes in the sensitivity of the corneal membrane were also investigated. The usual therapeutic methods were not used, and atropine was employed only in cases of pronounced hyperæmia or inflammation of the iris. In a number of cases where the patients were transferred to the clinic from the out-patients' department, they had already been treated by ordinary therapy. Its lack of success was a special incentive for employing our procedure.

In all, observations were made on 34 cases of various kinds of acute and chronic ceratitis, including 10 cases of herpetic ceratitis (4—*keratitis dendritica*, 3—*ulcus corneæ herpetica*, 2—*keratitis disciformis, and* 1—*keratitis superficialis punctata*).

In 7 of these cases, lumbar blockade resulted in rapidly extinguishing the disease. In 3, recovery was delayed.

The first consequence was usually a marked improvement in the general state of the patient which has to be connected with the cessation of tormenting pains, lachrymation and photophobia. In 2 cases, a brief intensification of the symptoms was noted immediately after the operation.

[1] I. E. Barbel, A. A. Vishnevsky, L. A. Dymshits, R. K. Mikhaelyan, V. V. Chirkovsky. *Arkh. Biol. Nauk*, Vol. 34, No. 4, 1933.

The objective changes in the disease were as follows. In the first place, there was diminution and subsequently dissolution of infiltrates both in the superficial and deeper layers of the cornea. At the same time, the vascular reaction of the conjunctiva was weakened. Hyperæmia and inflammation of the irideal membrane was often abolished in the first few days. The pupils, which had shown no reaction to atropine, became dilated. In two cases hypopyon rapidly disappeared. Among these patients were some with ulcerous ceratitis of long standing who had been unsuccessfully treated by various methods and in whom the disease easily yielded to the above-mentioned form of operation.

There were 17 cases of purulent ceratitis. In 9 of them there was creeping ulcer, in 4 ulcerous ceratitis accompanied by trachoma, and in 4 peripheral ceratitis of the catarrhal ulcer type. The cases were diverse in ætiology, severity and stage of disease. Out of 9 cases of *ulcus corneæ serpens*, pneumococcus was found in 5 cases, diplobacillus MA in 1 and staphylococcus in 1 case. In 2 cases, no microbe was discovered.

The efficacy of lumbar blockade in this group of patients was even greater than in the first. However, besides rapid cure of the disease, there were three cases in which an intensification of the pathological symptoms was observed after the operation, and the useful effect was delayed.

In 4 cases of ceratitis, not of typical form, which had developed on the basis of trachoma and had been treated for a long time without result, our operation caused a marked turn towards recovery. One case of purulent ceratitis, resembling a round abscess, was especially convincing. The disease had involved a considerable portion of the periphery of the cornea and threatened to destroy it. During the days immediately following blockade, the patient had a restful night for the first time in 2 weeks. The depressed condition gave way to cheerfulness. The purulent globular infiltrate quickly dissolved and was only maintained a little in the lower part of the cornea. A second injection of novocaine in the lumbar region on the opposite side of the body quickly resulted in the abolition of the pathological symptoms.

One of the 2 cases of *keratitis parenchymatosa* which had been unsuccessfully treated for a long period was also very significant. Within 14 days after the blockade, the acuity of vision, which on entry of the patient to the clinic had been equal to the movement of the hand before the eye, increased to 0.5. The second case also yielded to the action of blockade, but only on repetition of the latter.

Out of 2 cases of *rosacea keratitis*, in one a positive effect was observed within 2 days from the operation, and within 9 days the patient was discharged with a healthy eye. In the other case, rapid reabsorption of the infiltrate in the cornea and weakening of all the inflammatory symptoms also began within 2 days. The patient was discharged after 9 days, but returned after a week with a relapse of the disease. A second blockade was required to strengthen the effect.

The last group contained 5 cases of scrofulous ceratitis, of various ages and intensity. In 3 of them, we observed rapid dissipation of the disease very soon after the blockade.

In all forms of ceratitis, there were changes of sensitivity, both decrease and increase; the former, however, occurring more frequently. *It was not possible to establish any parallelism between the process of extinction of ceratitis and the restoration of sensitivity.* There were cases where the inflammatory process came to an end while the sensitivity still remained unchanged for a long period. *Hence, there is apparently no direct connection between these processes.*

Coming to a general appraisal of the data obtained, it must be especially emphasised that *in many cases the success of the operation was achieved after the usual local and, in part also, general therapy had been employed for a long time not only without result but with marked progress of the disease.* In those few cases where the blockade remained without effect and even resulted in progressive development of the disease, the alteration in the nervous system had probably already attained a degree at which any new operation acted as a "second blow."

An interesting point is the fact of the intensification of pathological symptoms in the first period after the blockade. We have repeatedly encountered this phenomenon in other spheres of our work. Before the requisite form of transformation of nerve interrelations is achieved, the operation acting as a direct trauma raises the excitability of the pathologically altered elements.

It must be mentioned that we achieved indubitable successes not only in regard to acute but sometimes also in regard to chronic affections of the corneal membrane. Blockade here quickly removed the symptoms of accentuation.

It is interesting to note that an absolutely identical form of operation yielded results in cases of ceratitis of diverse ætiology. We took no account of the original cause of the disease; nevertheless *its different forms yielded to the action of one and the same operation, directed, not to the cause of the disease, but to the dialectics of its development.*

In the same clinic (Professor V. V. Chirkovsky) observations were made on adaptation of the eye to darkness after lumbar blockade (experiments of Drs. L. A. Dymshits, L. N. Lukova, L. V. Rokitskaya[1]). In all cases a positive effect was obtained, sometimes very pronounced, but always temporary.

[1] L. A. Dymshits, L. N. Lukova and L. V. Rokitskaya. *Arkh. Biol. Nauk*, Vol. 34, No. 4, 1933.

CHAPTER XXXI
SEPTIC PROCESSES

THE data obtained during the study of local inflammatory processes naturally raised the problem of septic diseases.

What is properly to be understood by this conception remains altogether
unknown. In some cases it is often difficult even to answer the question of
whether we are confronted by miliary tuberculosis, polyneuritis, septic endo-
carditis, rheumatism, or something else. Moreover, I have already pointed out
that the presence of a microbe in the blood *can only be an indicator and not the
cause of a pathological state*. This makes it comprehensible that we should
endeavour to study septic processes independently of their formal cause.

We carried out two series of investigations along this line: one in regard
to pulmonary gangrene, the other in regard to sepsis in its pure form.

The study of the influence of lumbar blockade on the course of pulmonary
gangrene was made by my collaborators S. V. Kurakin and I. A. Pigalev.[1] In
the Obukhov Hospital in Leningrad, 8 cases of this disease, of from 5 days' to
2½ months' standing, were under their observation. For the time being, 4
of the patients were not given any other treatment, the remainder for more
than a month received salvarsan therapy, internal injections of hypertonic
sodium chlorate solution, dietetic therapy (dry diet, etc.) without success. In
6 cases, the disease was present in a severe form. Lumbar blockade was carred
out in the usual way.

The following factors were taken into account in estimating the results:
1) subjective state of the patient, pains, sleep, appetite; 2) changes in regard
to sputum; 3) temperature chart; 4) X-ray data; 5) weight.

The operation resulted in the first place in an improvement of the general
state of the patient, and also in lessening the pain felt. The changes in the
sputum were very constant both qualitatively and quantitatively. The quantity
usually increased considerably even during the first 2-3 days. In some cases it
amounted to 600-800 c.c. in 24 hours. From this moment, *the three layers
of the sputum begin to change: the lower, purulent layer increases and the
upper, serous layer decreases*. It will not be out of place here to compare these
changes with those observed in regard to trophic ulcers of the extremity, treated

---

[1] S. V. Kurakin and I. A. Pigalev. *Arkh. Biol. Nauk*, Vol. 34, No. 4, 1933.

by operating on the nerves (Molotkov). In the days immediately following neurotomy of one or other of the spinal nerves, the meagre serous secretion of these ulcers is replaced by an abundant thick pus which almost invariably signalises the favourable result of the operation.

In the majority of our cases of pulmonary gangrene, the temperature began to fall soon after the operation and returned to normal. Rarely, brief periods of rise were noted, coinciding with delay in expectoration.

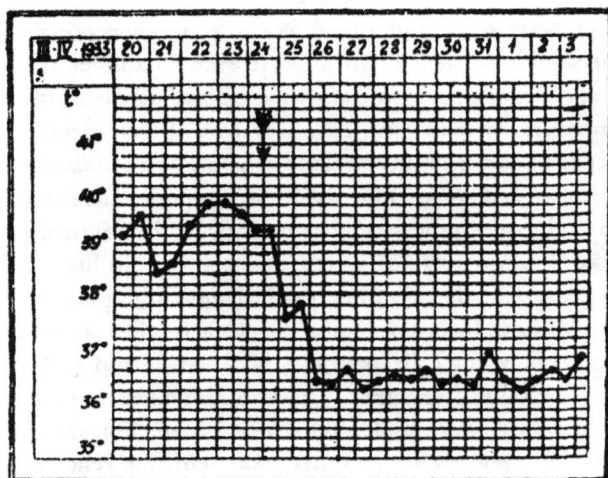

Fig. 20. Tonsilar Sepsis. The Effect of Lumbar Blockade. (The arrow in this and the following diagrams indicates the injection of a 0.25 per cent solution of novocaine into the retro-peritoneal tissue.)

The changes in the lungs were confirmed by X-ray examination. In 6 out of 8 cases, healing proceeded very rapidly. In one case, where X-rays revealed a cavity of the size of a large apple, even within 20 days after blockade it was possible only to observe some opacity. In another patient, almost the same result was achieved after 50 days. In a third, the diffuse opacity which occupied four inter-costal spaces decreased within 15 days to a single intercostal space. In the fourth, fifth and sixth patients, after 25-30 days only a shadow could be noted at the place of the former cavity.

Two of the patients died. Both were neglected cases. In one of them, diagnosis of pulmonary gangrene was made on February 9, 1933. During the following weeks, injection of salvarsan was carried out five times without any signs of improvement, the disease obviously progressing. Lumbar blockade was carried out only on April 1 of the same year (180.0 c.c. of 0.25 per cent

novocaine solution). At first there were certain indications of a favourable turn
in the disease. The temperature went down, the general state improved, the
quantity of sputum considerably increased, but the effect was not lasting, expectoration of blood continued, sometimes reaching the degree of pulmonary
hæmorrhage, and the patient died two weeks after our operation.

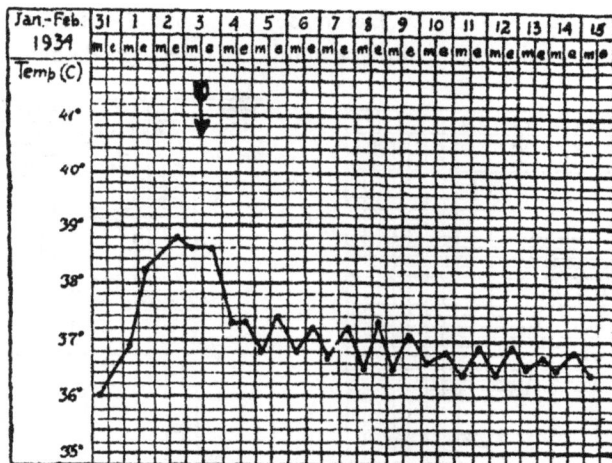

Fig. 21. Temperature curve of patient I. Diagnosis: *ulcera
puerperalia et pyelitis sinistra.*

The second case was even more severe. The patient entered the hospital
with a diagnosis of spotted typhus. After 1½ months, he left to go to work and
again became ill. The diagnosis was pneumonia and pulmonary gangrene. On
several occasions, the patient received internal injections of salvarsan without
result. There was heavy expectoration of blood throughout the course of the
disease. Novocaine blockade was performed two months after the beginning of
the second illness and at first gave a positive effect, but this proved of short duration. A second blockade again improved the general state and removed some
symptoms. Nevertheless, hæmorrhage from the lungs was periodically repeated
and the patient succumbed.

Sepsis was investigated in the same hospital by my collaborators V. S. Galkin
and G. V. Davidov.[1] The material consisted of 12 cases. The cause of the
septic symptoms lay in various kinds of injury (frost-bite, lesions, fractures) or
diseases with the formation of local inflammatory foci (angina, carious affections
of the teeth with subsequent peridentitis, erysipelas). The observation included
cases of septico-pyæmia. Half of the material consisted of severe cases.

[1] V. S. Galkin and G. V. Davidov. *Arkh. Biol. Nauk*, Vol. 34, No. 4, 1933.

In the majority of cases, *our operation produced a definite turn for the better, the disease sometimes being interrupted almost instantaneously, although it had continued previously for a number of days or even weeks*. In other cases, recovery was protracted, its commencement, however, clearly coincided with the time of operation. Two cases ended fatally.

A certain number of observations were made by my other collaborators, A. S. Vishnevsky and G. D. Derchinsky, on septic diseases developing after childbirth or abortion. Here also in a number of cases a good effect was obtained

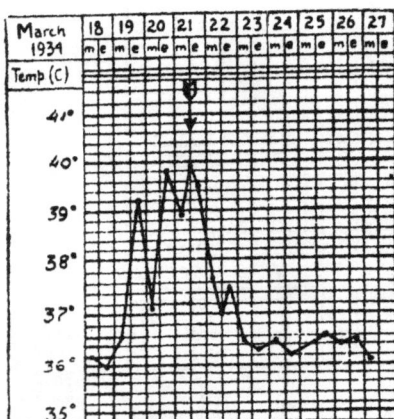

Fig. 22. Temperature curve of Patient C. Diagnosis: *Endometritis post abortum*.

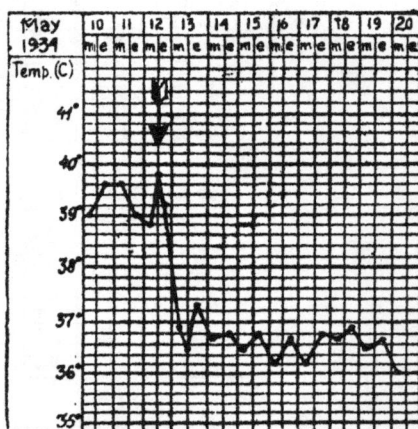

Fig. 23. Temperature curve of Patient Ts. Diagnosis: *Salpingo-ophoritis bilateralis post abortum*.

both in light and severe forms of the process. I am not able to give any details at present as the investigations are not concluded. It was discovered that the earlier the operation was made, the greater was its effect. Here also one of the constant features was improvement of the subjective state of the patient, cessation of pain and decrease or even cessation of hæmorrhage. The temperature fell, sometimes critically, sometimes in the form of a more or less prolonged lysis, but its commencement clearly coincided with the performance of the operation. Septic affections of the sexual organs after abortion yielded more readily to the operation than the same process developing after childbirth.

CHAPTER XXXII

OTHER DISEASES

Skin diseases form one of the most obscure fields of pathology. The ætiology and pathogenesis of most of them remain unknown. At the same time, the connection between skin affections and diseases of the nervous system often stands out so clearly, that long ago it evoked the efforts of many investigators to introduce greater precision in this question. I shall not attempt to give a historical review of these efforts.

In our clinical experiments, we studied skin affections from the point of view of the nervous component of the processes, and for this purpose we established contact with Professor O. N. Podvysotskaya working in the Tarnovsky Hospital in Leningrad. A large number of investigations of various kinds were carried out there during the last $1\frac{1}{2}$ years. It is still too early to give a summary of them. I shall only mention that among other methods of treatment novocaine blockade of the nerves was also employed, most frequently in the form of lumbar blockade.

As was to be anticipated, it gave a curative effect in many cases, but in others, on the contrary, it was accompanied by progress of the disease. *The most constant therapeutic effect was noted in deep forms of dermatitis,* expressed in nodular affections of the skin (erythematic nodes, the deep form of lupus, elephantiasis, leprosy, etc.). Sometimes the effect was exhibited very rapidly and was maintained for a long time. It consisted in a decrease in the density of infiltrates, in an increase in their mobility and the abolition of vascular derangements. *Not infrequently, the operation resulted in restoration of sensitivity in places where this had been lost for a long time.*

As regards superficial dermatitis, in 2 cases of Dühring's herpetic dermatitis the disease was abolished. In 5 cases of red lupus, an almost complete cure was obtained, and in 4 cases there was a considerable improvement. In 4 cases of tuberculous lupus, the disease became worse. Here the local process became intensified and the patients began to lose weight progressively, with activisation of the lung process.

Improvement of the general state was especially clearly shown in cases of pellagra. Depression gave way to cheerfulness, sleep improved, diarrhœa decreased, the headaches passed off and the patients put on weight. These data are supplemented by the investigations of Dr. Kuimov of the Nervous Diseases Clinic of the Perm Medical Institute. On the basis of an analysis of a number of cases he came to the conclusion that pellagra is a neuro-trophic disease and that it is necessary to take the nervous system into account in its prophylaxis and treatment.

In superficial affections of the skin such as eczema, prurient eruptions, etc., an effect was either not obtained or it was only transient.

A certain number of observations on leprosy were made by my collaborators A. A. Vishnevsky and M. I. Shcheperin in the Krutye Ruchi Lazar-hospital. *In cases that had not been neglected, novocaine blockade had a good and lasting therapeutic effect.* We had a number of patients who almost regained their working capacity, chiefly owing to the restoration of sensitivity. Levelling, and in some cases, disappearance of skin nodes was also noted, as well as healing of chronic ulcers and removal of contractures. The fingers of the patient, after being contracted for a number of years, regained sensitivity and mobility, even becoming capable of performing certain forms of fine work (embroidery). Similar improvement occurred in regard to the general state (subjective state, weight, appetite, sleep, etc.). It must be mentioned that in some cases it was possible by means of the novocaine blockade to do away with the sudden intense attacks experienced by leper patients, a process which is frequently the cause of death. A detailed report on this work will be given in a separate article.

Of other diseases, we must mention bronchial asthma which my collaborators I. A. Pigalev and Y. G. Evzerov frequently treated with success by means of lumbar blockade.

Professor V. A. Vorobyev and Dr. V. N. Domarev in the Zakharino Sanatorium of the Central Tuberculosis Institute of the People's Commissariat for Health in Moscow employed the novocaine blockade for treating pulmonary tuberculosis. The method worked out by them consisted in injection of 0.25 per cent novocaine solution into the cervical region of the sympathetic chain with the object of affecting the stellate ganglion. The technique was elaborated by Dr. V. N. Domarev. The investigators come to the conclusion that the form of novocaine blockade mentioned can be employed in treatment of pulmonary tuberculosis. At the moment they are not prepared to define exactly the indications and limits of employment of this method, but they point out that a number of serious symptoms in regard to the intestines and circulatory system and also temperature, chest pains, racking cough, laboured breathing, sleeplessness, general weakness, etc., can be abolished or diminished by its means. However, their observations include also cases which terminated in an intensification of the pulmonary symptoms.

For experimental study, they employed novocaine blockade by itself, but express their view of the need to combine it with other methods of treatment.

In the department for diseases of the ear, throat and nose at the Ryazan City Hospital, Dr. Aleksandrin worked out a convenient and technically simple method for pharyngal vago-sympathetic blockade of the nervous system. Together with Dr. N. A. Ivanova he carried out a number of observations on the effect of this method on various kinds of illnesses: gastric and duodenal ulcer, trophic ulcers of the lower extremities, spontaneous gangrene, etc.

Recently, during the course of the year 1934, Leriche and René Fontaine published the data of their observations on anæsthesia of *g. stellatum*. The technique of the operation is also described in their article. Among their patients are a number of cases where a single employment of anæsthesia had a curative effect, which, for instance, in bronchial asthma and *angina pectoris* lasted for many months. The authors note that it is impossible to explain these facts on the basis of existing views.

Not long ago a method was introduced of treating acute, hysterical and cyclothymic psychoses by subcutaneous injections of substances which cause the formation of an abscess (Jacobi, Azemar, Catola). In the Soviet Union, Drs. A. A. Epstein, S. N. Braines and E. M. Palei have published data on the employment of turpentine abscesses obtained from material of the Balinsky Hospital in Leningrad. It was found that incoherence, delirium, motor-agitation reaching the degree of frenzy, and other symptoms may be caused to disappear in a comparatively short period and very often do not return. In my opinion, the production of the phenomena described must also be connected with the mechanism to the study of which this book is devoted.

In conclusion, I consider it necessary to point out *the need for a different attitude to the method of novocaine blockade from that which has become usual in medical practice.*

It is not a means to abolish the disease. If novocaine blockade does not produce an effect at once, a second blockade often proves to be useful. On the other hand, if the first operation produces an effect, a second is frequently harmful. If we were actually dealing with a means acting on the particular disease, the reverse should be the case. *The cure is effected, not by our operation itself, but by what takes place in the organism after it.* When the effect is immediately positive, a repetition of the operation alters the favourable situation into another one, the character of which is unknown in advance. On the contrary, if the first blockade does not create the required form of nerve relations, we are justified, of course, in altering these relations further. Hence, we obtain the rule—*if the effect of the operation is immediately positive then the interval before it is repeated must be more prolonged.*

CHAPTER XXXIII
SUMMARY

WITH this I shall conclude the account of the data from clinical experiments. They demonstrate that the clinic is already in a position to utilise some of the theses put forward here. To what extent and in what form the actual procedures selected by us will be confirmed, and when and by what they will be replaced, is a matter for the future to decide. From various parts of the Soviet Union, I receive letters from physicians who are endeavouring to apply our form of approach to the understanding of the genesis of pathological processes. A number of new observations have been made, which is evidence that the drawing in of new forces will widen the scope of the work and deepen the means for its investigation. Practice, keenly sensitive to its successes and failures, will have the final word in the matter.

The theorist still has his task to perform. Medicine as yet has no theory. The genuinely scientific study of medical theory began only recently, from the time when experiment became a basic method of physiological work. Hence, the development of scientific medical thought did not proceed independently. It depended on the development of biology in general. Medicine constructed its views by adapting itself to the results obtained in neighbouring fields. The endeavour to unite all streams into a single, general biological channel is, of course, entirely natural and absolutely correct as an ideal. However, before this synthesis can be achieved, it is necessary not only to collect material but to make an appropriate characterisation of its special features, *to carry the analysis of the subject to the utmost perfection.* Passive subordination to a foreign leadership can easily be ruinous, for it is bound up with obligatory acceptance of verbal analogies, with grouping together of qualitatively distinct phenomena according to an accidental characteristic. As a result, *instead of synthesis we lose the possibility of manœuvring and end by appealing for the help of specialists in other branches of science.*

This has already happened more than once with pathology. Who has not considered himself master of the house here? What petty facts have served as the impulse for creating the principles on which this science is built! Each of these facts was expected to create a synthetic pathology, each of the claimants has striven to give *an exhaustive and final definition of the concept of disease.*

Not one of them has succeeded in doing so: up to now as soon as such a definition is brought forward tedious discussion arises immediately, without any hope of arriving at even temporary agreement.

We exhaust ourselves in new efforts for finally discovering the required formula, while in point of fact the question that should be decided is why this formula is unobtainable. The cause is very simple: disease was never looked upon as an independent quality, as a special form of biological processes; the starting point has always been formed by conceptions of a contrary nature. Taking as an indicator one or more groups of complex reactions that go to make up the conception of normality, disease was conceived as a distortion or alteration of these conditions. From this, it was rightly concluded that to understand a disease, it is necessary to know what is normal.

But we have also no suitable means of approaching the concept of normality. Everything is still in the stage of accumulation. The work is still expanding in volume, and is mainly of a quantitative character. Until now, there have been very few principles capable of embracing and governing the whole material. It is natural that under these circumstances, the task, even though correctly formulated, becomes simply impossible to fulfil. We cannot define disease as the antithesis of health, since neither side of such a medal bears any imprint.

At the present stage of science, what has to be done is to look for the qualitative distinguishing features within each of these conceptions. It seems to me, that as far as disease in a complicated organism is concerned, we have succeeded in solving this task. The form in which the nervous component of pathological processes makes its appearance *does not occur under normal conditions.* The pathological conditions are characterised by *new reactions.* The presence of the latter is evidence that we are dealing with a real pathological process. Consequently, it is neither the disharmony of phenomena existing in normality, nor the disorganisation of correlation in the functioning of separate parts of the organism, that defines its pathological state, *but the emergence of new qualitatively distinct processes.* The disorganisation of correlations, disharmony, etc., are only a consequence of these last.

There is no doubt, of course, that the basis for the development of neuro-dystrophic processes in the organism lies in the peculiarities of structure and function of the nervous system, *i.e.,* in its physiological properties. But their distortion creates, as it were, a new type of nervous activity, the appearance of new reactions, not only unnecessary but directly harmful to the life of the individual. *Hence, the question is one, not of degree, but of form, in other words of qualitatively new biological phenomena.*

This also decides the old dispute as to whether medicine is to be regarded as an independent science. We must undoubtedly recognise it as such, since it has *its own* tasks and aims, has *its own* material at its disposal, and *its own* technical methods, and investigates phenomena which are not known to biology in other spheres. Finally, it has *its own* technical application. All this marks out an independent place for the science of medicine among the biological sciences. The designation morbid physiology not only offends the ear on account of its crude and somewhat contradictory association of terms, but is also incorrect in essence. *The old term "general pathology," discarded owing to the fear that it would not be justified by independent research, ought now to be revived.*

We have seen that whenever our procedures enabled us to influence the nervous component of any complex pathological process, this resulted in changes not only of the nervous component itself but of the whole complex of the phenomena manifested. *Further research ought to be directed towards an all-embracing study of the details of standard and special forms of neuro-dystrophic processes and should aim at discovering new means for actively interfering in their course.* The ancient methods of treatment in the form of such devices as cauterisation by hot iron, setons, fontanelles, cupping glasses, poultices, smearing with irritating substances, etc., equally with more recent methods—subcutaneous injections of milk and other protein substances, radium, X-rays, diathermy and all that is included under the term *"Reiztherapie,"* and finally "pumping" and temporary disconnection of parts of the nervous system by means of anæsthesia—all these find the explanation of their action in those characteristic changes which the nervous system undergoes *on encountering processes of irritation.* There is every reason to believe that drugs such as sodium salicylate, quinine, arsenic, mercury, and perhaps many others as well, owe their action to the same mechanism. This provides a foundation for understanding the directions along which clinical research work has to be carried out. The differences in the forms of the neuro-dystrophic process and the peculiarities of individual nervous systems call in each case for the search for new forms of interference. *This shows that medicine can never have a panacea.* It also shows that research is indispensable.

It should not be thought, however, that the diversity of therapy must correspond to that of pathology, that every disease must have its particular form of treatment. We have seen that the various forms of neuro-dystrophic processes despite their diversity have a group character. Moreover, every act of interference on our part has not one but many consequences. *The effect may depend both on the sum total of all the parts and on each part in particular.* This is the reason why different kinds of ceratitis, gastric ulcer, gangrene of the extremities, septic and many other pathological processes, may yield to externally identical forms of action.

At the same time, one and the same procedure, applied in one and the same disease, often gives different effects. The cause lies in the fact *that in our diagnosis we actually fasten on the result and do not take into account the mechanism of the pathological process.* Let us take sepsis as an example. In its first stages, sepsis starting from the uterine cavity has little in common as regards the mechanism of its development with sepsis starting from sore throat, since the *primary locus determines at least for a time the form of the neuro-dystrophic process.* Under these circumstances, it is clear that a single form of operation cannot have the same effect on the course of the disease in all cases. Subsequently, when the process has assumed the standard form of development, any new action may serve to aggravate it. *In such cases, it is often too late.*

But whatever turn the process may take, whether towards aggravation or, on the contrary, towards extinction, it remains a fact that the basic constituent feature of the process, its "leading link," is the nervous component.

The second condition for a theory of medicine is, as was mentioned above, the union of all the varied data of pathology around a common centre. I shall not repeat here either the reasons making this task a very urgent one at the present moment or the data which testify to the fact that the desired centre has been found by us in the nervous component of pathological processes.

The investigation of this aspect is not only interesting on its own account but also *makes it possible to give a suitable arrangement to all the other facts, to find the proper place for each constituent and to determine the order of functioning of the separate parts.*

It is necessary to dwell a little on this point.

Six years ago I published the first summary of our data in a book entitled *The Nervous System in Pathology.* During recent years, a large number of works issued from my laboratory and devoted to the same subject have appeared in the Soviet and foreign press. In 1933, I published two articles on neuro-trophic processes and a symposium devoted to our clinical observations and experiments in the new direction.[1] During the following months I gave several lectures in Moscow and Leningrad on the same theme. In the discussion that developed, and to some extent in the periodical press, some objections were raised.

It is characteristic that the criticism was hardly at all concerned with de-

[1] A. D. Speransky. *Arkh. Biol. Nauk*, Vol. 33, No. 5-6, 1933; *Arkh. Biol. Nauk*, Vol. 34, No. 4, 1933.

fence of the old views. Fundamentally, it consisted of warnings against being led into simplifying complex phenomena, and reducing many-sided reality to a series of elementary formulæ.

I venture to think that there is a misunderstanding here. In the first place, the formulations at which I have arrived are not elementary; in the second place, *they do not make any claims to exhaust the subject or to do away with the necessity of other ways of studying it.* The whole character of our work is evidence of this.

We never began with an attack on existing propositions; on the contrary, *we always took the past for our starting point and based ourselves on it.* It is not our fault if this support proved hopeless. In addition, during the investigations we made use of all available and suitable methods—instrumental physiology, bacteriology, morphology, chemistry, etc.; consequently, there are no grounds for saying that these sciences are under the threat of being ousted. On the contrary, they should now obtain a wide field of application *since anarchic development will be replaced by work in a definite direction and according to a definite system.*

We are also unable to admit the justice of the reproach, because the *tendency to schematism is an old failing of pathology* and it is precisely with this tendency that we have come into conflict. Especially great confusion has been introduced here by clinical experiment, which has been in turn under the fascination of specific therapy, of *therapia sterilisans magna,* of endocrinology in its most primitive forms, of acidosis and alkalosis, and of the "mutual struggle" of potassium and calcium in the organism. On achieving a success in one field, the clinic naturally endeavoured to extend it. For this purpose it had recourse to generalisations, and constructed theories in haste, forgetting that *such a procedure is permissible only as a temporary measure, and is harmless only so long as its temporary character is understood.* As a result, many petty schemes were produced, incompatible with one another.

Along with these, important systems have also been created which have held their ground in pathology for many years. One must mention here the morphological tendency, whose authority is now considerably weakened, and the chemical tendency which is at present endeavouring to assume the leading position.

It is essential to be quite clear on this subject. We are passing through an epoch of impetuous development in physics and in all forms of chemistry and other so-called exact sciences. Their achievements during the last decades have been very great. Much of this new knowledge has found application in biology, and particularly in physiology and medicine. And it is the merit of these innovations that they are distinguished precisely by *the exact-*

ness of the methods with the aid of which they were obtained. The difference from the old position is so striking that it has already almost done away with any desire to undertake biological research work with the old methods.

As a result, both the clinic and the laboratory are passing through a period which can be termed that of *fascination by chemistry*.

It is not surprising that the chemists have calmly assumed the leadership; but it is strange that the physicians have not only become reconciled to it but seem to be convinced that this position is inevitable.

Well, let us even suppose this is correct. Let us suppose that the time will come when the complicated problems of medicine will be simplified to such an extent that they can be understood by the aid of chemical formulæ and equations. Be that as it may, *at the present moment we can count only on a substitute for what will be finally established in the future.*

Pathology is turning to chemistry because, not having good methods of its own, it hastily seizes on methods which may be good but are foreign to it, without always taking into account the limits of their applicability. This is not the first time that pathology is passing through such a period. Quite recently, the leadership in this science was in the hands of pathological anatomy. Virchow's cellular pathology provided the investigator with a simple method for estimating structural changes in affected tissues. By its aid very great achievements were accomplished in systematising pathological processes. The morphological method became a universal weapon and its achievements marked an epoch in pathology. But, by employing the same method, attempts were made to construct a theory of the dynamics of a number of pathological processes. The actual value of such theories is doubtful, since they were often merely logical conclusions from morphological observations, a rearrangement of static phenomena in an artificially dynamic series.

By concentrating our whole attention on the study of physico-chemical change in separate tissues or in the whole organism, *we risk exactly the same thing; only the external form will be different.*

When biology does homage to the accuracy of chemical methods, it frequently forgets about the object of its study. *Contemporary chemistry can only deal with small things.* Its possibilities must not be exaggerated. It must be remembered that where the task arises of preparing a more complicated product, as in industrial production, *scientific chemistry has frequently to make way for the methods of industrial chemistry.* Along with the simple factors that are easily taken into account and can be accurately measured, it employs a number of practical *recipes and procedures*, the scientific significance of which is not always clear. In such cases it reproduces modestly and faithfully a number of conditions in a definite order, without being capable of assessing the actual significance of each of them.

The same thing is done in biology. Hence, the recourse to physics and chemistry is comprehensible in all those cases where it is a question of comparatively simple things, amenable to exact analysis even at the present time. But the fact that a method has made it possible to explain part of the minute details of a complex process affords no justification for constructing a general conception by means of the same method.

The best example is the work of Academician I. P. Pavlov, who laid the foundations for the physiological study of higher nervous activity in animals. Thanks to his work, we now have a real physiology of the big hemispheres. Its basic propositions, as well as many apparently altogether elusive details, are presented in such clear formulations that contemporary, instrumental, physical physiology might envy them. Nevertheless, not only was all this obtained by the method of conditioned reflexes, but *it could not have been,* and still cannot be, achieved by any other method of research. Physics and chemistry will inevitably participate in the further working out of the questions raised, *but they could not have put these questions.* This was done by biological experiment.

The data assembled in this book were obtained by the aid of just such experiments, and therefore they cannot lay claim to exactness. One of the most difficult problems of technique, *viz.,* to find a simple and constant indicator, is almost insoluble in biology, and we have often had to base ourselves on such indicators, for instance, as the life or death of the animal, which in themselves are very complex processes and until now have not been defined even in words. *Nevertheless, the generalisations arrived at by their aid have enabled us to take up new questions and to subject them to the test of experiment, permitting us to establish relationships which had previously escaped observation.* Hence the justification for this form of work and for the appearance of this book.

The application of chemistry, as one of the methods for the analysis of biological processes, is undoubtedly of great benefit, but it is still impossible to achieve their synthesis by this method, and consequently it is impossible to regard chemistry as being capable of organising pathology, of becoming its central, unifying point.

There remains the road along which physiology is travelling. It is true that this also has not yet been able to rise above the level of elementary (working) synthesis, *i.e.,* above an understanding of the mere mechanics of vital processes. Basically, the subject with which it is concerned is *the sequence in the functioning of separate parts of a complex organism and their inter-*

dependence. These parts themselves, and the essence of the processes comprising them, are still far from having been adequately estimated. However, no one doubts that physiology arranges its data in systematic order, and that it forms an independent branch of science. It does not owe this to the greater accuracy of its methods, or to a clearer formulation of its aims, but to the uniform and harmonious development of the separate parts. *It is terrifying to think what would have happened to physiology if, in the processes which it studies, nervous influences were ignored as persistently as they have been until recently in pathology.*

Pathology also has chosen the path of comprehensive analysis. But analysis alone is not enough for setting the data in order, for systematising them and creating working hypotheses. Synthesis is required. In pathology, this became absolutely indispensable from the moment when it became clear that the confusion in its views did not depend on lack of details.

Consequently, one more obstacle remains to be overcome in order to achieve the desired aim. We have to define the principles which *at the given moment* are best capable both of unifying the data and of putting pathology on the path of effective work.

The difficulty of the task consists in finding these principles, since up to now pathology has not had time to acquire an independent character. The blame for this must be laid on that view of the science which regards it as physiology plus an accessory irritating agent. But if this were so, logic demands that the cause for *its special character should be sought precisely in the accessory feature.* It has been demonstrated more than once in this book that it is this that has given rise to the chief confusion.

Pathology is not merely the disorganisation of physiological co-ordination, not merely the derangement of normally existing connections, but the creation of new conditions unknown to physiology. *This characteristic feature, this new quality, which makes pathology an independent branch of science, is introduced into it by the nervous component of pathological processes.* We have seen that although the diversity of the special manifestations may attain a very high level, they are all subject to a number of general laws.

Where then is the danger of over-simplification of which we have been accused? Do we not define theory as "experience . . . taken in its general form"? (J. Stalin.) Hence what is first of all necessary is experience, the work of collection and careful analysis of data. This part of the work must now proceed on a still greater scale. But the scope of the work depends directly on the general prospects, and *the latter necessitate a "general form," a general plan, where details are a hindrance, obscuring the true meaning of the generalisations made.*

It remains to say a few words in answer to objections of a more concrete character. It has been said that by reducing "everything" (?) to the nervous system, we leave out of account such well-established active factors as constitution, endocrine and neuro-humoral factors, etc.

This is not correct. We do recognise them; still more, we use them and will continue to use them in our work no less than others. But, surely, our main task is to find the principles unifying the material, to create a point of view by means of which it can be evaluated.

What can be unified at the present time by the theory of the constitution? The principles on which it is based are derived from observations and calculations. Statistics tell us that, as a response to different influences, a black rabbit differs from a white one, a tall, thin man from a fat, short one, an Englishman from an Italian. If we use more subtle means of determination, such as the morphology and chemistry of the blood, the velocity of reactions, the predominance of a particular internal secretory function in the general endocrinological make-up, we still in essence preserve the same statistical principle.

The constitution controls a large number of all kinds of indicators, which would undoubtedly be of interest for theory, *if it were known what exactly they indicate*. But it is precisely on this account that no progress is being made. The theory of the constitution enables so-called "forecasts" to be compiled such as are necessary to the clinic and perhaps for insurance, *i.e.*, they satisfy a certain number of practical requirements. But surely one could use also peasants' weather forecasts, since here also *the foundation consists of omens, in other words, of accompanying signs*. The essential nature and the mechanism of the phenomena themselves escape us in both cases.

What can be unified in a system which lives in perpetual expectation of aid from outside for introducing order within itself? The data that we have described contain many examples where, by acting on a particular part of the nervous system, we changed the whole "constitution" of an animal in the most radical fashion. *The presence of all the other factors did not ensure the preservation of the previous state.* In consequence, one can consider that the action of all those influences which in their sum total go to make up the content of the word "constitution" are also determined by the nervous part of the process, that it is actually just at this point that all the lines intersect. The decision of the question we are dealing with would give possibilities of new development to the neglected theory of the constitution and would put an end to prejudice and stagnation in the use of indicators by setting the task of determining what each of these indicators actually indicates in the highly complex system of relations under consideration.

The same thing has to be said of humoral factors, both of endocrine and nervous origin. These factors form part of the general conditions of life of the organism and ensure the associated activity of its constituent parts. *But how they could serve as a basis for unifying the complex data of pathology is absolutely incomprehensible.* If it is proper to use for this purpose the endocrine function of the thyroid gland, suprarenal or testicle, why should we not use for the same purpose the liver, bones or muscles? *And if, in spite of everything, we agree to work of this nature, what could possibly result from it except disconnected conceptions?*

It is still more strange that nervous and neuro-humoral influences should be contrasted with one another. The latter result from the formation of special substances in the tissues. *But is not irritation of the nerve the cause of their formation?* It has proved to be advantageous to the general functioning of the organism that the maintenance of a particular function begun by nervous excitation should be subsequently entrusted to other mechanisms. A nerve stimulus creates in the tissues a definite substance which afterwards acts as an irritating agent, as the originator of other, but quite definite, reactions.

We cannot be reproached with underestimation of the neuro-humoral factor. We observe with interest the work begun by Loewi and now continued in many other places. The investigations in this field of Professor I. P. Razenkov and of the laboratories and clinics connected with him have also given results of great interest and practical value. *But we cannot accept an overestimation of the significance of this factor for unifying the data of physiology, and still more of pathology.* Neither now nor later will this be successful, for the simple reason that the neuro-humoral functions do not exist apart from the nervous functions. The humoral factor is the reflection of nervous influences in the peripheral tissues, *without which not a single nervous function is known to us.*

With this our book comes to a close. It does not claim as yet to expound general pathology in the light of the new principles. *Its object is to give a systematic account of the data that have come into our hands and to draw the basic conclusions which can serve for constructing the theory of medicine.* The remainder has to be left to the future.

Whatever attitude is taken towards our exposition, it must be recognised that the appearance of the book is timely. During the post-war history of medicine, everyone has experienced a certain dissatisfaction and weariness in the face of verbal mysticism, a disillusionment in wealth consisting of unreal values. The medicine of Virchow, Pasteur and Ehrlich is approaching exhaustion and cannot cope with the contradictions that have arisen. Along with the part that is still firmly based, there has been accumulated much that is unsuccessful, doubtful and paradoxical. All these doubts are also based on the observation of facts. To call these facts exceptions is merely to close one's eyes to reality, to dismiss the question. A way out has been sought in new verbal definitions. By frequent repetition words acquire an apparently real meaning; it is enough to refer to such terms as allergy and anergy. The analysis of a phenomenon is carried just far enough to make it possible to apply one of the above-mentioned words, and when this is done, the study of the phenomenon is considered practically concluded—although the conceptions expressed by these words are entirely chaotic.

The system of views put forward by us will undoubtedly encounter some resistance. This is understandable and entirely legitimate. By this means it will be purified from all that is accidental, not firmly based and insufficiently tested in practice. *But in this struggle the past also will have to abandon the protection of verbal constructions and at last reveal its real countenance.*

A. P. Chekhov, in a conversation on the technique of writing, once expressed himself in approximately the following words: "If in the first chapter of your novel, a weapon is hanging on the wall, then some time later on it must be fired, otherwise there was no use in its hanging there."

The theory of medicine has on its walls such a number of weapons incapable of being fired that it produces the impression rather of a museum than of an arsenal.

A way out of this position must be found. Criticism alone, however merciless, will not save the situation. Before pulling down the old edifice, one must have a plan of the new one, one must assess and collect the means. *This is the reason why our experiments have had to embrace such a number of questions.*

In regard to a revision of pathology, the time has come for a revolution; it has matured, it must begin, the more so because in this revolution there is indeed nothing to be lost but *"chains."*

BIBLIOGRAPHY

A. Works from the Laboratory of A. D. Speransky [1]

Alisov, P. A.: "The Significance of Neuro-Trophic Changes in Certain Chronic Illnesses," 1934. (Manuscript.)

Aristovsky, V. M. and Ponomarev, A. V.: "The Pathogenesis of Local Tetanus." Lecture to the All-Russian Conference of Micro-Biologists in Leningrad, Dec. 7-11, 1934.

Astapow, N. A. und Bobkow, J. P.: "*Beobachtungen über experimentelle Epilepsie nach Vereisung der Hirnrinde bei Katzen,*" *Zeitschr. f. d. ges. exp. Med.*, Vol. 80, pp. 829-35, 1932.

Astapov, N. A. and Bobkov, I. P.: "On Certain Conditions of Alcoholic Sleep." (Manuscript.)

Astapov, N. A. and Bobkov, I. P.: "On the Question of the Nature of Tissue Affections Resulting from the Action of Poisonous Substances Used in War," *Medico-Hygienic Questions of Anti-Chemical Defence*, Symposium, No, 1, 1932.

Astapov, N. A., Vishnevsky, A. A. and Skoblo, M. C.: "The Action of Mustard Gas on Subarachnoid Introduction into the Animal Organism." (Manuscript.)

Babkova, A. A. and Kanarevskaya, A. A.: "Clinical Experience of Subarachnoid Injection of Serum from Convalescents in Typhus Exanthematicus," *Archive of Biological Sciences*, Vol. 34, No. 5-6, 1933.

Babkova, A. A. and Kanarevskaya, A A.: "The Role of the Nervous System in Gastro-Intestinal Diseases." (Manuscript.)

Bank, I. L.: "The Treatment of Malaria by Pumping." (Manuscript.)

Barbel, I. E., Vishnevsky, A. A., Dymshits, L. A., Mikaelyan, P. K. and Chirkovsky, V. V.: "The Nerve Clinic in the Pathogenesis and Clinical Treatment of Ceratitis," *Archive of Biological Sciences*, Vol. 34, No. 4, 1933.

Bobkov, I. P. and Fenelonov, A. L.: "Conditions for the Development of Sagittal Tetanus in Cats." (Manuscript.)

Bokhon, N. F.: "Consequences of experimental Irritation of the Frontal Sinuses." (Manuscript.)

Buschmakina, M. und Pigalew, J.: "*Experimentelle Beiträge zur Frage des Mechanismus der direkten Affektionen der Oblongata bei diffuser Peritonitis,*" *Zeitschr. f. d. ges. exp. Med.*, Vol. 63, pp. 117-24, 1928.

Cheshkov, A. M.: "The Role of Cerebro-Spinal Fluid in the Mechanism of Development of Rabies," *Archive of Biological Sciences*, Vol. 27, No. 4-5, 1927.

Chirkovsky, V. V.: "The Nervous Component in the Pathogenesis of Ceratitis," *Archive of Biological Sciences*, Vol. 34, No. 4, 1933.

Doinikov, B. S.: "Morphological Changes of the Nervous System on Chemical Trauma of a Peripheral Nerve by Formalin," *Archive of Biological Sciences*, 1935.

Dolinskaya, A. T. and Chetvertak, D. S.: "The Influence of the Place of Primary Irritation on the Form of Development of Dystrophic Processes." (Manuscript.)

---

[1] In this section all Russian works have been cited in English. The titles of Russian journals, in English transliteration together with English equivalents, will be found on page 417.

Dymshits, L. A., Luk-va, L. N. and Rokitskaya, L. V.: "Accommodation of the Eye to Dark on Novocaine Blockade of Nerves at a Distance from the Eye," *Archive of Biological Sciences*, Vol. 34, No. 4, 1933.

Entin, D. A.: "The Neuro-Trophic Factor in the Pathology of the Organs of the Oral Cavity," *Archive of Biological Sciences*, Vol. 34, No. 4, 1933.

Fedoroff, L. N.: "*Über die wechselseitige Beteiligung der Hirnrinde und der subkortikalen Abschnitte des Gehirns beim Entstehen des epileptischen Anfalls,*" *Zeitschr. f. d. ges. exp. Med.*, Vol. 72, pp. 82-89, 1930.

Fedoroff, L. N.: "*Versuchsmaterial u. Methode zur Frage der Genese des epileptischen Anfalls,*" *Zeitschr. f. d. ges. exp. Med.*, Vol. 72, pp. 72-81, 1930.

Galkin, W. S.: "*Über die Bedeutung der Nasebahn für den Abfluß aus der subarachnoidalraum,*" *Zeitschr. f. d. ges. exp. Med.*, Vol. 72, pp. 65-71, 1930.

Galkin, W. S.: "*Zur Methodik der Injektion des Lymphsystems von Subarachnoidalraum aus (Bedeutung der Injektionstelle),*" *Zeitschr. f. d. ges. exp. Med.*, Vol. 74, pp. 482-89, 1930.

Galkin, W. S.: "*Weitere Beobachtungen an experimenteller, durch partielle Vereisung der Hirnrinde hervorgerufener Epilepsie,*" *Zeitschr. f. d. ges. exp. Med.*, Vol. 77, pp. 476-89, 1931.

Galkin, W. S.: "*Über die Form der Beteiligung der Hirnrinde an der Organisation des epileptischen Anfalls,*" *Zeitschr. f. d. ges. exp. Med.*, Vol. 78, pp. 527-44, 1931.

Galkin, W. S.: "*Die Schwankungen der Erregbarkeit der Nervenzelle und der epileptische Anfall,*" *Zeitschr. f. d. ges. exp. Med.*, Vol. 81, pp. 374-89, 1932.

Galkin, W. S.: "*Über der Abbau des Hirngewebes in der Zerebrospinalflüssigkeit,*" *Zeitschr. f. d. ges. exp. Med.*, Vol. 84, pp. 510-17, 1932.

Galkin, W. S.: "*Über die Bedeutung der rezeptorischen Apparate für die Arbeit der höheren Anteile des Nervensystems,*" *Zeitschr. f. d. ges. exp. Med.*, Vol. 88, pp. 316-49, 1933.

Galkin, W. S.: "*Die Gesetzmäßigkeit in der Reihenfolge der Affektion der Abdominalorgane,*" *Zeitschr. f. d. ges. exp. Med.*, Vol. 94, pp. 127-29, 1934.

Galkin, W. S. and Davidov, G. V.: "Data on the Question of the Genesis and Therapy of Sepsis," *Archive of Biological Sciences*, Vol. 34, No. 4, 1933.

Galkin, V. S. and Kotov, N. G.: "Data on the Question of the Composition, Genesis and Therapy of Typhus Exanthematicus," *Archive of Biological Sciences*, Vol. 36, No. 3, 1935.

Galkin, W. S. und Tscheschkow, A. M.: "*Der Erregbarkeitszustand der Nervenzelle und das Lyssabild,*" *Zeitschr. f. d. ges. exp. Med.*, Vol. 82, pp. 445-50, 1932.

Gantt, W. H. und Ponomarew, A. W.: "*Über den Mechanismus der Verbreitung des Tollwutwirus (virus fixe) im Organismus,*" *Zeitschr. f. d. ges. exp. Med.*, Vol. 66, pp. 583-95, 1929.

Glushkov, P. A.: "On the Question of the Neuro-Trophic Nature of 'Alveolar Pyorrhœa,'" *Archive of Biological Sciences*, Vol. 34, No. 4, 1933.

Golysheva, K. P.: "Experimental Data on the Question of the Genesis of the Toxic Form of Epileptic Seizures," *Archive of Biological Sciences*, Vol. 32, No. 4, 1932.

Gorstchkow, M. A. und Babkowa, A. A.: "*Zur Frage der Pathogenese des akuten Rheumatismus,*" *Zeitschr. f. d. ges. exp. Med.*, Vol. 67, pp. 278-92, 1929.

Halperin, S. J.: "*Die Entfaltung des dystrophischen Prozess bei Affektionen der oberen sympathischen Halsganglien,*" *Zeitschr. f. d. ges. exp. Med.*, Vol. 90, pp. 115-19, 1933.

Ilinsky, V. I. and Evzerov, Y. D.: "The Role of the Nervous System in the Pathogenesis of Rheumatism." (Manuscript.)

Iwanow, G.: "*Über die Abflusswege aus den submeningealen Räumen des Rückenmarks,*" *Zeitschr. f. d. ges. exp. Med.*, Vol. 58, pp. 1-21, 1927.

Iwanow, G.: *"Über die Abflusswege aus den Subarachnoidalräumen des Gehirns und Rückenmarks und über die Methodik ihrer Untersuchung," Zeitschr. f. d. ges. exp. Med.,*Vol. 64, pp. 356-75, 1929.

Iwanow, G.: *"Die Beschädigung des* Tuber cinereum *als ursächliches Moment einer Destruktion der Zellen des oberen sympathischen Halsganglions," Zeitschr. f. d. ges. exp. Med.,* Vol. 74, pp. 773-86, 1930.

Iwanow, G. und Romodanowsky, K.: *"Über den anatomischen Zusammenhang der cerebralen u. spinalen submeningealen Räume mit dem Lymphsystem (J. Mitteil., Methodik u. wichtigste Beobachtungen)," Zeitschr. f. d. ges. exp. Med.,* Vol. 58, pp. 596-607, 1927.

Jefimow, K.: *"Zur Frage der Genese des epileptischen Anfalls," Zeitschr. f. d. ges. exp. Med.,* Vol. 62, pp. 662-70, 1928.

Jowelew, B. M.: *"Über einige Bedingungen der Impfung mit Tollwut aus dem Blute," Zeitschr. f. d. ges. exp. Med.,* Vol. 74, pp. 217-23, 1930.

Kaminsky, S.: *"Der nervöse Mechanismus der Tetanusintoxikation," Zeitschr. f. d. ges. exp. Med.,* Vol. 88, pp. 804-15, 1933.

Kartashev, P. N.: "Trophic Disturbances on the Action of Diphtheria Toxin in Branches of *n. trigeminus," Archive of Biological Sciences,* Vol. 34, No. 4, 1933.

Kartashev, P. N. and Matveyeva, L. M.: "Trophic Disturbances on Injury to Nerves of the Dental Apparatus," *Archive of Biological Sciences,* Vol. 34, No. 4, 1933.

Kotlyarenko, B. N.: "On the Genesis of Skin Reactions," *Journal of Microscopic Pathology and Infectious Diseases,* Vol. 6, No. 2, 1928.

Kotow, N. und Kotljarenko, B.: *"Zur Frage der Pathogenese und Behandlung von Scharlach im Zusammenhang mit Versuchen einer Subduralen Einführung von antitoxischen Serum," Verhandl. d. Deutsch. Russ. Scharlach-Kongress vom 11-14 Juni 1928 in Königsberg.*

Kurakin, S. V. and Pigalev, I. A.: "The Pathogenesis and Therapy of Pulmonary Gangrene," *Archive of Biological Sciences,* Vol. 34, No. 4, 1933.

Kusayev, I. A.: "The Treatment of Persian (Recurrent) Typhus by 'Pumping.' " (Manuscript.)

Lebedinskaya, S. I.: "Data, on the Mechanism of Action of Specific Toxins," *Archive of Biological Sciences,* Vol. 34, No. 4, 1933.

Lebedinskaya, S. I.: "The Pathogenesis of Local Tetanus." (Manuscript.)

Lebedinskaya, S. I. and Osipov, M. O.: "The Locus of Irritation in the Syndrome of Tetanus Symptoms." (Manuscript.)

Malinovsky, Z. A.: "Clinical Experience of Subarachnoid Injection of Blood in Some Forms of Affection of the Nervous System," *Archive of Biological Sciences,* Vol. 32, No. 5-6, 1932.

Manenkow, P. W.: *"Zur Frage des Mechanismus einer sekundären Affektion paariger Organe nach einseitiger Erkrankung," Zeitschr. f. d. ges. exp. Med.,* Vol 63, pp. 688-98, 1928.

Manenkow, P. W.: *"Experimentelle Befunde zur Frage des Mechanismus einer direkten Affektion der Oblongata bei diffuser Peritonitis," Zeitschr. f. d. ges. exp. Med.,* Vol. 64, pp. 239-48, 1929.

Manenkow, P. W.: *"Experimentelle Beiträge zum Mechanismus der direkten Affektion der Oblongata bei akuter diffuser Peritonitis," Zeitschr. f. d. ges. exp. Med.,* Vol. 66, pp. 338-54, 1929.

Nikitin, N. und Ponomarew, A.: *"Über die passive und aktive Immunisierung des Zentralen Nervensystems gegen Diphtherie-Intoxikation," Zeitschr. f. d. ges. exp. Med.,* Vol. 70, pp. 551-63, 1930.

Petrunkina, A. und Petrunkin, M.: *"Über die Bedingungen des Magnesium- und Bromschlafes," Zeitschr. f. d. ges. exp. Med.,* Vol. 68, pp. 720-36, 1929.

Pigalew, J.: "*Methoden z. Trennung der Subarachnoidalraumes bei Hunden im chronischen Experiment,*" *Zeitschr. f. d. ges. exp. Med.*, Vol. 61, pp. 1-4, 1928.

Pigalew, J.: "*Über die Bedingungen der Entstehung 'lokaler' Erscheinungen bei Anwendung von Diphtherietoxin,*" *Zeitschr. f. d. ges. Exp. Med.*, Vol. 63, pp. 643-51, 1928.

Pigalew, J.: "*Über den Mechanismus der Entstehung von 'Teerkrebs,'*" *Zeitschr. f. d. ges. exp. Med.*, Vol. 63, pp. 662-76, 1928.

Pigalew, J. A.: "*Zur Methodik der Injektionen des Lymphsystems vom Subarachnoidalraum aus,*" *Zeitschr. f. d. ges. exp. Med.*, Vol. 66, pp. 454-58, 1929.

Pigalew, J. A.: "*Reihenfolge und Bedingungen der Erkrankung der Bauchhöhlenorgane bei experimenteller Tuberculose,*" *Zeitschr. f. d. ges. exp. Med.*, Vol. 80, pp. 356-61, 1932.

Pigalew, J. A.: "*Zur Frage der Genese geschwüriger Prozesse im Magen-Darmkanal,*" *Zeitschr. f. d. ges. exp. Med.*, Vol. 82, pp. 617-32, 1932.

Pigalew, J. A. und Epstein, G. S.: "*Die Rolle des Nervensystems in der Entwicklung und dem Verlauf des tuberkulosen Prozesses beim Kaninchen,*" *Zeitschr. f. d. ges. exp. Med.*, Vol. 70, pp. 417-37, 1930.

Pigalev I. A. and Epstein, G. S.: "The Role of the Nervous System in the Development of Genito-Urinary Tuberculosis Produced by Experimental Means in Rabbits," *Archive of Biological Sciences*, Vol. 32, No. 2, 1932.

Pigalew, J. A. und Fedoroff, L. N.: "*Über eine der Methoden zur experimentellen Erzeugung Reflektorischer Epilepsie,*" *Zeitschr. f. d. ges. exp. Med.*, Vol. 70, pp. 564-70, 1930.

Pigalew, J. und Kusnetzowa, Z.: "*Über die Bedingungen der Entwicklung begrenzter und diffuser Affektionen trophischen Charakters,*" *Zeitschr. f. d. ges. exp. Med.*, Vol. 67, pp. 265-77, 1929.

Pigalev, I. A. and Pukhidsky, A. K.: "Certain Forms of Local Reaction to Mustard Gas and Lewisite," *Medico-Hygienic Questions of Anti-Chemical Defence*, Symposium, No. 1, 1932.

Ponomarev, A. V.: "The Capacity of Cerebro-Spinal Fluid to Cause the Separation of a Mixture of Tetanus Toxin and Brain Tissue," *Archive of Biological Sciences*, Vol. 26, No. 4-5, 1926.

Ponomarev, A. V.: "The Role of the Cerebro-Spinal Fluid in the Mechanism of Action of Tetanus Toxin on Brain Tissue," *Archive of Biological Sciences*, Vol. 26, No. 4-5, 1926.

Ponomareff, A.: "*Sur les conditions qui modifient la vitesse de propagation de la toxine tétanique dans le nerf,*" *Compt. rend. Soc. Biol.*, Vol. 97, p. 503, 1927.

Ponomarew, A. W.: "*Zur Frage der Pathogenese des Tetanus und des Fortbewegungsmechanismus des Tetanustoxin längs dem Nerven,*" *Zeitschr. f. d. ges. exp. Med.*, Vol. 61, pp. 93-106, 1928.

Ponomarew, A. W.: "*Zur Frage des Mechanismus der 'lokalen Immunisation,'*" *Zeitschr. f. d. ges. exp. Med.*, Vol. 63, pp. 52-63, 1928.

Ponomarew, A. W.: "*Über die Folgen der Einführung von Steinkohlenteer unmittelbar in den Subarachnoidalraum bei Kaninchen,*" *Zeitschr. f. d. ges. exp. Med.*, Vol. 63, pp. 652-61, 1928.

Ponomarew, A. W.: "*Über einige Bedingungen der Wirkung von Antidiphtherie- und Antidysenterieserum im Organismus,*" *Zeitschr. f. d. ges. exp. Med.*, Vol. 64, pp. 126-32, 1929.

Ponomarew, A. W.: "*Der suboccipitale Durchstich als Methode der Impfung des Lyssavirus durch den Subarachnoidalraum,*" *Zeitschr. f. d. ges. exp. Med.*, Vol. 64, pp. 650-57, 1929.

Ponomarew, A. W.: "*Zur Frage der Beteiligung des Nervensystems am tuberkulosen Prozess,*" *Zeitschr. f. d. ges. exp. Med.*, Vol. 70, pp. 403-16, 1930.

Ponomarev, A. V. and Kanarevskaya, A. A.: "The Hemato-Encephalitic Barrier and Sensibilisins," *Archive of Biological Sciences,* Vol. 36, No. 3, Series B.

Ponomareff, A. et Tchechkoff, A.: "*Les conditions de l'action du sérum antirabique dans l'organisme,*" Comptes rend. Soc. Biol., Vol. 97, pp. 376-78, 1927.

Skoblo, M. S.: "*Materialien und Untersuchungsmethoden zur Physiologie des* Tuber cinereum," *Zeitschr. f. d. ges. exp. Med.,* Vol. 73, pp. 57-82, 1930.

Speransky, A.: "*La congélation de tissus. Procédés d'obtention de l'autoneurotoxine et d'autres autatoxines cellulaires (note préliminaire),*" Ann. Inst. Pasteur, Vol. 40, pp. 213-31, 1926.

Speransky, A.: "*L'influence du liquide céphalo-rachidien sur l'évolution des processus physiologiques et pathologiques du cerveau,*" Ann. Inst. Pasteur, Vol. 40, pp. 156-86, 1926.

Speransky, A.: "*Faits nouveaux sur la pathogénie et la prophilaxie de la rage,*" Ann. Inst. Pasteur, Vol. 41, pp. 166-88, 1927.

Speransky, A.: "*Contribution à l'étude de l'action des anticorps spécifiques dans l'organisme,*" Ann. Inst. Pasteur, Vol. 41, pp. 1063-77, 1927.

Speransky, A.: "*Le rôle du système nerveux central dans les processus morbides locaux,*" Ann. Inst. Pasteur, Vol. 42, pp. 179-95, 1928.

Speransky, A. D.: "*Mécanisme des lésions segmentaires du cerveau et leur rôle dans la pathogénie de certains processus généraux et locaux,*" Ann. Inst. Pasteur, Vol. 43, pp. 1021-45, 1929.

Speransky, A. D.: "*Epileptic Seizures,*" Leningrad, 1932.

Speransky, A. D.: "The Mechanism of Segmentary Affections of the Brain and on its Significance in the Pathogenesis of Certain General and Local Processes," *Messenger of Surgery and Related Fields;* No. 45-46, 1929; Ann. Inst. Pasteur, May-June, 1929.

Speransky, A. D.: "How the Theory of Neuro-Trophism Arose," *Archive of Biological Sciences,* Vol. 33, No. 5-6, 1933.

Speransky, A. D.: "The Nervous System in Pathology," 1930.

Speransky, A. D.: "Neuro-Trophism in the Theory and Practice of Medicine," *Archive of Biological Sciences,* Vol. 34, No. 4, 1933.

Spirov, M. S.: "The Subarachnoid Space of the Cerebrum and Spinal Cord and Its Relation to the Cerebro-Spinal Fluid," *Russian Archive of Anatomy, Histology and Embryology,* Vol. 6, No. 2, 1927.

Spirov, M. S.: "The Paths of Distribution of Cerebro-Spinal Fluid and of Injection Masses from the Subarachnoid Space of the Cerebrum and Spinal Cord," *Ibid.,* Vol. 6, No. 2, 1927.

Suslow, G. W.: "*Das chemische Trauma des Nervensystems durch Formalin, dessen Folgen und Bedeutung,*" Zeitschr. f. d. ges. exp. Med., Vol. 83, pp. 386-95, 1932.

Uljanow, A. M.: "*Über die Bedingungen des Eindringens von Tollwutvirus in die Tränendrüsen,*" Zeitschr. f. d. ges. exp. Med., Vol. 78, pp. 143-46, 1931.

Uljanow, P.: "*Über den Mechanismus des Eindringens verschiedener Substanzen in das Hirngebiet, längs den Scheiden der Blutgefäße u. Nerven,*" Zeitschr. f. d. ges. exp. Med., Vol. 64, pp. 78-81, 1929.

Uljanow, P. N.: "*Zur Frage der Verbindungen zwischen den Subarachnoidalräumen des Gehirns und der Lymphsystem des Körpers,*" Zeitschr. f. d. ges. exp. Med., Vol. 65, pp. 621-26, 1929.

Uljanow, P. N.: "*Experimentelle Befunde über die Bewegung der zerebrospinalen Flüssigkeit im Zentralkanal des Rückenmarks,*" Zeitschr. f. d. ges. exp. Med., Vol. 78, pp. 695-99, 1931.

Wassilenko, F. D.: "*Über die vasomotorischen Reflexe bei experimentellen trophischen Geschwüren,*" Zeitschr. f. d. ges. exp. Med., Vol. 74, pp. 769-72, 1930.

Vishnevsky, A. A. and Glushkov, P. A.: "The Pathogenesis and Therapy of Alveolar Pyorrhœa," *Archive of Biological Sciences*, Vol. 34, No. 4, 1933.

Wischnewsky, A. A. and Golyschewa, K. P.: "*Zur Frage der Prädisposition,*" *Zeitschr. f. d. ges. exp. Med.*, Vol. 89, pp. 105-12, 1933.

Vishnevsky, A. A. and Shcheperin, M. I.: "The Pathogenesis and Therapy of Leprosy." (Manuscript.)

Vishnevsky, A. S.: "The Role of Cerebro-Spinal Fluid in the Mechanism of Action of Absinthe on the Brain," *Archive of Biological Sciences*, Vol. 26, No. 4-5, 1926.

Vishnevsky, A. S.: "Certain Conditions of the Formation of Experimental Ulcers in Dogs after Nerve Injuries," *Messenger of Surgery and Related Fields*, Vol. 39, 1928.

Wischnewsky, A. S.: "*Eine Methode zur Blutstillung bei Schädeltrepanation und Sinusverletzungen,*" *Arch. f. klin. Chir.*, Vol. 146, pp. 544-49, 1927.

Wischnewsky, A. S.: "*Über die Bedingungen einer verschiedenen Schnelligkeit der Fortbewegung von Farbstoffen im Nerven,*" *Zeitschr. f. d. ges. exp. Med.*, Vol. 61, pp. 107-13, 1928.

Wischnewsky, A. S.: "*Über den Mechanismus segmentärer Gehirnaffektionen bei 'trophischen' Störungen,*" *Zeitschr. f. d. ges. exp. Med.*, Vol. 63, pp. 677-87, 1928.

Wischnewsky, A. S.: "*Experimentelle klinische Untersuchungen zur Frage der Genese u. Behandlung chronischer trophischer Geschwüre beim Menschen,*" *Arch. f. klin. Chir.*, Vol. 154, pp. 195-247, 1929.

Wischnewsky, A. S.: "*Über die Rolle nervöser Einflüsse auf den Prozeß der Regeneration des Nervenstammes,*" *Zeitschr. f. d. ges. exp. Med.*, Vol. 76, pp. 193-209, 1931.

Vishnevsky, A. S. and Derchinsky, G. D.: "Infection of the Genital Paths." (Manuscript.)

Zacharowa, A. E.: "*Über histolytische Eigenschaften der flüssigen Augenmedien,*" *Zeitschr. f. d. ges. exp. Med.*, Vol. 93, pp. 236-41, 1934.

Zakaraja, E. P.: "*Zur Frage des Mechanismus der segmentären Affektionen des Nervensystems und deren Folgen,*" *Zeitschr. f. d. ges. exp. Med.*, Vol. 80, pp. 670-83, 1932.

Zhabotinsky: "Changes of the Nervous System in Chemical Trauma of Nerves of the Fore Extremity in Rabbits," *Archive of Biological Sciences*, 1935.

B. OTHER LITERATURE

Aschoff u. Robertson: *Med. Klinik*, 1905.

Baatard: "*Le barrière hémato-encéphalique, etc.,*" *Thèse de Génève*, 1924.

Balo, J. and Gal, E.: *Virch. Arch. f. path. Anat.*, Vol. 265, pp. 386-402, 1927.

Baum, H. und Trautmann, A.: *Anatom. Anzeiger*, Vol. 60, No. 7-8, 1925.

Becht and Groer: *Journal of Inf. Dis.*, Vol. 7, p. 127, 1910.

Berghaus, W.: *Zentralbl. f. Bakt.*, Vol. 48, p. 450, 1908.

Besredka: "*Immunisation locale,*" Masson, Paris, 1925.

Bingel, D.: *Arch. f. klin. Med.*, Vol. 104, pp. 370-93, 1911.

Boer de: *Pflügers Arch. für die ges. Physiol.*, Vol. 190, 1921.

Brucke: *Arch. f. exp. Path.*, Vol. 63, 1910.

Brüning: *Zbl. f. Chir.*, 1921.

Brüning: *Arch. f. klin. Chir.*, Vol. 117, 1921.

Brüning: *Klin. Woch.*, 1923, Vol. II.

Bykov: *Messenger of Surgery*, 82-84, 1932. (Russian.)

Carlson and Hektoen: *Journal of Inf. Dis.*, Vol. 7, 1910.

Centanni: *Riforma med.*, Vol. 5, p. 14, 1900.

Charcot, J. M.: "*Leçons sur les maladies du système nerveux,*" Paris, 1874.

Chirkovsky, V. V. and Dymshits: *Kazan Med. Journal*, Vol. 24, p. 1351, 1928. (Russian.)

Courmont et Doyon. "*Le tétanos,*" Paris, 1899.

Cushing: The Cameron Prize Lectures. Lecture I, "The Third Circulation," 1925.

Delezenne, C.: *Ann. Inst. Pasteur*, Vol. 14, pp. 686-704, 1900.
Descombey: *Ann. Inst. Pasteur*, Vol. 43, No. 5, 1929.
Dogiel: *Anat. Anz.*, Vol. 11, 1896.
Dogiel: *Arch. f. Anat. u. Physiol., Anat. Abt.* 1899.
Enriquez, E. et Sicard, A.: "*Sérums neurotoxiques,*" *Compt. rend. soc. Biol.*, Vol. 52, pp. 905-06, 1900.
Epstein, Braines and Palei. *Collected Papers of the Balinsky Psychiatrical Hospital*, Leningrad, Vol. 1, 1934. (Russian.)
Fermi, Cl.: *Zentralbl. f. Bakt.*, Vol. 52, pp. 576-86, 1909-10.
Friedberger, E.: *Med. Klin.*, Vol. 24, p. 767, 1928.
Fujibayashi, K.: *Jap. J. M. Sc. Tr., IV, Pharmacol.*, 4, pp. 203-17, 1930.
Gellhorn, Ernst: "*Das Permeabilitätsproblem,*" Berlin, Springer, 1929.
Gibier: *Compt. rend. soc. Biol.*, Paris, 1896.
Goldscheider: *Zeitschr. f. klin. Med.*, Vol. 26, p. 175, 1894.
Gottlieb u. Freund: *Münch. med. Woch.*, p. 141, 1916.
Gozzano, M. e Rizzo, C.: *Boll. d. Soc. ital. di biol. sper.*, Vol. 4, pp. 497-500, 1929.
Gumprecht: *Pflügers Arch. für die ges. Physiol.*, Vol. 59, p. 105, 1895.
Hahn: "*Die Chirurgie d. vegetativen Nervensystems,*" 1923.
Horsber u. Whitman: *Zeitschr. f. Hyg.*, Vol. 113, 1931.
Itshikawa et Kotzareff: *Bull. Assoc. Franc. Étude Canc.*, Vol. 14, 1925.
Kafka: "*Die Zerebrospinalflüssigkeit,*" 1930.
Key u. Retzius: "*Anatomie des Nervensystems u. des Bindegewebes,*" Stockholm, 1875.
Khoroshko, V. K.: "Reactions of the Animal Organism to the Introduction of Nerve Tissue," Thesis, 1912. (Russian.)
Kraus-Gerlach-Schweinburg: "*Lyssa bei Mensch u. Tier,*" Berlin-Wien, Urban u. Schwarzenberg, 1926.
Kraus u. Doerr. *Wien. klin. Wochenschr.*, No. 7, 1905; No. 30, 1906.
Lacker u. Magnus: *Zeitschr. f. d. ges. exp. Med.*, Vol. 13, 1921.
Lawrentjew: *Zeitschr. mikr. anat., Forsch.*, Vol. 23, p. 527, 1931.
Le Filliatre, G.: *Vie méd.*, Vol. 9, pp. 1319-27, 1928.
Leporsky: "The Problem of the Pathogenesis of Acute Arthritic Rheumatism and its Treatment," *Proceedings of the Third All-Ukrainian Therapeutical Congress*, Kharkov, 1933. (Russian.)
Leriche, R. et Fontaine, R.: *Presse méd.*, Vol. 42. pp. 849-50. 1934.
Levaditi, C. et Muttermilch, St.: *Compt. rend. Soc. Biol.*, Vol. 74, pp. 379-82, 1913.
Lewandowsky: *Zeitschr. f. klin. Med.*, Vol. 40, p. 480, 1900.
Loeb: "Proteins and the Theory of Colloidal Behaviour," New York, 1924.
Loewi: *Pflügers Arch. für die ges. Physiol.*, Vol. 189, p. 233, 1921.
Magendie: *Journ. de Physiol. exp.*, Vol. 4, 1824.
Magnus, R.: "*Körperstellung. Experimentell-physiologische Untersuchungen über die einzelnen bei der Körperstellung in Tätigkeit tretenden Reflexe, über ihr Zusammenwirken u. ihre Störungen,*" Berlin, 1924.
Magnus-Alsleben u. Hoffmann: *Biochem. Zeitschr.*, Vol. 127, p. 103, 1922.
Marie, A. et Morax, V.: *Ann. Inst. Pasteur*, Vol. 16, pp. 818-32, 1902.
Marie, A. et Tiffeneau, M.: *Ann. Inst. Pasteur.*, Vol. 22, pp. 289-99, 1908.
Mathey-Cornat: "*Chirurgie du sympathique periart. des membres,*" 1926.
Markov, S. N.: *Clinical Medicine*, 1928. (Russian.)
McCartney, J. E.: *Journal. of Exper. Med.*, Vol. 39, pp. 51-61, 1924.
Meissner: *Zeitschr. f. rat. Med.*, 1867.
Metalnikov: "*Rôle du système nerveux et des facteurs biologiques et psychiques dans l'immunité,*" Masson, Paris, 1934.
Meyer u. Ramson: *Arch. f. exper. Pathol.*, Vol. 49, 1903.

Molotkov: "The Trophic Function of the Nervous System as the Basis of Pathological Processes in Surgery," *Journal of Physiology*, Vol. 8. No. 5-6, 1925. (Russian.)

Morozkin, N. I.: "The Treatment of Scarlatina by Intra-lumbar Injection of Antitoxin," *Physician's Journal*, No. 3, 1930. (Russian.)

Moschowitz: *Ann. of Surgery*, 1901.

Mott: "The Oliver Sharpey Lectures on the Cerebro-Spinal Fluid," *Lancet*, Vol. 179, pp. 1-79, 1910.

Muttermilch, St. et Salamon, E.: *C. r. Acad. d. Sc.*, Vol. 188, pp. 205, 1929.

Muttermilch, St. et Salamon, E.: *Ibid.*, pp. 350-52,.

Nikolayev: "Rheumatism," *Clinical Medicine*, Vol. 9, 1931. (Russian.)

Nicolau, S., Cruveilhier, L. et Kopciowska, L.: *C. r. Soc. de Biol.*, Vol. 108, pp. 871-75, 1931.

Nicolau, S., Cruveilhier, L. et Kopciowska, L.: *Ibid.*, pp. 937-40.

Ogata, H.: *Jap. J. M. Sc. Tr.*, IV, Pharmacol. 4, pp. 219-44, 1930.

Openchowski. *C. r. Soc. Biol.*, Paris, Vol. 5, No. 2, 1883.

Orbeli: "The Sympathetic Innervation of the Skeletal Musculature," *Bulletin of the Lesgaft Scientific Institute*, Vol. 6, p. 187, 1923. (Russian.)

Orbeli a. Fursikov: *Ibid.*, Vol. 8, 1924. (Russian.)

Papilian, V. et Stanescu-Jippa, V.: *Compt. rend. Soc. de Biol.*, Vol. 91, 1465-66, 1924.

Rachmanov: "The Spreading of Toxins Through the Nervous System." Thesis, 1910. (Russian.)

Radetsky. "The Subarachnoid Space," *Russian Physician*, 1917. (Russian.)

Rasenkov: *Trans. of Internat. Physiolog. Congress*, Rome, 1932.

Remlinger et Bailly: *C. r. Soc. Biol.*, Paris, 1928.

Ricker, Gust: "*Pathologie als Naturwissenschaft—Relationspathologie—für Pathologen, Physiologen, Mediziner und Biologen*," Berlin, Springer, 1924.

Rizzo: *C. Riv. di pat. nerv.*, Vol. 35, pp. 212-16, 1930.

Rivela Greco, A.: *Ann. Inst. Pasteur*, Vol. 51, pp. 265-72, 1933.

Rivela Greco, A.: *Zeitschr. f. die ges. Neurol. u. Psychiat.*, Vol. 147, pp. 145-52, 1933.

Rivela Greco, A.: *Note e riv du psichiat.*, Vol. 61, pp. 1-40, 1932.

Rivela Greco, A.: *Ibid.*, pp. 361-83.

Roux, E. et Borrel, A.: *Ann. Inst. Pasteur*, Vol. 12, pp. 225-39, 1898.

Shamov: *New Surg. Arch.*, Vol. 1, 1921. (Russian.)

Shamov: *Messenger of Surgery*, Vol. 1, 1922. (Russian.)

Samuel: "Die trophischen Nerven," Leipzig, 1860.

Samuel: "Trophoneurosen," *Real-Enzyklop.*, 1890.

Schiff: *Zeitschr. f. rat. Med.*, 1867.

Scholer: *Zeitschr. f. Immun. Forschg.*, Vol. 79, p. 99, 1933.

Schweinburg, F.: *Zbl. f. Bakt. (Abt. 1)*, Vol. 124, pp. 426-53, 1932.

Seifried, O.: *Zeitschr. f. Infektionskr. par. Krankh. u. Hyg. d. Haustiere*, Vol. 36, pp. 18-30, 1929.

Sepp: "*Die Dynamik der Blutzirkulation im Gehirn*," Berlin, 1928.

Shimura: *Virch. Arch. für Path. Anat.*, Vol. 251, 1924.

Sozon-Yaroshevich: "Trophic Ulcers of the Extremities," *Gosmedizdat*, 1931. (Russian.)

Spiegel, E. A.: "*Experimentelle Neurologie (Physiologie und Pathologie des Nervensystems)*," Teil 1, Berlin, Karger, 1928.

Spiess: *Münch. med. Woch.*, 1906, p. 345.

Stepanov: *Bulletin of the Lesgaft Scientific Institute*, Vol. 6, 1923. (Russian.)

Stern et Gautier: *Arch. intern. de physiol.*, Vol. 17, 1921-22.

Stern et Gautier: *Ibid.*, Vol. 20, 1923.

Teale and Embleton: *Journal of the Royal Army Med. Corps*, Vol. 35, 1920.

Tizzoni u. Cattani: *Arch. f. exp. Path.*, Vol. 27, p. 432, 1890.

Trendelenburg: *Pflügers Arch.*, Vol. 133, p. 305, 1910; Vol. 135, p. 469, 1910; Vol. 136, p. 429, 1910; Vol. 139, p. 515, 1910.

Tschudnosowjetow: *Acta oto-laryngolog.*, Vol. 19, 1931.

Tsunoda, I.: *Zeitschr. f. Krebsforschung*, Vol. 25, pp. 423-30, 1927.

Ukhtomsky, A.: "Parabiosis and the Dominant," 1927. (Russian.)

Vishnevsky, A. A. and Rupasov, N. F.: *Collected Papers of the Kazan Surgical Clinic*, Vol. I, 1932. (Russian.)

Vishnevsky, A. V.: *Archive of Biological Sciences*, Vol. 34, 1933. (Russian.)

Vishnevsky, A. V.: "Questions of Neuro-Trophism and Surgery," *Collected Papers of the Kazan Surgical Clinic*, Vol. II, 1934. (Russian.)

Walter, F. K.: "*Die Blut-Liquorschranke: eine physiologische u. klinische Studie*," Leipzig, Thieme, 1929.

Wassermann u. Takaki: *Berlin. Kl. Woch.*, 1898.

Wedensky: *Arch. de physiol.*, Vol. 4, 1892.

Weed: *Journal Medical Research*, Vol. 31, p. 21, 1914.

Weed: *Anat. Record*, Vol. 10, p. 475, 1916.

Weed: *J. Hopkins Hosp. Rep.*, Vol. 31, p. 342, 1920.

Weed: *Physiol. Rev.*, Vol. 2, p. 171, 1922.

Weed: *Amer. Journ. Anat.*, Vol. 31, p. 191, 1923.

Weiss, Paul: (Wien) *Ergebn. d. Biol.*, Vol. 3, pp. 1-151, 1928.

Weiss, Paul: (Berlin) *Naturwissenschaften*, Vol. 16, pp. 626-36, 1928.

Weiss, P.: (Berlin) *Pflügers Arch. f. d. ges. Physiol.*, Vol. 226, pp. 600-658, 1931.

Widal, F. et Sicard, A.: *Ann. Inst. Pasteur*, Vol. 11, pp. 353-432, 1897.

Widal, Sicard et Lesné: *C. r. Soc. Biol.*, Paris, 1898.

Zdrowski, P. et Golinewitch, H.: *Ann. Inst. Pasteur*, Vol. 53, pp. 120-55, 1934.

RUSSIAN JOURNALS CITED

1. *Arkh. Biol. Nauk (Archive of Biological Sciences)*.
2. *Izv. Inst. im. Lesgafta (Bulletin of the Lesgaft Scientific Institute)*.
3. *Kazansk. Med. Zhurn. (Kazan Medical Journal)*.
4. *Klin. Med. (Clinical Medicine)*.
5. *Med.-San. Vopr. Protivokhim. Zashch. (Medico-Hygienic Questions of Anti-Chemical Defence)*.
6. *Nov. Khirurg. Arkhiv (New Surgical Archive)*.
7. *Russk. Arkhiv Anat., Hist. i Embr. (Russian Archive of Anatomy, Histology and Embryology)*.
8. *Russk. Fiziol. Zhurn. (Russian Journal of Physiology)*.
9. *Russk. Vrach. (Russian Physician)*.
10. *Vestnik Khirurg. i Pogr. Obl. (Messenger of Surgery and Related Fields)*.
11. *Vrach. Gaz. (Physician's Journal)*.
12. *Zhurn. Exp. Biol. (Journal of Experimental Biology)*.
13. *Zhurn. Mikr. Path. i Inf. Bolez. (Journal of Microscopic Pathology and Infectious Diseases)*.

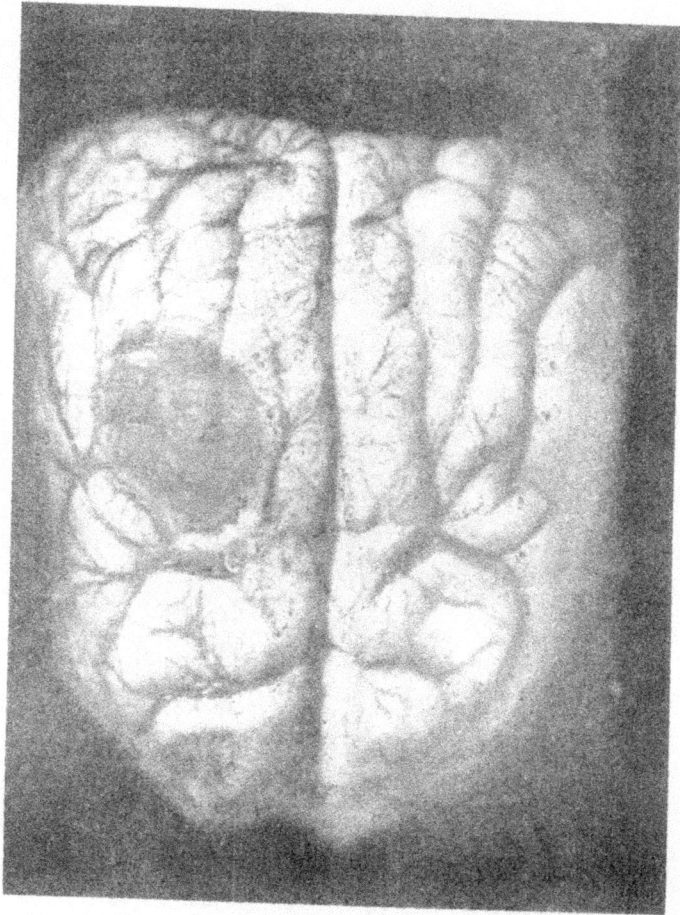

PLATE 1. The brain of a dog after freezing a portion of the cortex

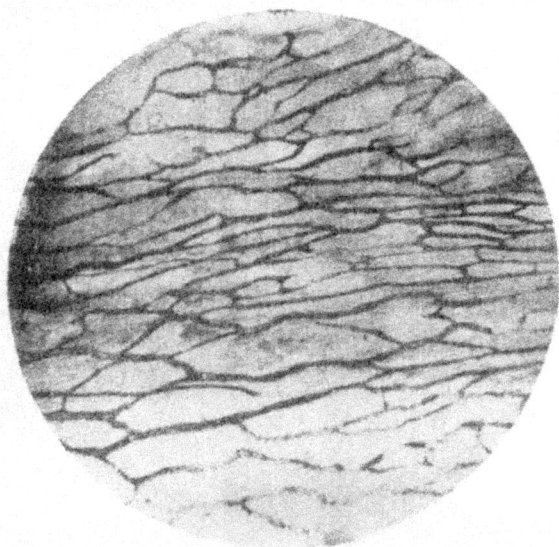

PLATE 2. Nasal mucous membrane of a dog. Vital injection of the lymphatic vessels carried out from the subarachnoid space

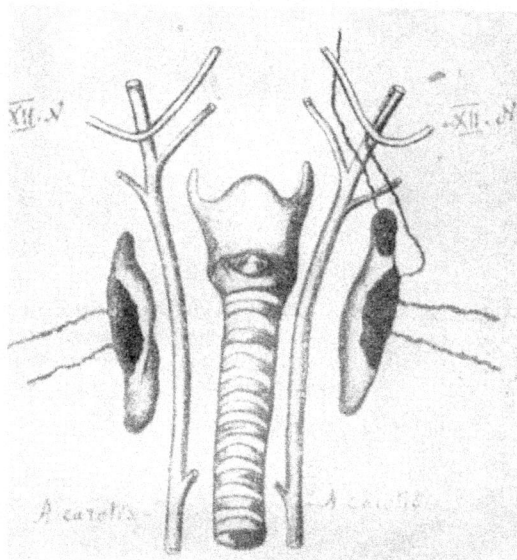

PLATE 3. Injection of the deep pharyngeal lymphatic
glands and vessels in the middle cervical region, carried
out from the subarachnoid space on the freshly-killed
body of a normal dog

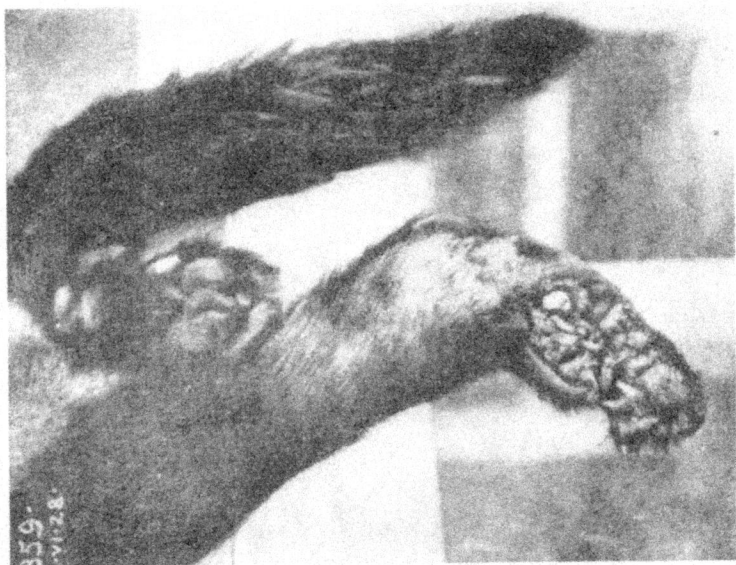

PLATE 4. Gangrenous ulcer with sequestration of the phalanges and meta-tarsal bones after section of the corresponding sciatic nerve and introduction of a drop of pus into its centripetal end (with subsequent extraction of the cerebro-spinal fluid)

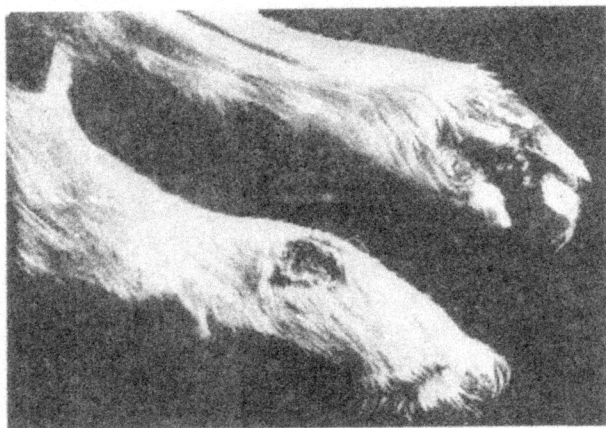

PLATE 5. Symmetrical ulcers on both hind extremities after section of the left sciatic nerve and injection of a drop of pus into its centripetal end (with subsequent extraction of the cerebro-spinal fluid)

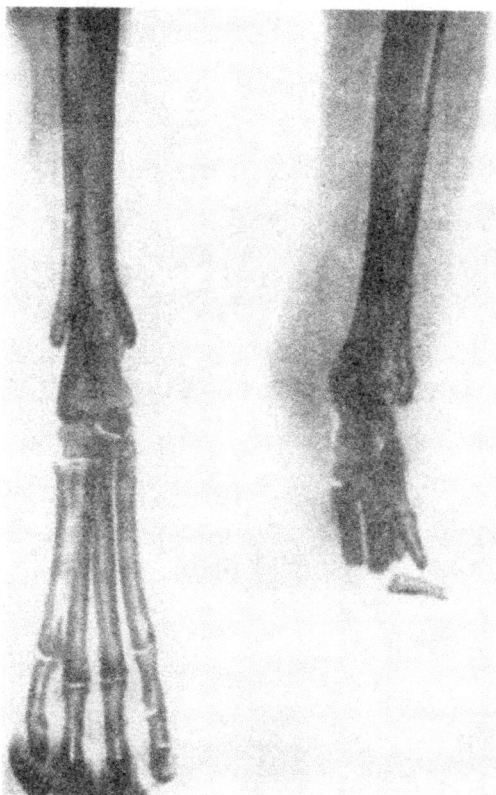

PLATE 6. X-ray photograph of the extremity shown
in Plate 4, and of the contralateral extremity

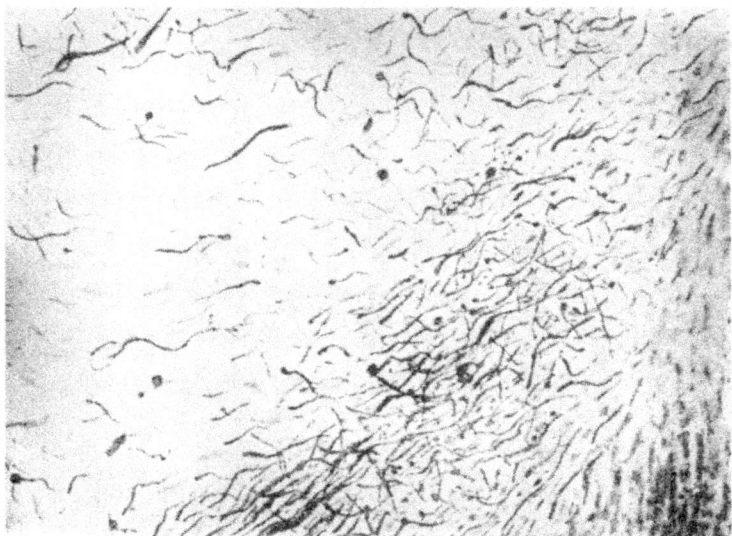

PLATE 7. Experimental group. Portion of the sciatic nerve in the region of the suture, six weeks after the operation

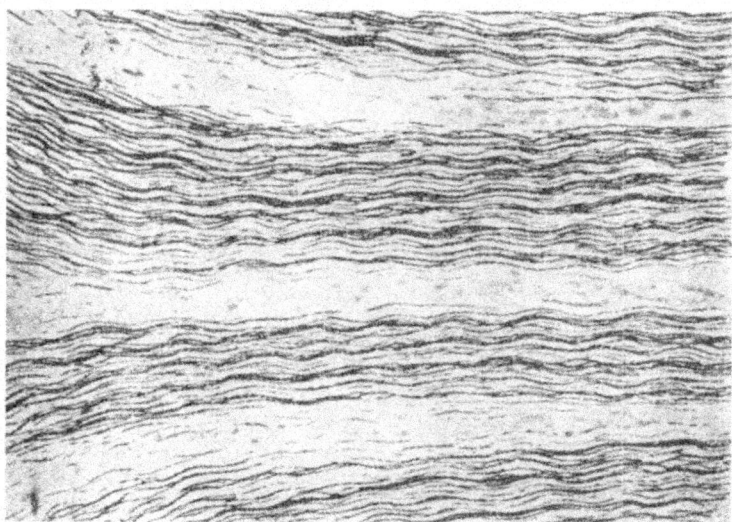

PLATE 8. Control group. Portion of the sciatic nerve in the region of the suture, six weeks after the operation

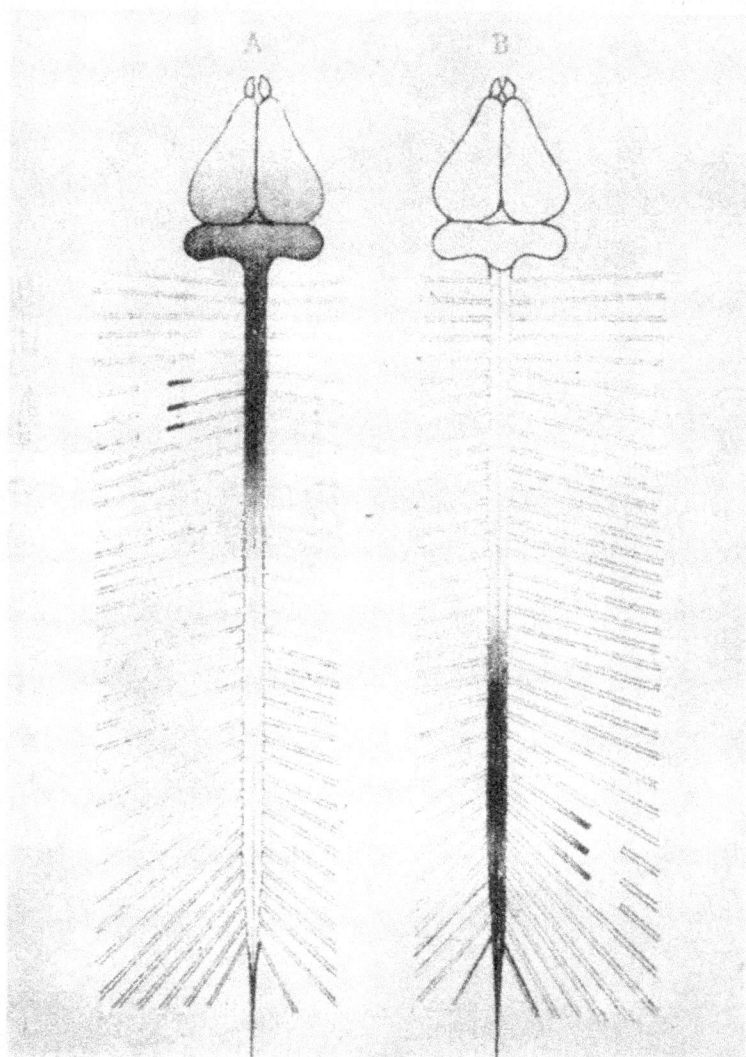

PLATE 9. The effect of trypan blue in dyeing the spinal cord, arachnoidea and pia mater. a) On continuous irritation of the centripetal end of the severed brachial nerve with croton oil; b) on continuous irritation of the centripetal end of the sciatic nerve

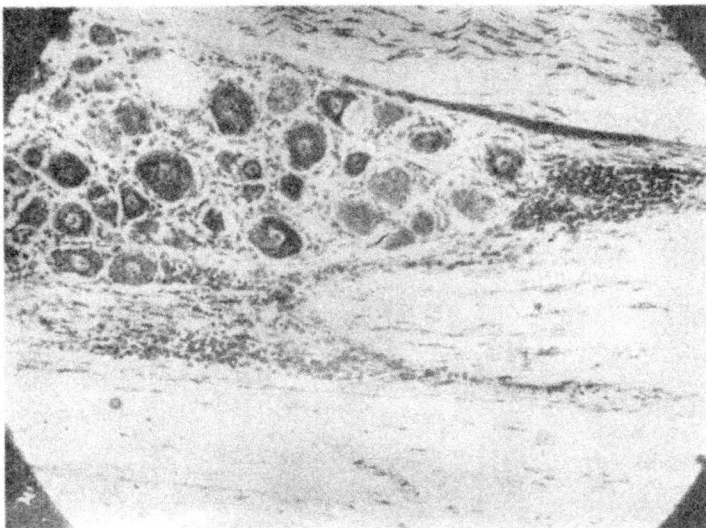

PLATE 10. Infiltration of the perineurium in the region of the distal end of the lower lumbar inter-vertebral ganglion on the side of chemical trauma of the sciatic nerve produced by formalin. Fourteen days after trauma. Nissl method

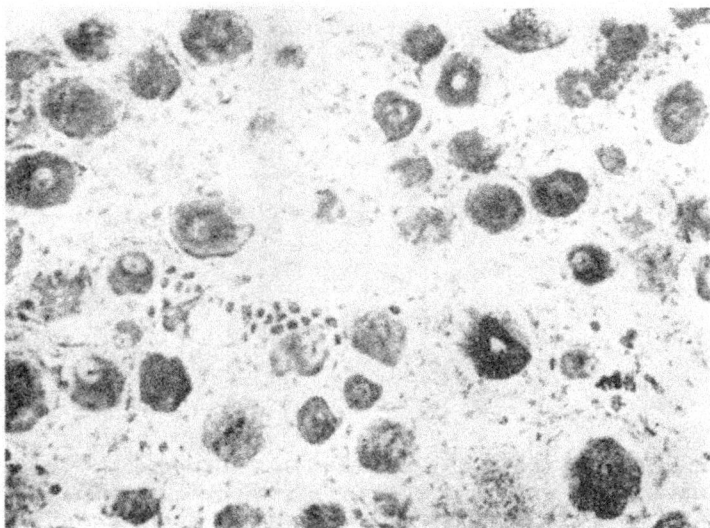

PLATE 11. Inter-vertebral ganglion of the cervical region on the side of trauma of *n. medianus* by formalin. Degenerating nerve cells (microphotograph of a Nissl preparation)

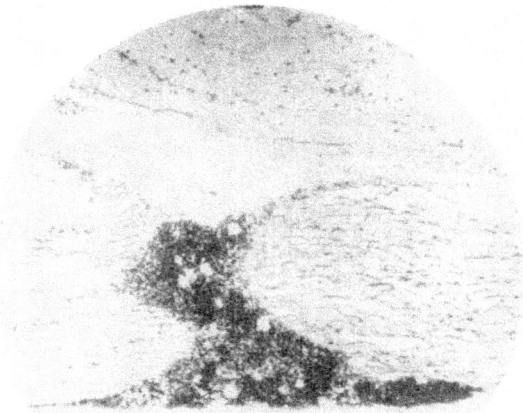

PLATE 12. Ring of inflammatory infiltrate in the sheath of a nerve root immediately above a sacral inter-vertebral ganglion on the side of chemical trauma of the sciatic nerve caused by formalin

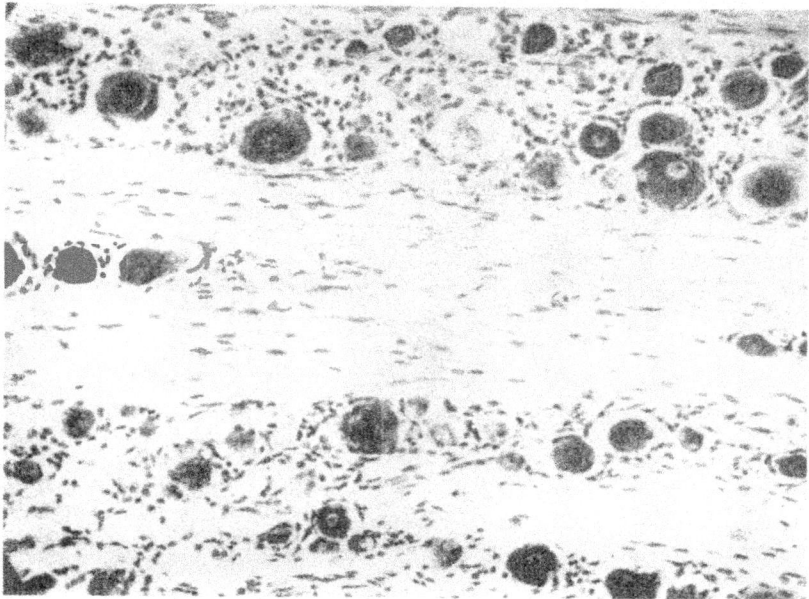

PLATE 13. Alteration of some of the nerve cells of a lumbar inter-vertebral ganglion on the side of chemical trauma of the sciatic nerve by formalin. Perinuclear accumulation of Nissl substance

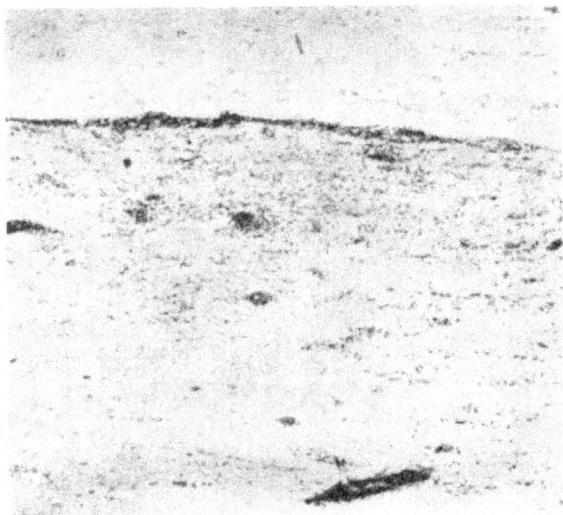

PLATE 14. Numerous infiltrates of polvblasts in the cervical region of the spinal cord on the side of the injection of 5 per cent formalin into the trunk of *n. medianus*. Microphotograph of a Nissl preparation

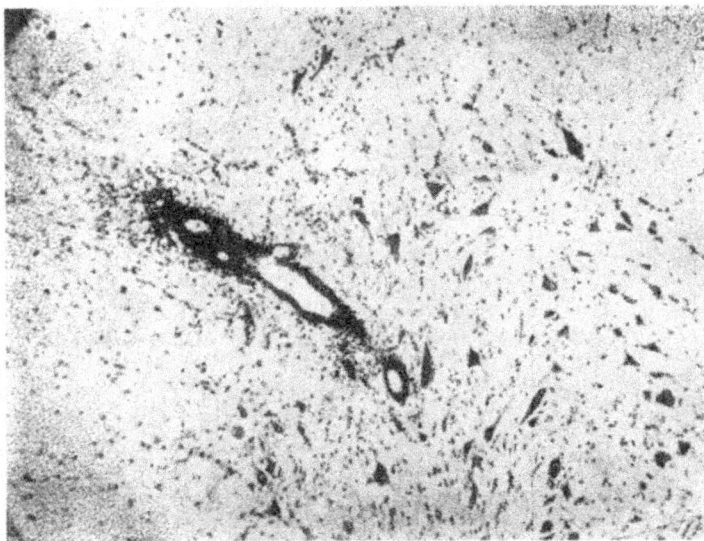

PLATE 15. Cervical region of the spinal cord. An inflammatory focus is seen at the border of the anterior horn and of the anterior lateral column. Seventeen days after chemical trauma of the sciatic nerve by formalin. Nissl method

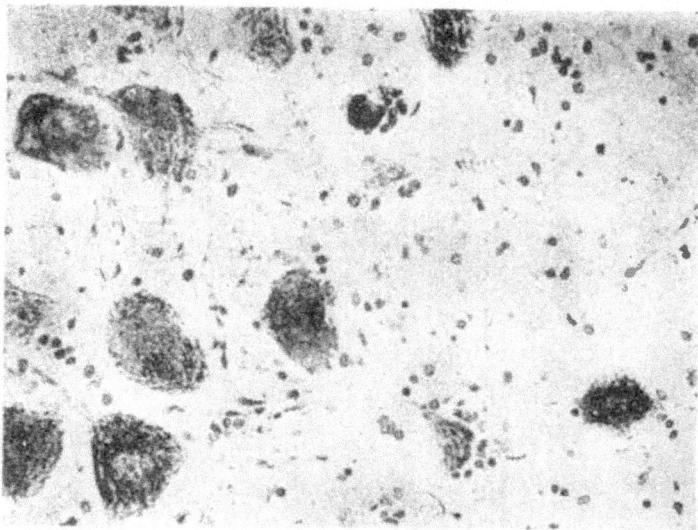

PLATE 16. Motor cells of the lumbar region of the spinal cord on the side of chemical trauma of a nerve. Perinuclear accumulation of Nissl substance; pericellular gliosis around isolated nerve cells. Seventeen days after chemical trauma of the sciatic nerve by formalin. Nissl method

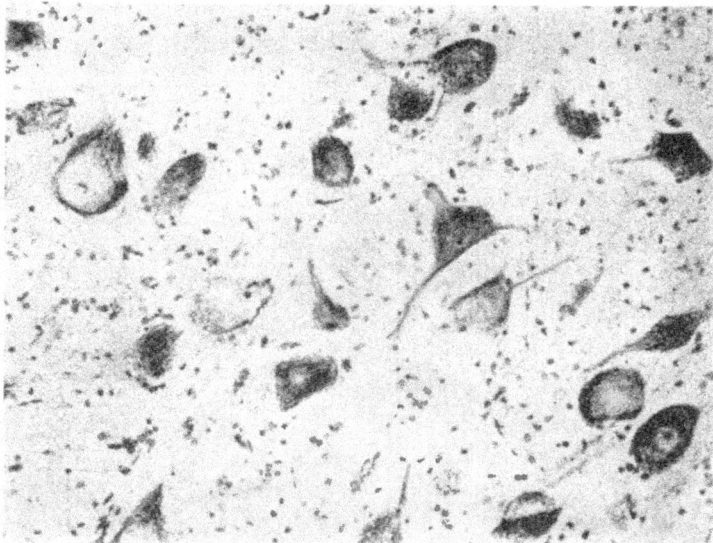

PLATE 17. Nerve cells of the contralateral anterior horn of the lumbar region of the spinal cord twelve days after chemical trauma by formalin. "Serious affection" and "primary irritation." Nissl method

431

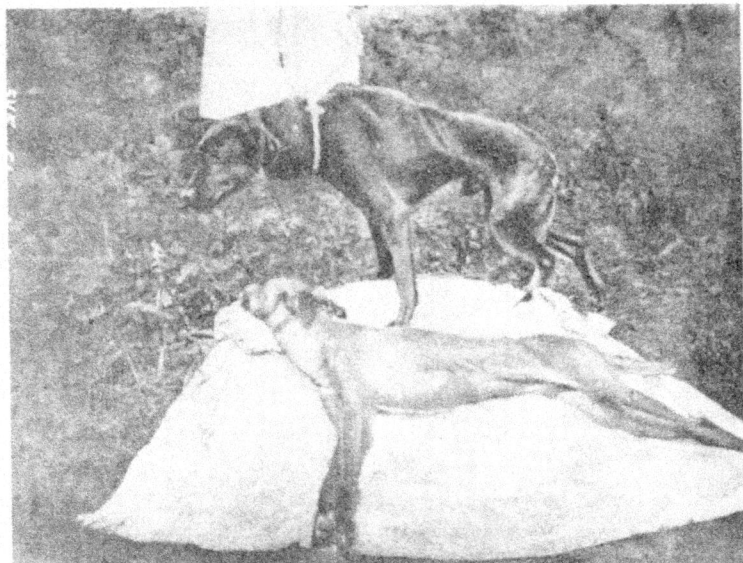

PLATE 18. Infection by tetanus shortly after the operation of removing the sympathetic chain. The control dog is lying down, the experimental animal is standing

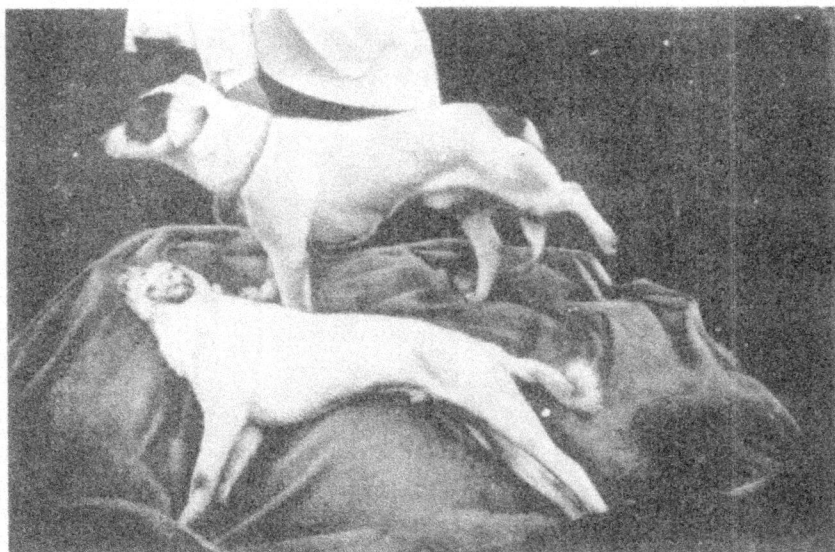

PLATE 19. Infection by tetanus some time after the operation of removing the sympathetic chain. The control dog is standing, the experimental animal is lying down

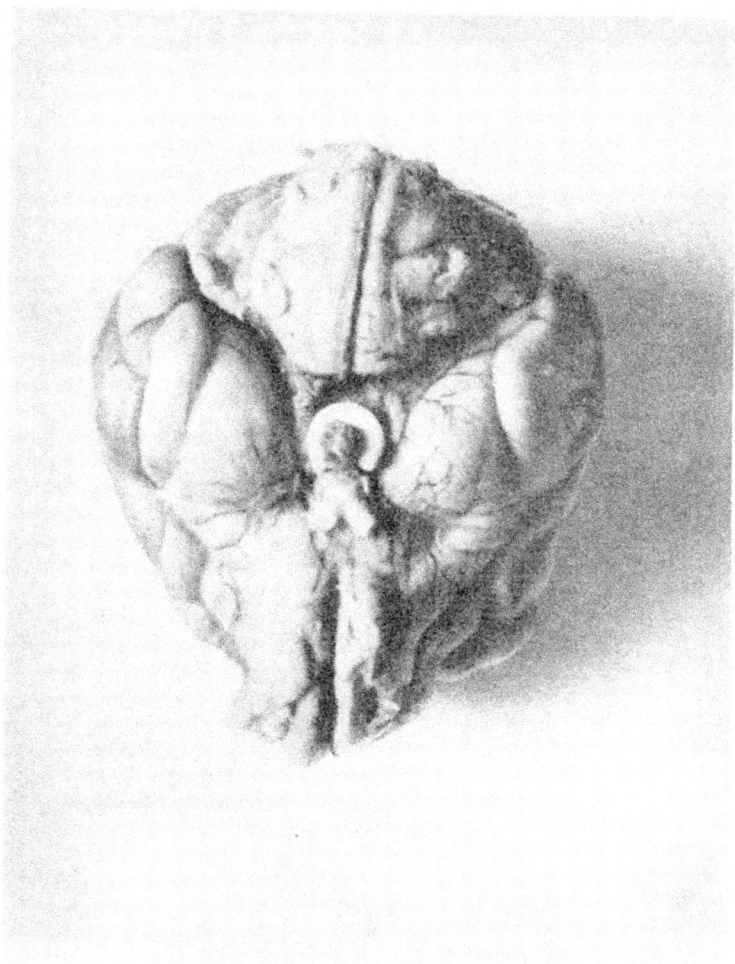

PLATE 20. Brain of a dog. A semi-circular glass ring has been placed
around the infundibulum

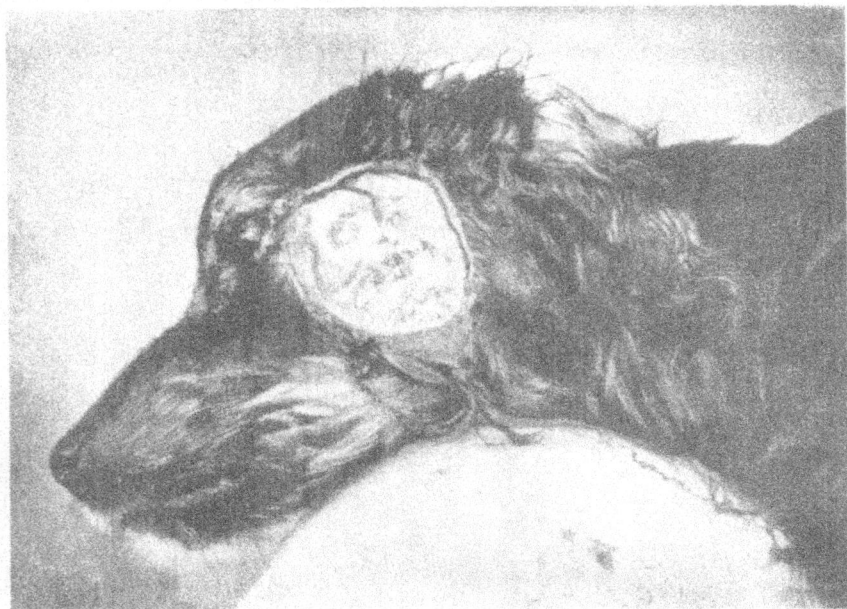

PLATE 21. A case of noma after the "glass sphere operation." Destruction of the cheek tissue

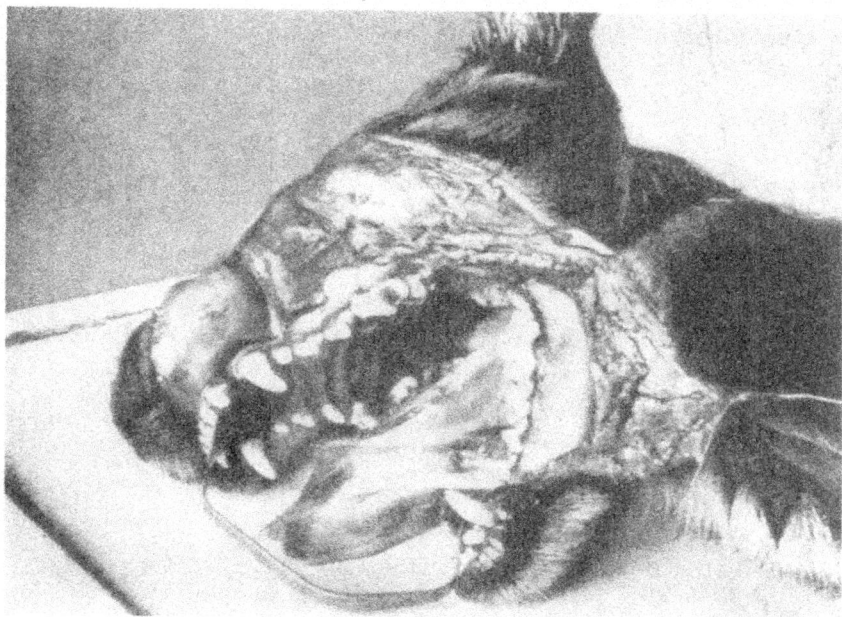

PLATE 22. A case of noma after the "glass sphere operation." The upper and lower jaws have been exposed almost throughout their extent

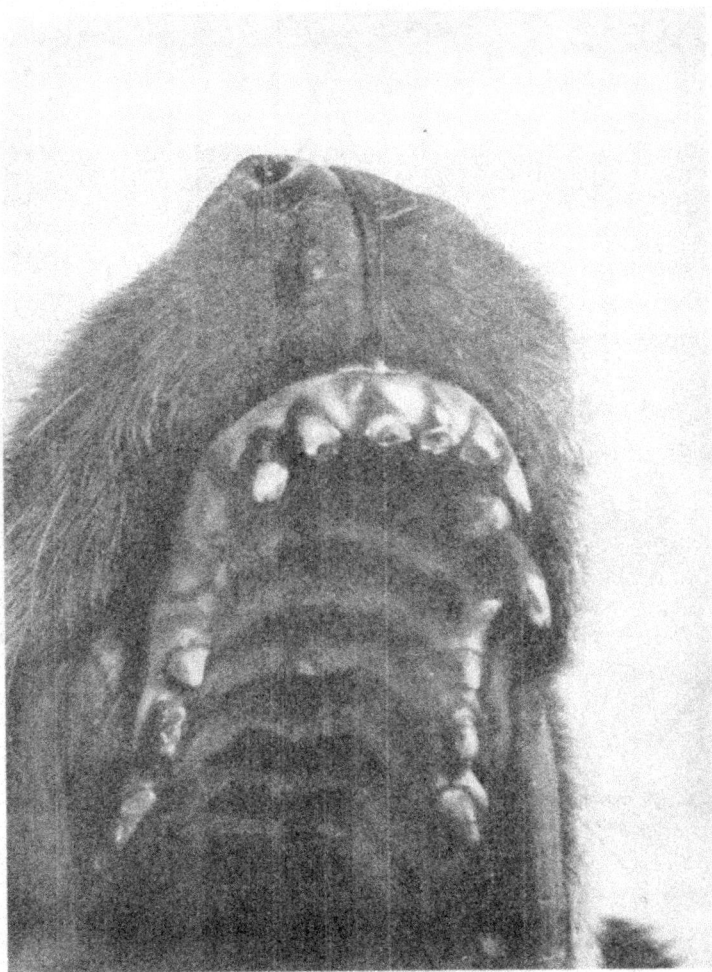

PLATE 23. Dental apparatus of dog No. 294, one and a half months after the "glass sphere operation"

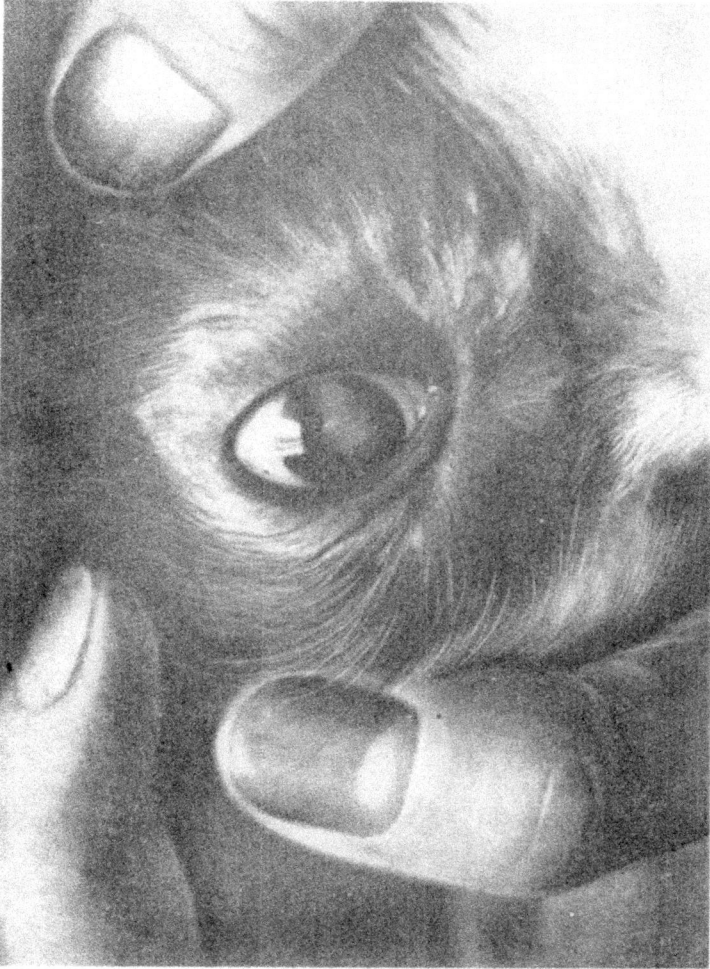

PLATE 24. Loss of hair round the eyes and opacity of the cornea after the "glass sphere operation"

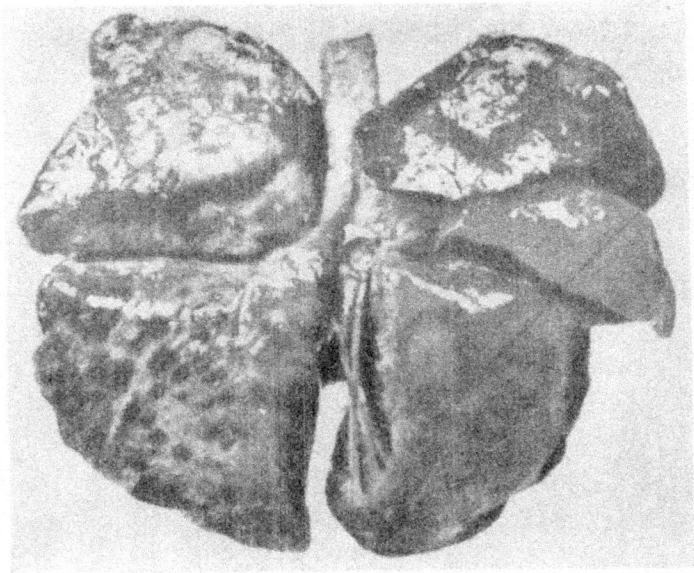

PLATE 25. Hæmorrhages in the lungs of a dog. Death here took place two and a half months after the "glass sphere operation"

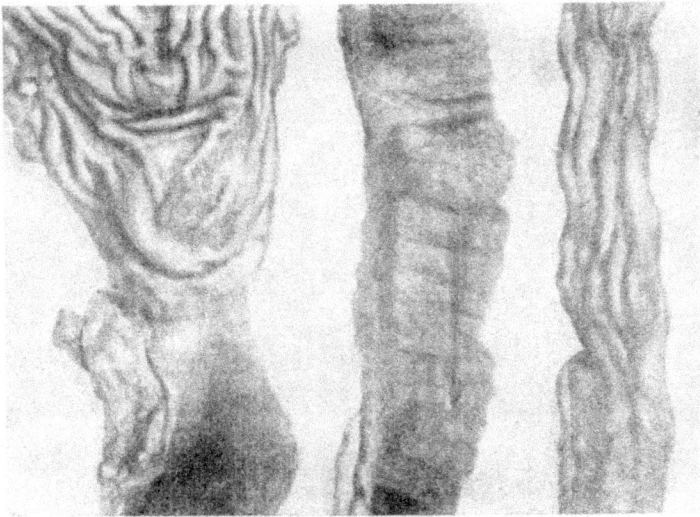

a   b   c

PLATE 26. Visceral organs of a dog dying seven and a half months after the "glass sphere operation." Hæmorrhage in the stomach (a) and in the duodenum (b). The small intestine (c) is unchanged

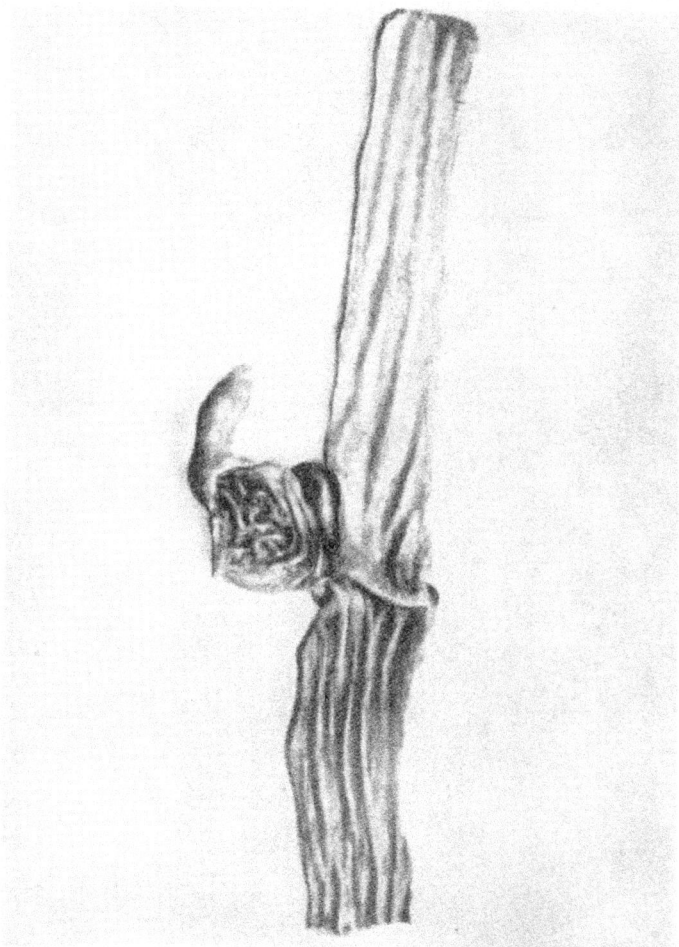

PLATE 27. Hæmorrhages in the valvula Bauhinii, cæcum and large intestine after the "glass sphere operation"

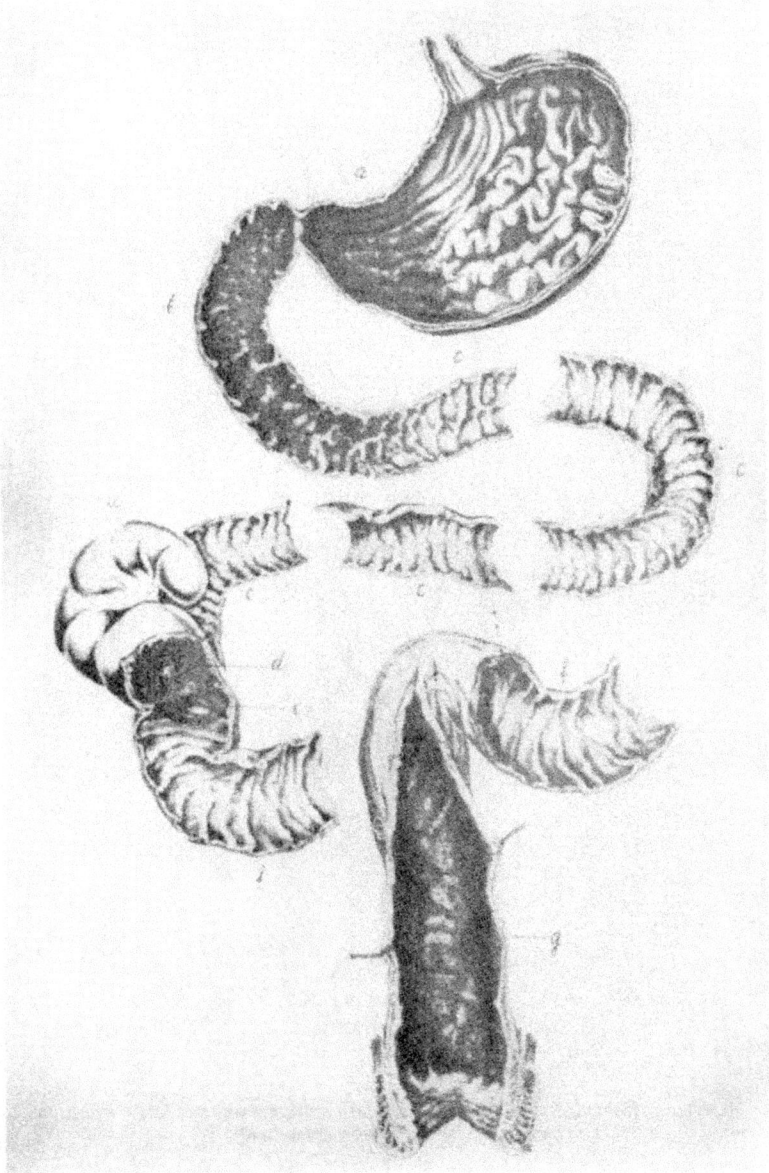

PLATE 28. Diagrammatic representation of the distribution of hæmorrhages along the gastro-intestinal tract: a) stomach; b) duodenum; c) small intestine; d) cæcum; e) valvula Bauhinii; f) large intestine; g) rectum

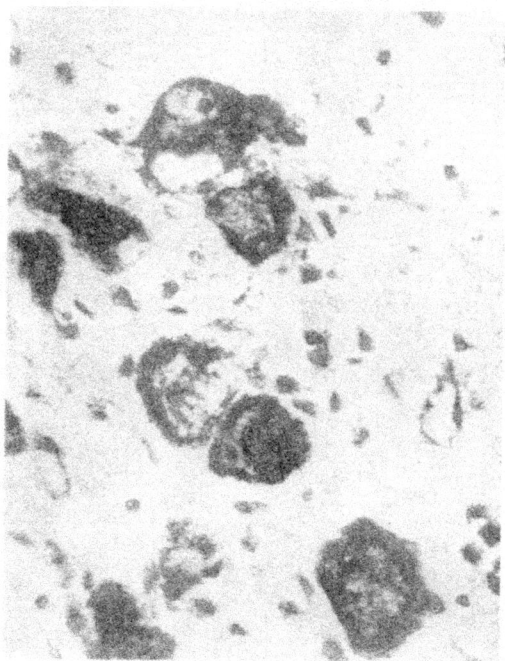

PLATE 29. Degenerative changes in cells of the upper
cervical ganglion after the "glass sphere operation"

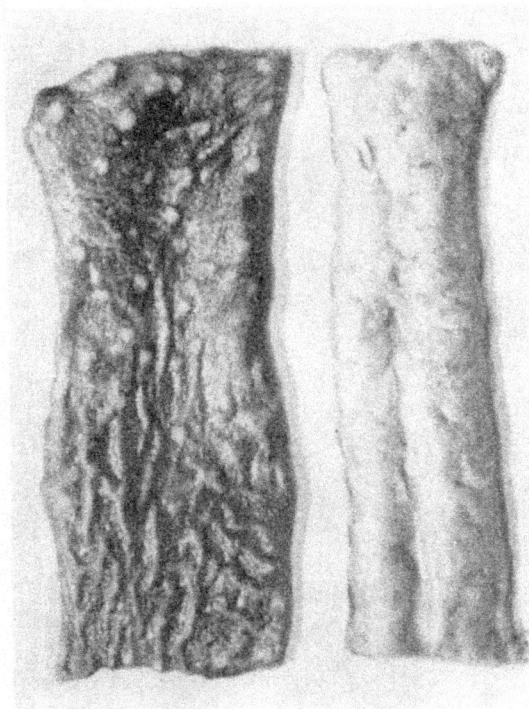

PLATE 30. Rectum and small intestine of a dog dying 24 hours after intravenal injection of a solution of mercuric chloride. Hæmorrhages are seen in the rectum, the small intestine is intact

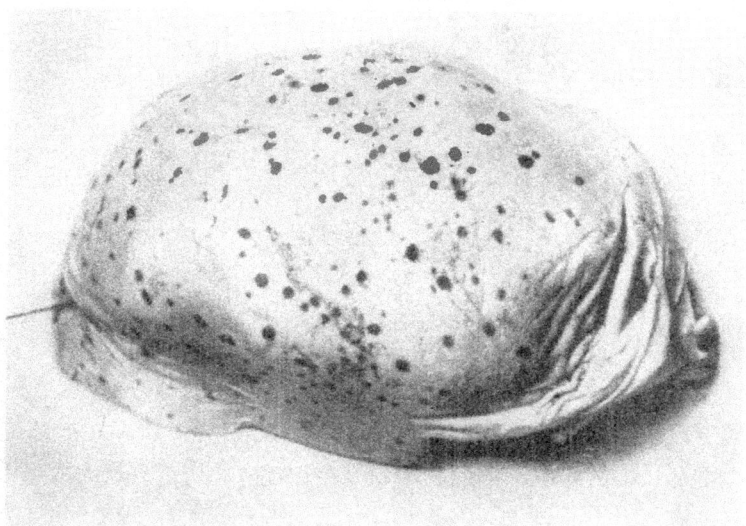

PLATE 31. Hæmorrhages in the mucous membrane of the stomach of a rabbit after injury to the sciatic nerve

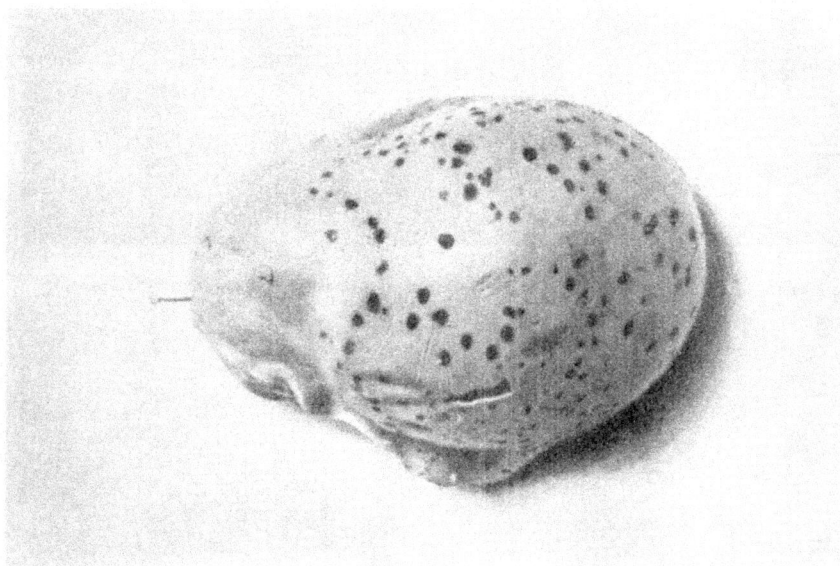

PLATE 32. Hæmorrhages in the mucous membrane of the stomach of a rabbit dying from rabies

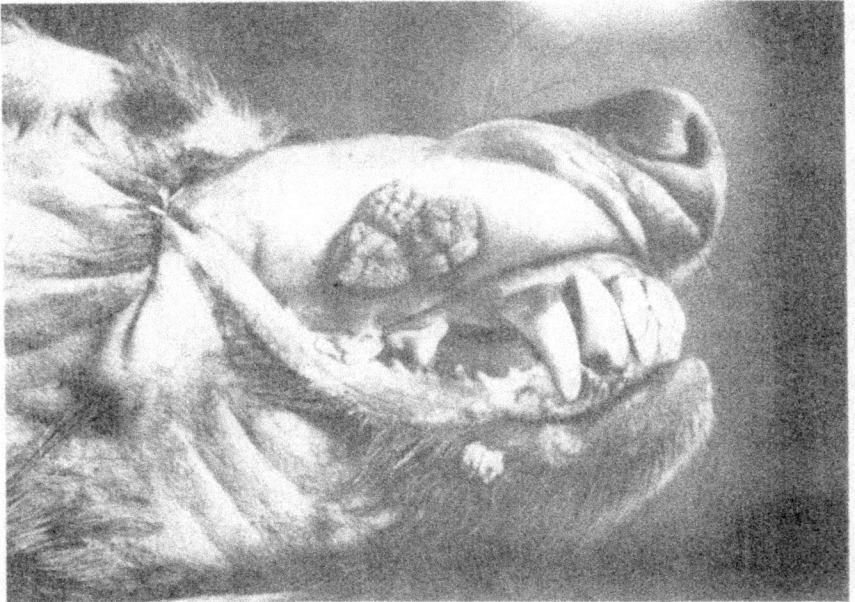

PLATE 33. Dog No. 378. Formation of papillomata on the mucous membrane
of the mouth

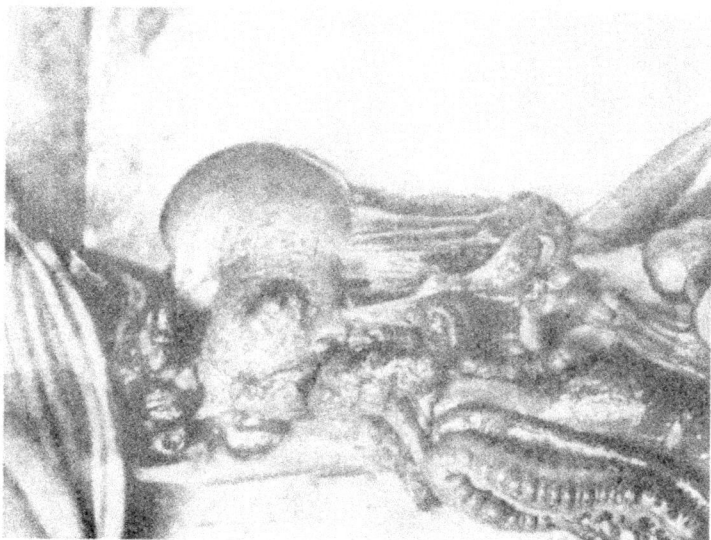

PLATE 35. Stomach of an experimental rabbit. Both *n. vagi* were severed below the diaphragm 22 days before infection with Vallée culture. The rabbit was killed 40 days after infection

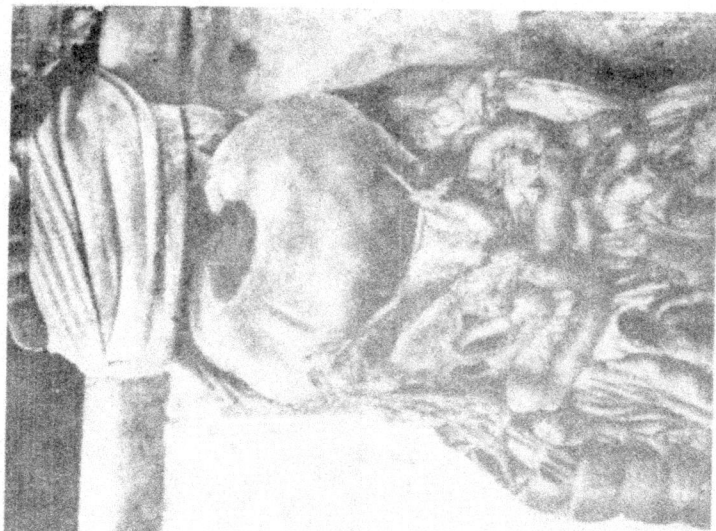

PLATE 34. Stomach of a control rabbit (normal) killed 40 days after inoculating the gastric wall with Vallée tuberculosis culture

445

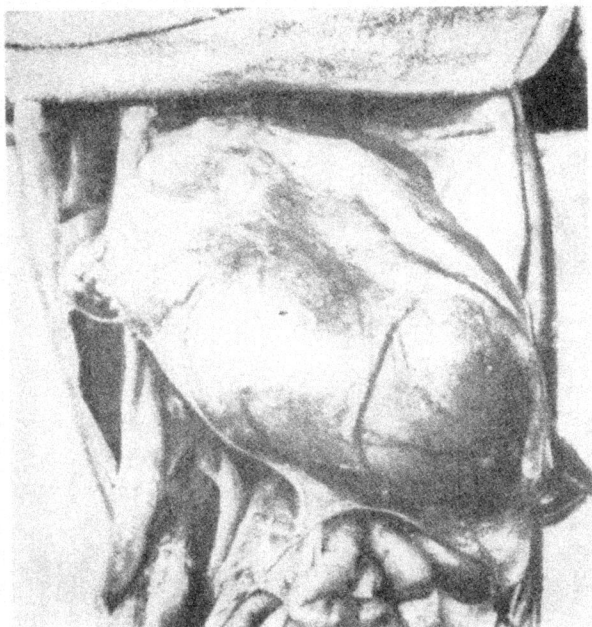

PLATE 36. Stomach of an experimental rabbit. Both *n. vagi* were severed below the diaphragm 27 days after infection by Vallée culture. The rabbit was killed 40 days after infection

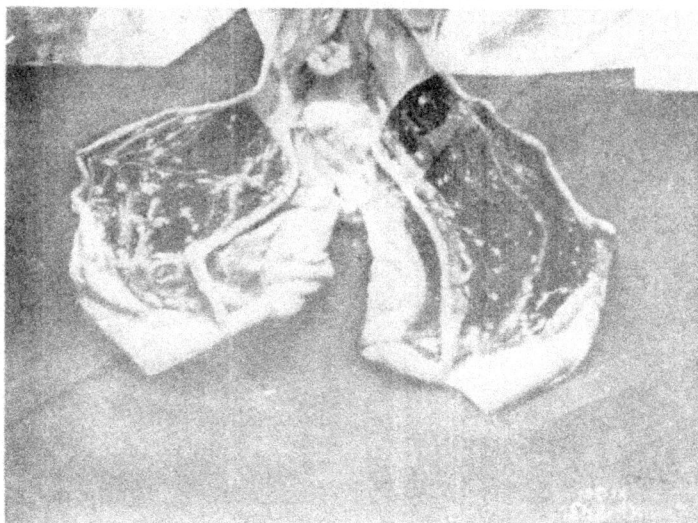

PLATE 37. First stage of tuberculous infection of the testicles and their mesenteries

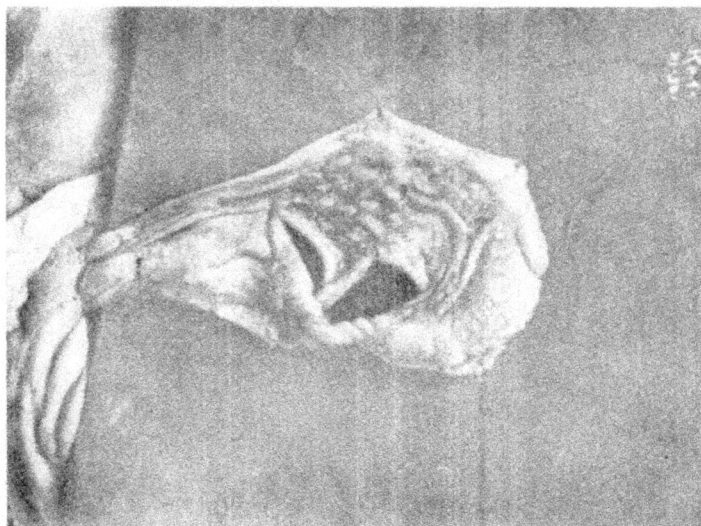

PLATE 38. Severe tuberculous affection of the testicle and its mesentery

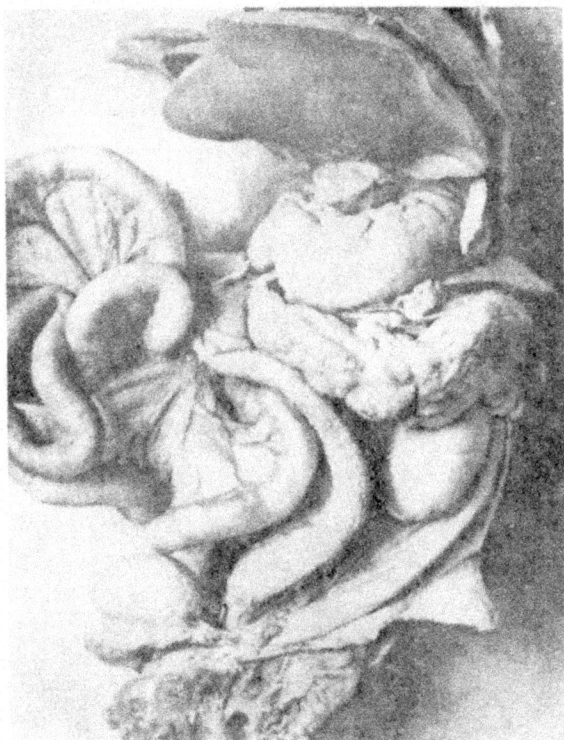

PLATE 39. Visceral organs of a cat infected by tuberculosis intra-peritoneally, and killed after six months twelve days. Pronounced tuberculous affection of the epiploon and serosa of the rectum

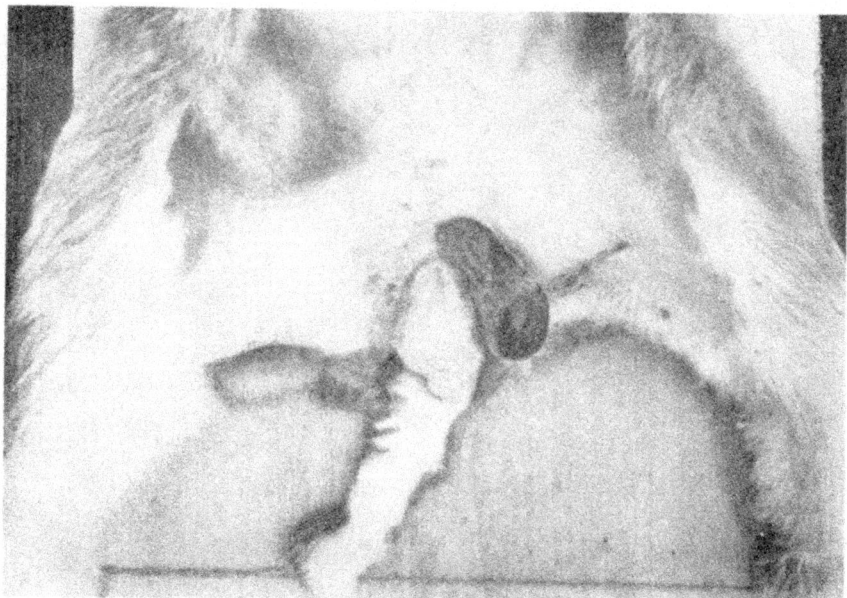

PLATE 40. Mortification of the skin of a rabbit's scrotum after applying a loop with lewisite to its distal end

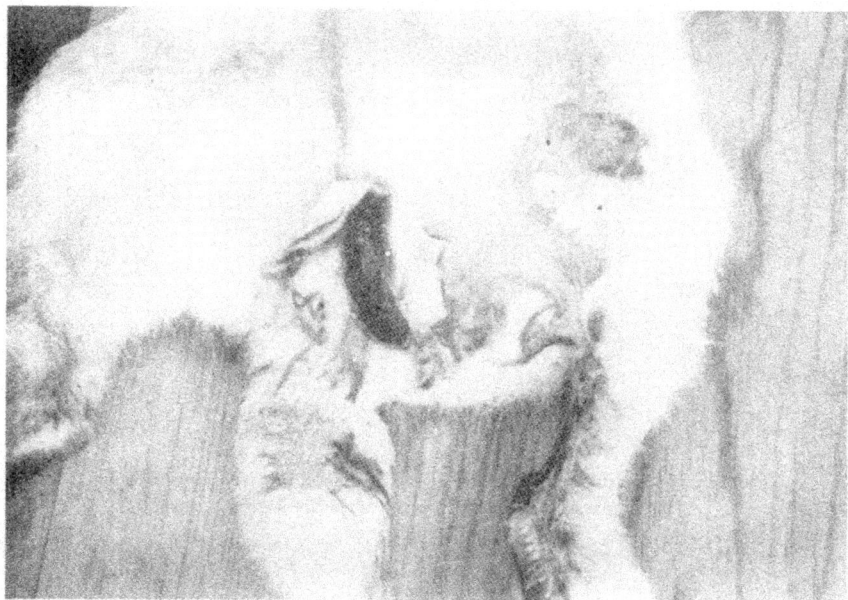

PLATE 41. Ditto, after applying a loop with lewisite to the root of the scrotum near the inguinal canal

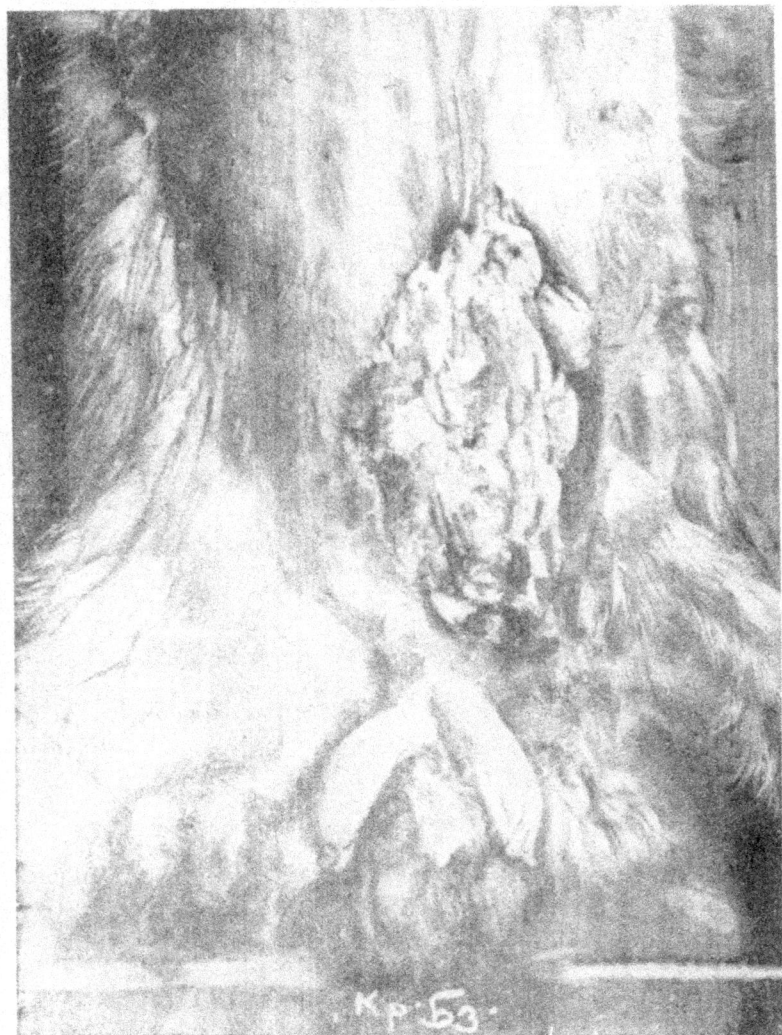

PLATE 42. Mortification of the skin of the belly after applying a loop
with lewisite to its lower portion near the inguinal canal

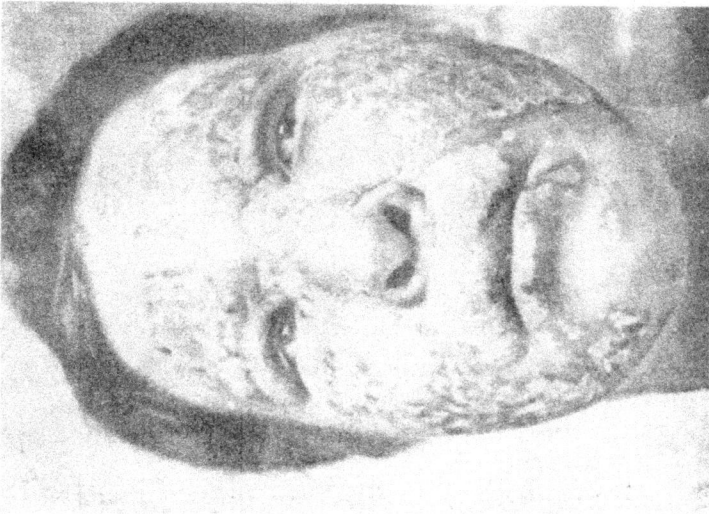

PLATE 43. A. M., suffering from red lupus. Duration of the disease ten years

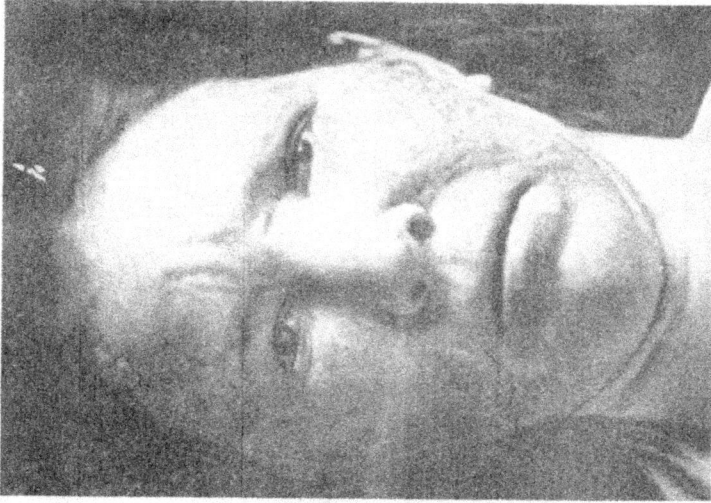

PLATE 44. The same patient one and a half months after blockade

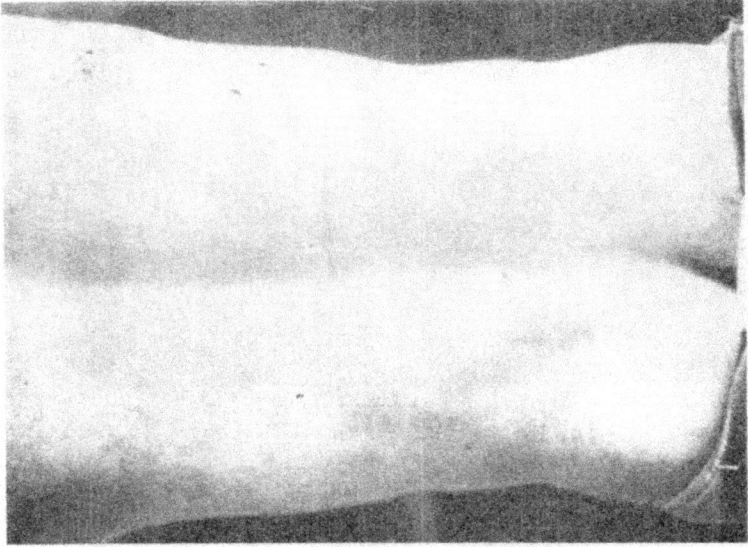

PLATE 46. The same patient twelve days after blockade

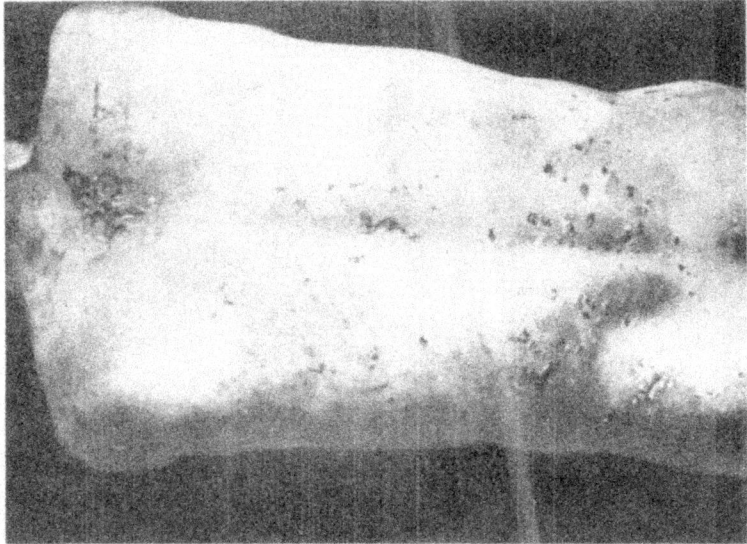

PLATE 45. Herpes-like Dühring's dermatitis before blockade

9780717807499